Telemedicine and Telehealth

Telemedicine and Telehealth

Edited by Brittany McGrath

hayle
medical

New York

Hayle Medical,
750 Third Avenue, 9th Floor,
New York, NY 10017, USA

Visit us on the World Wide Web at:
www.haylemedical.com

ISBN: 978-1-63241-624-7

Cataloging-in-Publication Data

Telemedicine and telehealth / edited by Brittany McGrath.
    p. cm.
Includes bibliographical references and index.
ISBN 978-1-63241-624-7
1. Telecommunication in medicine. 2. Medical telematics. 3. Medical informatics.
4. Medical care--Technological innovations. 5. Medical technology. I. McGrath, Brittany.
R119.9 .T45 2019
610.285--dc23

Table of Contents

Preface

This book has been an outcome of determined endeavour from a group of educationists in the field. The primary objective was to involve a broad spectrum of professionals from diverse cultural background involved in the field for developing new researches. The book not only targets students but also scholars pursuing higher research for further enhancement of the theoretical and practical applications of the subject.

The distribution of health-related services and information by using electronic information system and telecommunication technologies is known as telehealth. It facilitates long distance patient/clinician contact, intervention, education, monitoring and remote admissions. Telehealth involves two or more clinicians discussing a case over video conference, client to practitioner online conference, physical therapy via digital monitoring instruments, and robotic surgery occurring through remote access. The use of information technology and telecommunication to provide clinical health care from a distance is known as telemedicine. It is useful in overcoming distance barriers and in improving access to the medical services, which are not usually available in distant rural areas. The topics included in this book on telemedicine and telehealth are of utmost significance and bound to provide incredible insights to readers. It studies, analyzes and upholds the pillars of these fields and their utmost significance in modern times. This book will prove to be immensely beneficial to students and researchers in the fields of telemedicine and telehealth.

It was an honour to edit such a profound book and also a challenging task to compile and examine all the relevant data for accuracy and originality. I wish to acknowledge the efforts of the contributors for submitting such brilliant and diverse chapters in the field and for endlessly working for the completion of the book. Last, but not the least; I thank my family for being a constant source of support in all my research endeavours.

Editor

Application of Fractional Wave Packet Transform for Robust Watermarking of Mammograms

Pushpa Mala Siddaraju,[1] **Devappa Jayadevappa,**[2] **and Kaliyamoorthy Ezhilarasan**[1]

[1]*Research Scholar, Jain University and Department of Electronics and Communication Engineering, Sambhram Institute of Technology, Bangalore 560097, Karnataka, India*
[2]*Department of Electronic Instrumentation, JSS Academy of Technical Education, Bangalore 560060, Karnataka, India*

Correspondence should be addressed to Pushpa Mala Siddaraju; pushpasiddaraju@gmail.com

Academic Editor: Fei Hu

Exchanging of medical data requires efficient authentication and protection of medical data that can be illegally modified. Watermarking plays an important role in protecting, sharing, and securing medical data. In this work, a robust nonblind medical image watermarking scheme is proposed. The process involves two steps: the embedding and the extraction phase. During the embedding phase, l-level FRWPT is performed on the host image and the watermark is embedded into the modified reference image. In the second phase, inverse FRWPT is performed on the watermarked image to extract the watermark from the watermarked image. The proposed scheme is tested on mammograms images and is subjected to common attacks like Gaussian filtering, median filtering, compression, sharpening, and contrast adjustments. Experimental results show that the proposed scheme is robust.

1. Introduction

In the past few decades, there has been a tremendous growth in information and communication technology leading to easier access to any form of digital data including medical data. Modern health care systems produce a large amount of medical data. Medical data are those that are generated from Medical Information System (MIS), Hospital Information System (HIS), Radiology Information System (RIS), and Electronic Patient Records (EPR). Most of the medical diagnosis is based on images from CT scans, X-rays, MRI scans, mammography, and other forms of image modalities. Cancer is the most familiar disease that affects both men and women. The time factor is very important to discover the abnormality issues in target images, especially in various cancer tumors such as the breast cancer. Researchers at the January 1997 Consensus Development Conference presented data discussing the facts related to breast cancers detected by mammography. Their data showed that mammograms have more prognoses than cancers detected by other imaging modalities. Berry [1] has discussed the benefits and risks of mammography. Though the survival rate of a cancer patient is less, it makes a difference for a breast cancer patient. To increase the survival rate of breast cancer patients, mammography is used for earlier detection and treatment stages with reduced risk. These images were effective in detecting breast cancer early.

Doctors' advice and treatment are based on the data the doctor analyses from the mammogram. Nowadays, most of the patients prefer a second/third opinion on the medical analyses received from their doctor. The second/third opinion may be from a doctor located at a different place through telemedicine. There are many such circumstances where telemedicine exists.

Telemedicine applications are those that provide for diagnostics, prescription, consulting, and sometimes conferences to telesurgery. Telemedicine plays an important role in today's world, where the patient's medical data is transmitted over the Internet. The medical data considered may be medical images (mammogram) which has to be shared or transmitted over Internet. This medical data is crucial data and is at the risk of unauthorized access or manipulation. Authenticating as well as protecting it is essential since critical judgment is done on medical images especially mammograms during breast cancer detection.

Cryptography, steganography, and watermarking are such schemes that are used to protect digital data. Cryptography and steganography are less robust or partially robust to digital data modifications. This scenario is compensated in medical imaging through watermarking. Digital image watermarking is a technique of embedding a watermark (say logo) into the host image for dealing with security issues. Digital image watermarking can be extended to medical images too. Medical image watermarking deals with medical data authentication, ownership, security, source identification, and patient identification. When dealing with EPR, it is mandatory to consider confidentiality to access the information, availability of the data to be used when required, and reliability of the data. These are maintained through security issues, namely, integrity, availability, authentication, and confidentiality nonrepudiation [2]. Medical image watermarking provides for security at the origin reducing piracy of crucial medical data and also protects medical documents or images that can be illegally modified. The medical image watermarking scheme designed requires being robust, secure, and imperceptible. Part of the medical information, the Region of Interest (ROI), is crucial and must not be altered. This region provides the information for the doctor to diagnose and treat the patient. Hence this region has to be secured.

Watermarking schemes can be broadly classified as time domain and frequency domain schemes. Several watermarking schemes exist, and these schemes adopt both additive and multiplicative approaches in time domain. These schemes adopted SS (Spread Spectrum) [3], DCT (Discrete Cosine Transform) [4], DFT (Discrete Fourier Transform), DWT (Discrete Wavelet Transform) [5], SVD (Singular Value Decomposition) [6], Ridgelets [7], and contourlets [8] in frequency domain. Lim et al. [9] proposed a watermarking scheme to verify the integrity and authenticity of CT scan images. Here, the watermark was processed as an input to the hash function. Raúl et al. [10] proposed a pixel based watermarking embedding scheme using spiral scan.

Coatrieux et al. [11] have identified three different schemes to watermark a medical image:

(i) Embedding the information within the Non-Region of Interest (NROI): this method [12] generally places the watermark in the gray portions of the image. These methods were perceptible. During application of salt and pepper noise, this method may seem too annoying to the physician.

(ii) These schemes deal with reversible watermarking and were better suited for integrity control and data hiding [13].

(iii) These methods normally minimize distortion. This was achieved by replacing some of the image details.

Piva et al. [14] have proposed a method where the physician selects the maximum power of the watermark under the level of interference with diagnosis. This method was robust. Wakatani [15] proposed a scheme wherein the watermark

was embedded in the NROI (Non-Region of Interest) by adopting DWT. The nonwatermarked area was easily prone to attacks. Giakoumaki et al. [16] proposed a robust multiple medical image watermarking scheme using 4-level DWT. The watermark was embedded at different decomposition level and was tested on ultrasound images. Another multiple medical image watermarking was proposed by Memon et al. [17]. The watermark was embedded by separating the ROI and NROI. This scheme was both robust and fragile. Watermark embedded in the NROI is visible. Hence, another option is to embed the watermark in the ROI. This further preserves the ROI from unwanted manipulations. Medical image watermarking schemes must consider computational complexities which may lead to time delays for the physician and are still in the early stages of development. It is difficult to evaluate watermark interferences with diagnosis.

In this paper, a robust medical image watermarking scheme using fractional wavelets is proposed. The proposed scheme is divided into two stages, namely, the embedding stage and the extraction stage. FRFT (Fractional Fourier Transform) has good reconstruction capability compared to FFT (Fast Fourier Transform). When FRFT is combined with WPT (Wave Packet Transform), it has the capability to retain the coefficients after attacks. Three levels of security are provided. Firstly, Arnold Transform is applied to the host image and the host image is scrambled. Secondly, the value of the transform order β is used as the key. According to this key the reference image is generated. This provides for the security of the watermark. The transform order β is user defined and hence randomly chosen. Thirdly, the position of all frequency subbands is changed at each level using some secret rule known only to the user or creator. The adversary cannot extract watermark without accessing the reference image. Quality of the extracted watermark to the original watermark is directly proportional to degradation of the image quality.

A brief introduction on medical image watermarking is introduced in Section 1. This section also deals with some literature survey on the different schemes available. The paper is organized as follows. Sections 2 and 3 describe Fractional Wave Packet Transform and Arnold Transform, respectively. Section 4 describes the proposed method. Section 5 presents the results and discussions of the proposed method. In Section 6 we conclude the work presenting the future enhancements to obtain more robust medical image watermarking schemes.

2. Fractional Wave Packet Transform

Based on the idea of Fractional Fourier Transform (FRFT) and Wave Packet Transform (WPT), Fractional Wave Packet Transform (FRWPT) was introduced by Huang and Suter [18]. Mathematically, for an input signal $x(t)$ represented along the time axis and its Fourier Transform represented along the frequency axis, FRFT, $F_\alpha(t, u)$, of the input signal, $x(t)$, is given by

$$F_\alpha(t, u) = \int_{+\infty}^{-\infty} C_\alpha(t, u) x(t) \, dt, \qquad (1)$$

where $C_\alpha(t, u)$ is the Fourier transformation kernel. FRFT corresponds to a rotation by an angle.

The Wave Packet Transform (WPT) is a combination of Short Time Fourier Transform (STFT) and Continuous Wavelet Transform (CWT). WPT (W_α) of an input signal, $x(t)$, is given by

$$W_\alpha = \frac{1}{\sqrt{2\pi\alpha}} \int_{-\infty}^{+\infty} \exp\left(-jut\right) \psi\left(\frac{t - \beta}{\alpha}\right) x(t)\, dt. \quad (2)$$

WPT can also be defined as the FT of a signal windowed by a wavelet, dilated by α and translated by β.

FRWPT, $W_\alpha(u, a, b)$, for a given input signal $x(t)$ can be defined as

$$W_\alpha(u, a, b) = \frac{1}{\sqrt{a}} \int_{+\infty}^{-\infty} C_\alpha \psi\left(\frac{t - b}{a}\right) x(t)\, dt. \quad (3)$$

The FRWPT is a function of time, frequency, and scale.

The computation of FRWPT corresponds to the following steps as explained by Huang and Suter [18]:

(1) A product by a wavelet.

(2) A product by a chirp.

(3) A Fourier Transform.

(4) Another product by a chirp.

(5) A product by a complex amplitude factor.

For computational purposes, a simple implementation of FRWPT is used as shown in Figure 1.

The computational algorithm can be described as follows:

(1) The transform order of β is used for the FRWPT. This is obtained by trial and error method. If FRWPT is applied to the original signal, and the transformed signal is reconstructed from inverse FRWPT, then the transform order β is that value which results in minimum mean square error between the original and the reconstructed signal. The process may sometimes be long and cumbersome due to its trial and error approach, but it is limited only to once per signal.

(2) FRFT is performed on the input signal, with user defined transform order β, followed by Wavelet Packet Transform. This phase is the decomposition phase.

(3) Inverse Wavelet Packet Transform and inverse FRFT are performed on the transformed signal with transform order β. This phase is the reconstruction phase.

3. Arnold Transform

To further improve the security and improve the proposed watermarking scheme, the host image is preprocessed (scrambled) by applying Arnold Transform. 1-level FRWPT is applied to the Arnold Transformed image. One of the properties of the Arnold Transform is periodicity. Due to this property, the image can be easily recovered after n-permutations.

Consider an image of size $N \times N$; the Arnold Transform is defined by

$$\begin{bmatrix} x' \\ y' \end{bmatrix} = \begin{bmatrix} 1 & 1 \\ 1 & 2 \end{bmatrix} \begin{bmatrix} 1 & 1 \\ 1 & 2 \end{bmatrix} \begin{bmatrix} x \\ y \end{bmatrix} \mod (N), \quad (4)$$

where x, y are the coordinates of the image and x', y' are the coordinates after scrambling.

4. Proposed Work

The proposed scheme can be divided into two phases: the embedding phase and the extraction phase. In the embedding phase, the host image is converted to a reference image and the watermark is embedded on the reference image. During the extraction phase, the watermark is first extracted and then the host image is obtained from the reference image. The watermark used is a grey scale logo/image. The embedded watermark is smaller than the host image by a factor raised to the power of 2 along both the directions. The proposed embedding and extraction scheme is shown in Figures 2 and 3, respectively. Assuming that $I(x, y)$ represents the original image of size $P \times Q$, $W(x, y)$ represents the watermark of size $p \times q$; the embedding and the extraction phase can be detailed as follows.

4.1. Watermark Embedding. The proposed watermarking embedding process can be outlined as follows:

(1) Scramble the host image by applying Arnold Transform.

(2) Apply 1-level Fractional Wave Packet Transform to the Arnold Transformed image. The transform order β is chosen, defined by the creator. The subbands obtained are HH, HL, LH, and LL.

(3) Change the position of the subbands. The pattern to swap/change the image subband is defined by the creator.

(4) Apply 1-level inverse fractional wavelet transform to obtain the reference image $I_{\text{ref}}(x, y)$ and then divide the reference image into subblocks.

(5) Apply watermark to the subblocks to obtain the modified reference watermarked image.

The modified subblocks are represented by

$$W_{\text{ref}} = I_{\text{ref}}(x, y) + \beta W(p, q), \quad (5)$$

where α denotes the strength of the watermark. Integrate the subblocks to obtain the reference watermarked image, $W_{\text{ref}}^*(x, y)$.

(6) Perform 1-level fractional wavelet transform.

(7) Change the position of subbands. Perform 1-level inverse fractional wavelet transform.

(8) Apply Arnold Transform to scramble back the image to obtain the watermarked image, $W^*(x, y)$.

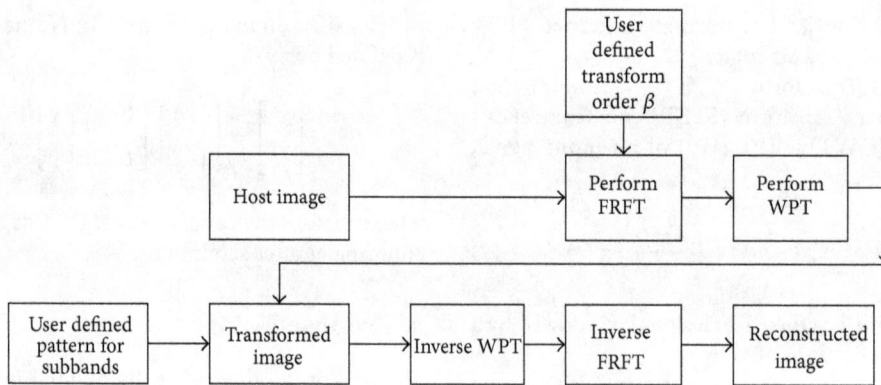

FIGURE 1: Simplified computation efficient FRWPT.

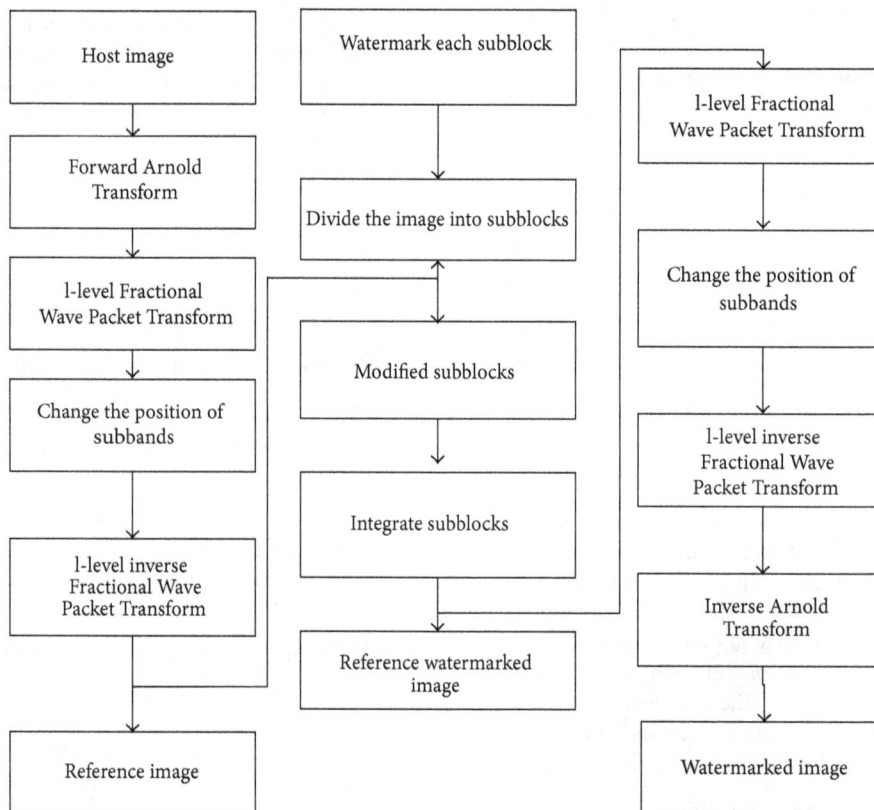

FIGURE 2: Watermark embedding.

4.2. Watermark Extraction. The watermark extraction process can be outlined as follows:

(1) Apply Arnold Transform on the watermarked image $W^*(x, y)$.

(2) Perform 1-level fractional wavelet transform on the Arnold Transformed image.

(3) Change the positions of all the subbands.

(4) Perform 1-level inverse fractional wavelet transform to obtain the watermarked reference image, $W_{\mathrm{ref}}^*(x, y)$.

(5) Extract the watermark, $W(x, y)$.

(6) Perform 1-level fractional wavelet transform on the watermarked image, $W^*(x, y)$.

(7) Change the positions of all the subbands.

(8) Perform 1-level inverse fractional wavelet transform to obtain the host image, $I(x, y)$.

5. Results and Discussions

The performance of the proposed scheme is explored and analysed using Matlab. A number of experiments are performed on mammogram images from the MIAS database. The images chosen are mdb001, mdb017, mdb054, and

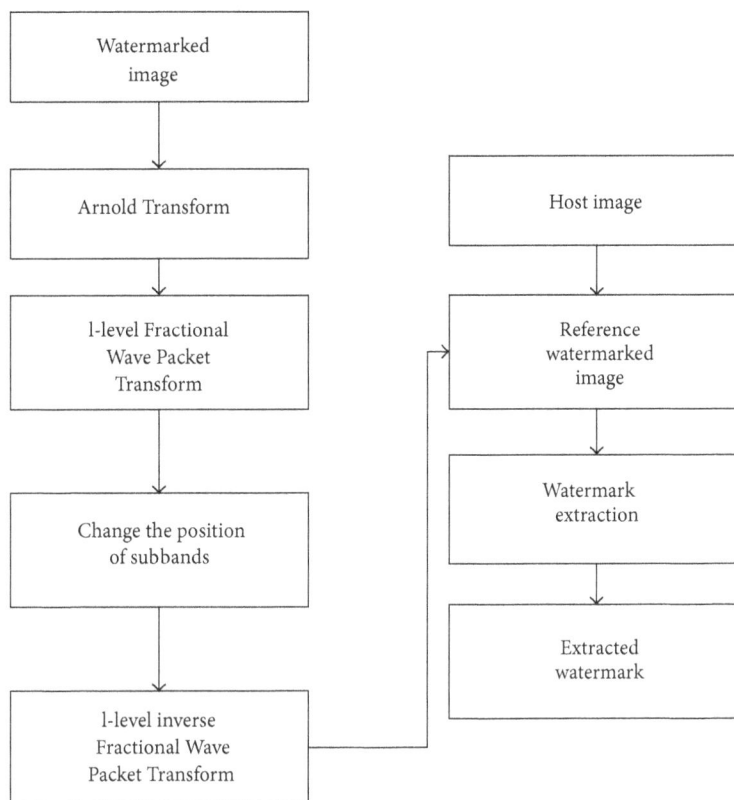

FIGURE 3: Watermark extraction process.

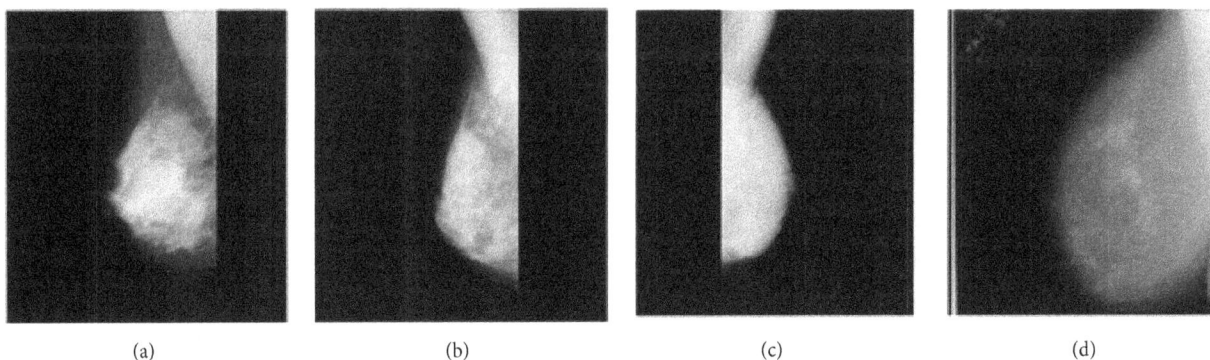

FIGURE 4: Host image: (a) mdb001, (b) mdb017, (c) mdb054, and (d) mdb153.

TABLE 1: Evaluation metrics of proposed algorithm.

Image	mdb001	mdb017	mdb054	mdb153
PSNR	51.9226	52.1666	52.1268	50.5253
SSIM	0.9876	0.9868	0.9863	0.9930

mdb153. Figure 4 shows the host images used. The watermark used is the BMW logo (any grey scale image can be used); reference image is obtained using 2-level decomposition of FRWPT. Since 2-level decomposition gives a block size of 64×64, the watermark is embedded 16 times into the modified reference image to get the watermarked reference image.

Figure 5 shows the watermarked image. The watermarked image quality is measured using the evaluation metrics PSNR and SSIM. Table 1 shows the values of PSNR and SSIM values of the watermarked image with reference to the original image without any attack. The watermarked image is subjected to common attacks to investigate the robustness of the proposed scheme. The attacks considered are average and median filtering, Gaussian noise, salt and pepper noise, cropping, resizing, rotation, and sharpening attacks. The extracted watermark is compared with the original watermark. The performance of the watermarking algorithm under these attacks is tabulated in Tables 2 and 3.

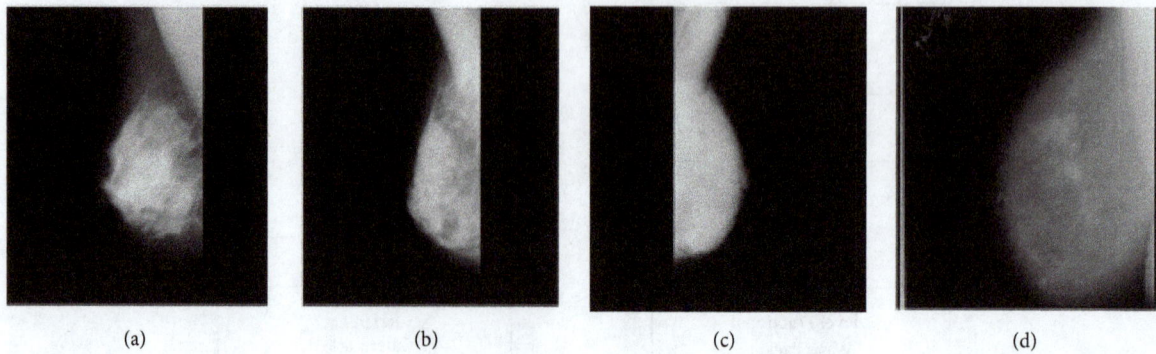

FIGURE 5: Watermarked image: (a) mdb001, (b) mdb017, (c) mdb054, and (d) mdb153.

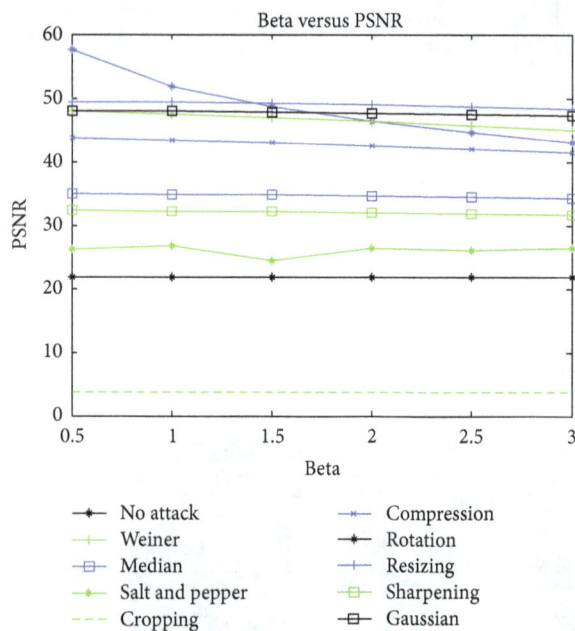

FIGURE 6: Relation between β and PSNR for various attacks.

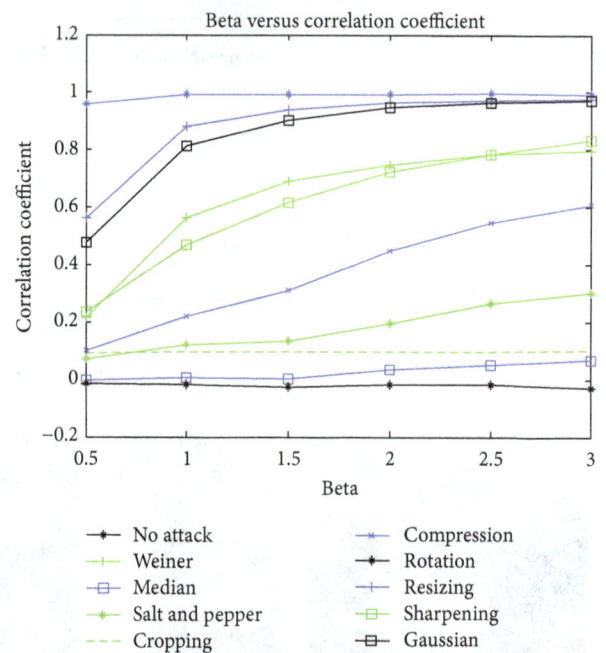

FIGURE 7: Relation between β and correlation coefficient for various attacks.

The watermarked image is subjected to 13×13 median filtering and Weiner filtering. Median filtering attack degrades the image quality. The extracted watermark quality is also degraded. When the image is subjected to Weiner filtering the image quality is not degraded and the watermark quality is recognizable. This is due to addition of noise which degrades the quality of the image and hence the watermark extracted is degraded. Similar effects are also seen when Gaussian noise and salt and pepper noise are added. Hence, the extracted watermarks under noisy environments are still recognizable.

Storage of medical image requires the images to be compressed. The proposed algorithm is observed to be robust under compression attack. Cropping is done by deleting certain number of rows and columns. Since a large part of the image was cropped (200×200 pixels towards upper left corner of the image), most of the medical information was removed. But this can be further modified to crop only the Non-Region of Interest, preserving important medical data.

The image was rotated by an angle of 5 degrees towards the left and right. The results for 5-degree left rotation are tabulated. The proposed scheme could also withstand rotation effect. The proposed algorithm was also tested for sharpening and contrast adjustments and results show that the proposed scheme could withstand these results. Graphical analysis of the proposed scheme under various common attacks discussed above is depicted in Figures 6 and 7. The graph shows the relation between PSNR and correlation coefficient for different values of β, where β denotes the strength of the watermark. It is observed that the proposed watermarking scheme is not image variant and maintains a linear relationship for most of the mammogram images used.

6. Conclusion

In this work, a robust nonblind medical image watermarking scheme for mammograms was proposed applying FRWPT.

TABLE 2: Correlation coefficients of extracted watermarks ($\beta = 1$).

Attack	mdb001 PSNR	Correlation coefficient	mdb017 PSNR	Correlation coefficient	mdb054 PSNR	Correlation coefficient	mdb153 PSNR	Correlation coefficient
No attack	51.9226	0.99167	52.1666	0.9911	52.1268	0.9863	50.5253	0.9990
Weiner	47.4623	0.56504	47.8532	0.5728	50.1466	0.6754	44.2345	0.5348
Median filtering	34.8623	0.00565	35.5175	0.0301	36.9109	0.03534	22.6301	0.0155
Salt and pepper noise	26.7163	0.12153	46.1605	0.7378	26.4035	0.1157	27.3673	0.1713
Cropping	3.84305	0.09536	3.4014	0.0762	3.3462	0.0764	3.6300	0.100
Compression	43.4441	0.21957	44.0487	0.1998	46.1554	0.2317	41.5755	0.2856
Rotation	21.8898	−0.0158	20.0117	−0.0046	19.6339	−0.0011	17.9435	0.0269
Resizing	49.4074	0.88312	47.210	0.8365	46.8850	0.8116	43.4394	0.8355
Sharpening	32.2288	0.46943	32.0762	0.4280	33.1590	0.4798	27.4106	0.4340
Gaussian filter	47.9443	0.81130	46.1605	0.7378	45.3153	0.7336	42.0658	0.7408

TABLE 3: Correlation coefficients of extracted watermarks (mdb001).

β	$\beta = 0.5$		$\beta = 1.5$		$\beta = 2.0$		$\beta = 2.5$	
Attack	PSNR	Correlation coefficient	PSNR	Correlation coefficient	PSNR	Correlation coefficient	PSNR	Correlation coefficient
No attack	57.6742	0.9586	48.7639	0.9951	46.4094	0.9946	44.5710	0.9970
Weiner	47.9247	0.2171	46.9645	0.6886	46.3327	0.7492	45.7129	0.7842
Median filtering	34.9318	0.0002	34.7781	0.0037	34.6527	0.0366	34.5133	0.05360
Salt and pepper noise	26.2601	0.0704	24.4059	0.1352	26.3242	0.1933	25.9943	0.2644
Cropping	3.8383	0.0932	3.8466	0.0956	3.8505	0.0972	3.8541	0.0981
Compression	43.7967	0.1001	43.0275	0.3107	42.5067	0.4475	42.0062	0.5454
Rotation	21.8911	−0.0137	21.8871	−0.0264	21.8810	−0.0165	21.8738	−0.0162
Resizing	49.458	0.5626	49.2708	0.9406	48.9864	0.9642	48.7016	0.9735
Sharpening	32.3031	0.2374	32.1365	0.6153	32.0112	0.7222	31.8713	0.7826
Gaussian filter	48.0211	0.4770	47.8309	0.9038	47.6739	0.9463	47.4890	0.9632

Experimental results show that the scheme is robust to common attacks like the compression attacks, interference attacks, and signal processing attacks. The experimental results are tabulated adopting watermark evaluation metrics PSNR and SSIM. The scheme can be further improved by embedding the watermarking in the NROI. But embedding the watermark in the NROI will make the watermark visible. It is vital to adopt imperceptible watermarks to ensure security issues of integrity and authenticity.

Acknowledgment

The authors would like to thank Dr. C. V. Ravishankar for his valuable suggestions on this paper.

References

[1] D. A. Berry, "Benefits and risks of screening mammography for women in their forties: a statistical appraisal," *Journal of the National Cancer Institute*, vol. 90, no. 19, pp. 1431–1439, 1998.

[2] C. D. Schou, J. Frost, and W. V. Maconachy, "Information assurance in biomedical informatics systems," *IEEE Engineering in Medicine and Biology Magazine*, vol. 23, no. 1, pp. 110–118, 2004.

[3] I. J. Cox, J. Kilian, F. T. Leighton, and T. Shamoon, "Secure spread spectrum watermarking for multimedia," *IEEE Transactions on Image Processing*, vol. 6, no. 12, pp. 1673–1687, 1997.

[4] C. I. Podilchuk and W. Zeng, "Image-adaptive watermarking using visual models," *IEEE Journal on Selected Areas in Communications*, vol. 16, no. 4, pp. 525–539, 1998.

[5] C.-S. Lu and H.-Y. M. Liao, "Multipurpose watermarking for image authentication and protection," *IEEE Transactions on Image Processing*, vol. 10, no. 10, pp. 1579–1592, 2001.

[6] R. Liu and T. Tan, "An SVD-based watermarking scheme for protecting rightful ownership," *IEEE Transactions on Multimedia*, vol. 4, no. 1, pp. 121–128, 2002.

[7] N. K. Kalantari, S. M. Ahadi, and M. Vafadust, "A robust image watermarking in the ridgelet domain using universally optimum decoder," *IEEE Transactions on Circuits and Systems for Video Technology*, vol. 20, no. 3, pp. 396–406, 2010.

[8] M. Jayalakshmi, S. N. Merchant, and U. B. Desai, "Digital watermarking in contourlet domain," in *Proceedings of the 18th International Conference on Pattern Recognition (ICPR '06)*, vol. 3, pp. 861–864, Hong Kong, August 2006.

[9] Y. Lim, C. Xu, and D. D. Feng, "Web based image authentication using invisible fragile watermark," in *Proceedings of the Pan-Sydney Area Workshop on Visual Information Processing (VIP '01)*, vol. 11, pp. 31–34, Sydney, Australia, 2001.

[10] R.-C. Raúl, F.-U. Claudia, and G. J. Trinidad-Blas, "Data hiding scheme for medical images," in *Proceedings of the IEEE 17th International Conference on Electronics, Communications and Computers (CONIELECOMP '07)*, Cholula, Puebla, Mexico, February 2007.

[11] G. Coatrieux, H. Maître, B. Sankur, Y. Rolland, and R. Collorec, "Relevance of watermarking in medical imaging," in *Proceedings of the IEEE EMBS International Conference on Information Technology Applications in Biomedicine (ITAB '00)*, pp. 250–255, Arlington, Va, USA, 2000.

[12] G. Coatrieux, H. Maître, and B. Sankur, "Strict integrity control of biomedical images," in *Security and Watermarking of Multimedia Contents III*, vol. 4314 of *Proceedings of SPIE*, pp. 229–240, San Jose, Calif, USA, January 2001.

[13] C. De Vleeschouwer, J.-F. Delaigle, and B. Macq, "Circular interpretation of bijective transformations in lossless watermarking for media asset management," *IEEE Transactions on Multimedia*, vol. 5, no. 1, pp. 97–105, 2003.

[14] A. Piva, M. Barni, F. Bartolini, and A. De Rosa, "Data hiding technologies for digital radiography," *IEE Proceedings—Vision, Image and Signal Processing*, vol. 152, no. 5, pp. 604–610, 2005.

[15] A. Wakatani, "Digital watermarking for ROI medical images by using compressed signature image," in *Proceedings of the 35th Annual Hawaii International Conference on System Sciences*, pp. 2043–2048, Big Island, Hawaii, USA, January 2002.

[16] A. Giakoumaki, S. Pavlopoulos, and D. Koutsouris, "Multiple image watermarking applied to health information management," *IEEE Transactions on Information Technology in Biomedicine*, vol. 10, no. 4, pp. 722–732, 2006.

[17] N. A. Memon, S. A. M. Gilani, and S. Qayoom, "Multiple watermarking of medical images for content authentication and recovery," in *Proceedings of the IEEE 13th International Multitopic Conference (INMIC '09)*, pp. 1–6, IEEE, Islamabad, Pakistan, December 2009.

[18] Y. Huang and B. Suter, "The fractional wave packet transform," *Multidimensional Systems and Signal Processing*, vol. 9, no. 4, pp. 399–402, 1998.

Is Telephysiotherapy an Option for Improved Quality of Life in Patients with Osteoarthritis of the Knee?

Adesola C. Odole[1,2] and Oluwatobi D. Ojo[1,3]

[1] Department of Physiotherapy, College of Medicine, University of Ibadan, Ibadan 200284, Nigeria
[2] School of Research and Postgraduate Studies, Faculty of Agriculture, Science and Technology, North West University, Mafikeng Campus, Mafikeng 2735, South Africa
[3] Department of Physiotherapy, Neuropsychiatric Hospital, Aro, Abeokuta 110251, Nigeria

Correspondence should be addressed to Oluwatobi D. Ojo; tobbyknow@hotmail.com

Academic Editor: Max Stachura

This study investigated effect of a 6-week telephysiotherapy programme on quality of life (QoL) of patients with knee osteoarthritis (OA). Fifty patients with knee OA were randomly and equally assigned into two treatment groups: clinic group (CG) and telephysiotherapy group (TG). The CG received physiotherapist-administered osteoarthritis-specific exercises in the clinic thrice weekly for 6 weeks while the TG received structured telephone monitoring with self-administered osteoarthritis-specific exercises for the same duration at home. Participants' QoL was assessed using WHOQoL-Bref at baseline, second, fourth, and sixth week of intervention. Data were analyzed using ANOVA and independent Student's t-test. Within-group comparison showed significant improvements in physical health domain ($P = 0.00^*$ for TG and CG) and psychological domain ($P = 0.02^*$ for TG; $P = 0.00^*$ for CG) of WHOQoL following six-week intervention. However, there were no significant differences ($P > 0.05$) in TG and CG's social relationship and environment domains. Between-group comparison showed no significant differences ($P > 0.05$) between CG and TG's physical health, psychological, and social relationships domains of WHOQoL following 6-week intervention. However, there was significant difference in the environment domain ($P < 0.05$). Telephysiotherapy using telephone medium improved QoL in patients with knee OA comparable to clinic based treatment.

1. Introduction

Osteoarthritis (OA) is the most common musculoskeletal disorder characterized by degeneration of articular cartilage, joint space narrowing, pain, and disability [1] with resultant poor quality of life [2]. Knee OA is a prevalent musculoskeletal condition affecting older people and causes pain and physical disability and reduces quality of life (QoL) with considerable economic burden on the health care system [3].

The worldwide prevalence estimates for symptomatic OA is about 13% in women and 10% in men aged 60 years and older. The proportion of people affected with symptomatic knee OA is likely to increase due to the aging of the population and the rate of obesity or overweight in the general population [4]. High prevalence rate of knee OA compared

with other types of OA has been documented [5]. The prevalence of knee OA increases rapidly in people aged ≥40 years [6]. In Nigeria, the prevalence of OA has been documented by several studies [7, 8] and the knee joint is the most frequently affected [7].

The management of knee OA is focused on optimizing the patient's QoL [9] and the term QoL references the general well-being of individuals and societies [10].

Physiotherapy treatment for knee OA involves therapeutic exercises which are used in almost all treatment sessions in the management of knee OA [11]. Exercise has been found to be an effective and well-tolerated treatment for knee OA [12].

The usual pattern of managing patients with knee OA requires patients to keep attending the clinic for one-on-one sessions with the physiotherapists. However, patients who live far away from the clinics may find it difficult to attend clinic regularly due to distance and cost of transportation [13, 14]. In order to address these problems which could make treatment ineffective, telephysiotherapy which entails the use of telecommunications technology as a medium for providing information for therapeutic exercises to patients at homes that are at a distance from the physiotherapy clinics [15] should be considered.

Telephysiotherapy is the development of telemonitoring systems to facilitate independent rehabilitations of patients within their own homes [16]. Telemonitoring is a convenient way for patients to avoid travelling and to perform some of the more basic work of healthcare for themselves [17]. The objective of telephysiotherapy is to allow patients and medical experts to carry on their sessions through telecommunication networks as if they are in the same place [18]. The applications of telephysiotherapy have been previously documented in some medical conditions. Its effectiveness has been documented in rehabilitation of stroke and patients with total knee replacement [19–21]. However, it appears that there is dearth of studies in developing countries like Nigeria on the effect of telephysiotherapy in the management of patients with osteoarthritis of the knee.

According to American Telemedicine Association, telemedicine is defined as the remote delivery of healthcare services and clinical information using telecommunications technology such as internet, wireless, satellite, and telephone media [22]. More so, it has been documented that the concept of telemonitoring can be carried out simply over a telephone or may be as complex as using satellite technology and videoconferencing to do a real-time consultation [23].

Therefore, this study is designed to investigate the effect of a 6-week telephysiotherapy programme on quality of life of patients with osteoarthritis of the knee using telephone medium which is widely available, affordable and relevant telecommunication in Nigeria.

2. Materials and Methods

2.1. Participants. Patients diagnosed with knee osteoarthritis were drawn from out-patient physiotherapy clinics in three hospitals in Southwestern Nigeria: University College Hospital, Ibadan, Neuropsychiatric Hospital, Aro, Abeokuta, and State Hospital, Ijaye, Abeokuta.

Inclusion criteria are as follows: patients that have been diagnosed with OA of the knee joint, patients that are literate in English or Yoruba language, and patients that have means of communication via mobile telephone.

Exclusion criteria are as follows: presence of comorbid medical conditions such as mental illness, diabetes, uncontrolled high blood pressure, and cancer that can influence overall well-being.

2.2. Outcome Measure. World Health Organisation Quality of Life-Bref (WHOQoL-Bref) and its Yoruba translated version. The 26-item WHOQoL-Bref is used in clinical trials to investigate changes in quality of life over the course of

interventions [24]. The WHOQoL-Bref was developed in the context of four domains of QoL: physical, psychological, social, and environment domain scores scaled in a positive direction; that is, higher scores denote higher quality of life [25]. It is self-administered by respondents but an experienced interviewer may assist the administration by reading items aloud where self-completion is not possible, usually for reasons of literacy or disability. The results of a study conducted by Skevington et al. [26] of WHOQoL group indicate that, overall, the WHOQoL-Bref is a sound, cross-culturally valid assessment of QoL, as reflected by its four domains: physical, psychological, social, and environment. The internal consistency shown by Cronbach's alpha for physical domain is 0.82, psychological domain is 0.81, social domain is 0.68, and environment domain is 0.80. Pearson's correlations (one-tailed test) between domains for the total sample were strong, positive, and highly significant ($P < 0.0001$), ranging from 0.46 (physical versus social) to 0.67 (physical versus psychological). The Yoruba version is a valid translation of the English WHOQoL-Bref. Stroke participants' domain scores on the Yoruba translated version of WHOQoL-Bref correlated significantly with those on its English version ($r = 0.695$–0.859; $P = 0.000$) [27].

3. Methods

3.1. Research Design. This study was a randomized clinical trial.

3.2. Sampling Technique. The calculated sample size (N) was fifty (50) patients with knee osteoarthritis. Simple random sampling using a computer generated table of random numbers was used to assign patients equally into telephysiotherapy group and clinic-based group.

3.3. Procedure. Ethical approval was sought and obtained from the Research Ethics Committee of University of Ibadan/ University College Hospital (UI/UCH), Nigeria. The patients were assessed and screened in line with the inclusion and exclusion criteria. The eligible patients were duly informed of the rationale and procedure for the study and were enlightened about the aim of the research in improving physiotherapy services to patients with knee OA. Thereafter, informed consent was obtained from each patient and confidentiality was ensured.

The patients were assigned equally into clinic-based group (25 patients) and telephysiotherapy group (25 patients) randomly using a computer generated table of random numbers.

3.4. Telephysiotherapy Group. Quality of life of this group of patients was assessed at baseline using WHOQoL-Bref. Standardized exercise programmes for patients with knee OA [28] were explained and performed for these patients. A copy of the standardized exercise programmes for patients with knee OA was given to each patient in this group to serve as a guide while performing the exercise at home, three times in a week for six weeks. Mobile telephone monitoring using uniform statements contained in structured telephone monitoring guide on the three occasions of the standardized exercise programmes in a week was done to monitor and coach them about the exercise programmes. They were also provided with exercise log-book for proper documentation of the exercise procedure. This group of patients only reported to the clinics at the end of the second, fourth, and sixth week for reassessment of their QoL.

3.5. Clinic-Based Group. The quality of life of this group of patients was also assessed at baseline using WHOQoL-Bref. However, the physiotherapists, not the patients, administered the same standardized exercise programme for patients with knee OA [28] to this group, three times in a week for 6 weeks in the clinic, and they were neither monitored nor coached on mobile telephone. These patients' QoL was also reassessed at second, fourth, and sixth week of clinic intervention.

English and Yoruba versions of WHOQoL-Bref were used for the assessment procedure in the two groups.

4. Data Analysis

Analysis of variance (ANOVA) was used to compare quality of life at baseline, second, fourth, and sixth week of intervention in clinic-based group and telephysiotherapy group, respectively.

Post hoc analysis of least square difference (LSD) was used to locate exactly where differences occur where there were statistical significant differences after using ANOVA.

Also, independent Student's t-test was used to compare quality of life between the two treatment groups (clinic-based and telephysiotherapy groups) at baseline, second, fourth, and sixth week of intervention.

Trends of quality of life in both groups were presented using graphs.

Level of significance was set at 0.05.

5. Results

5.1. Demographics of Participants. Fifty (50) patients (26 males and 24 females) with osteoarthritis of the knee in age range of 37–72 years with a mean age of 55.50 ± 7.55 years participated in the study. Twenty-five patients (12 males and 13 females) were in the clinic group (CG) with a mean age of 54.96 ± 7.81 years and also an equal number (14 males and 11 females) in the telephysiotherapy group (TG) with a mean age of 56.04 ± 7.40 years.

Both groups were comparable in their ages at baseline ($P = 0.62$) (Table 1).

5.2. Comparison of Physical Health Domain Scores of WHO-QoL of Participants in Telephysiotherapy Group across Baseline, Second, Fourth, and Sixth Week of Intervention. The mean physical health domain scores of WHOQoL of participants in telephysiotherapy group (TG) were significantly different across baseline, second, fourth, and sixth week of intervention (Table 2).

TABLE 1: Demographics of participants.

Group	N	Age Mean ± SD (Years)	t	P value
CG	25	54.96 ± 7.81	-0.502	0.62
TG	25	56.04 ± 7.40		

CG: clinic based group; TG: telephysiotherapy group.
* Significant level is at 0.05.

TABLE 2: Comparison of physical health domain scores of WHOQoL of participants in telephysiotherapy group across baseline, second, fourth, and sixth week of intervention.

Time point	N	PHD Mean ± SD	F	P value
Baseline	25	53.72 ± 11.40		
Second week	25	57.32 ± 9.70	11.208	0.00^*
Fourth week	25	64.08 ± 9.28		
Sixth week	25	69.28 ± 10.94		

PHD: physical health domain; WHOQoL: World Health Organization Quality of Life scale.
* Significant level is at 0.05.

TABLE 3: Post hoc test of physical health domain scores of WHOQoL of participants in telephysiotherapy group across baseline, second, fourth, and sixth week of intervention.

Week	P value
Baseline–second week	0.22
Baseline–fourth week	0.00^*
Baseline–sixth week	0.00^*
Second–fourth week	0.02^*
Second–sixth week	0.00^*
Fourth–sixth week	0.08

* Significant level is at 0.05.

The result of post hoc test (least square difference) shows that there were significant differences in physical health domain scores of WHOQoL of participants in telephysiotherapy group between baseline and fourth week, baseline and sixth week, second and fourth week, and second and sixth week. However, there were no significant differences between baseline and second week and fourth and sixth week (Table 3).

5.3. Comparison of Physical Health Domain Scores of WHOQoL in Clinic Group across Baseline, Second, Fourth, and Sixth Week of Intervention. The mean physical health domain scores of WHOQoL of participants in clinic group (CG) were significantly different across baseline, second, fourth, and sixth week of intervention (Table 4).

The result of post hoc test (least square difference) shows that there were significant differences in physical health domain scores of WHOQoL of participants in clinic group between baseline and fourth week, baseline and sixth week, second and fourth week, and second and sixth week. However, there were no significant differences between baseline and second week and fourth and sixth week (Table 5).

TABLE 4: Comparison of physical health domain scores of WHOQoL of participants in clinic group across baseline, second, fourth, and sixth week of intervention.

Time point	N	PHD Mean ± SD	F	P value
Baseline	25	51.48 ± 15.61		
Second week	25	55.68 ± 14.00	10.214	0.00*
Fourth week	25	64.08 ± 13.05		
Sixth week	25	71.16 ± 12.00		

*Significant level is at 0.05.

TABLE 5: Post hoc test of physical health domain scores of WHOQoL of participants in clinic group across baseline, second, fourth, and sixth week of intervention.

Week	P value
Baseline–second week	0.28
Baseline–fourth week	0.00*
Baseline–sixth week	0.00*
Second–fourth week	0.03*
Second–sixth week	0.00*
Fourth–sixth week	0.07

*Significant level is at 0.05.

TABLE 6: Comparison of psychological domain scores of WHOQoL of participants in telephysiotherapy group across baseline, second, fourth, and sixth week of intervention.

Time point	N	PD Mean ± SD	F	P value
Baseline	25	64.48 ± 10.03		
Second week	25	67.04 ± 9.10	3.464	0.02*
Fourth week	25	69.72 ± 7.97		
Sixth week	25	71.96 ± 7.55		

PD: psychological domain; WHOQoL: World Health Organization Quality of Life scale.
*Significant level is at 0.05.

TABLE 7: Post hoc test of psychological domain scores of WHOQoL of participants in telephysiotherapy group across baseline, second, fourth, and sixth week of intervention.

Week	P value
Baseline–second week	0.30
Baseline–fourth week	0.04*
Baseline–sixth week	0.00*
Second–fourth week	0.28
Second–sixth week	0.05*
Fourth–sixth week	0.37

*Significant level is at 0.05.

TABLE 8: Comparison of psychological domain scores of WHOQoL of participants in clinic group across baseline, second, fourth, and sixth week of intervention.

Time point	N	PD Mean ± SD	F	P value
Baseline	25	61.04 ± 10.45		
Second week	25	66.60 ± 10.74	5.399	0.00*
Fourth week	25	69.64 ± 9.45		
Sixth week	25	71.40 ± 8.23		

*Significant level is at 0.05.

TABLE 9: Post hoc test of psychological domain scores of WHOQoL of participants in clinic group across baseline, second, fourth, and sixth week of intervention.

Week	P value
Baseline–second week	0.04*
Baseline–fourth week	0.00*
Baseline–sixth week	0.00*
Second–fourth week	0.27
Second–sixth week	0.09
Fourth–sixth week	0.53

*Significant level is at 0.05.

5.4. Comparison of Psychological Domain Scores of WHOQoL of Participants in Telephysiotherapy Group across Baseline, Second, Fourth, and Sixth Week of Intervention.

The mean psychological domain scores of WHOQoL of participants in telephysiotherapy group (TG) were significantly different across baseline, fourth, and sixth week of intervention (Table 6).

The result of post hoc test (least square difference) shows that there were significant differences in psychological domain scores of WHOQoL of participants in telephysiotherapy group between baseline and fourth week, baseline and sixth week, and second and sixth week. However, there were no significant differences between baseline and second week, second and fourth week, and fourth and sixth week (Table 7).

5.5. Comparison of Psychological Domain Scores of WHOQOL of Participants in Clinic Group across Baseline, Second, Fourth, and Sixth Week of Intervention.

The mean psychological domain scores of WHOQoL of participants in clinic group (CG) were significantly different across baseline, second, fourth, and sixth week of intervention (Table 8).

The result of post hoc test (least square difference) shows that there were significant differences in psychological domain scores of WHOQoL of participants in clinic group between baseline and second week, baseline and fourth week, and baseline and sixth week. However, there were no significant differences between second and fourth week, second and sixth week, and fourth and sixth week (Table 9).

5.6. Comparison of Social Relationship Domain Scores of WHOQOL of Participants in Telephysiotherapy Group across Baseline, Second, Fourth, and Sixth Week of Intervention.

The mean social relationships domain scores of WHOQoL of participants in telephysiotherapy group (TG) were not significantly different across baseline, second week, fourth week, and sixth week of intervention (Table 10).

5.7. Comparison of Social Relationship Domain Scores of WHOQOL of Participants in Clinic Group across Baseline, Second, Fourth, and Sixth Week of Intervention.

The mean social

TABLE 10: Comparison of social relationship domain scores of WHOQoL of participants in telephysiotherapy group across baseline, second, fourth, and sixth week of intervention.

Time point	N	SRD Mean ± SD	F	P value
Baseline	25	64.80 ± 8.92		
Second week	25	64.52 ± 9.41	0.560	0.64
Fourth week	25	66.80 ± 8.29		
Sixth week	25	67.04 ± 8.44		

SRD: social relationships domain; WHOQoL: World Health Organization Quality of Life scale.
*Significant level is at 0.05.

TABLE 11: Comparison of social relationship domain scores of WHOQoL of participants in clinic group across baseline, second, fourth, and sixth week of intervention.

Time point	N	SRD Mean ± SD	F	P value
Baseline	25	65.76 ± 12.37		
Second week	25	67.04 ± 11.62	0.350	0.79
Fourth week	25	67.00 ± 11.22		
Sixth week	25	69.04 ± 10.58		

*Significant level is at 0.05.

relationships domain scores of WHOQoL of participants in clinic group (CG) were not significantly different across baseline, second, fourth, and sixth week of intervention (Table 11).

5.8. Comparison of Environment Domain Scores of WHOQoL of Participants in Telephysiotherapy Group across Baseline, Second, Fourth, and Sixth Week of Intervention. The mean environment domain scores of WHOQoL of participants in telephysiotherapy group (TG) were not significantly different across baseline, second week, fourth week, and sixth week of intervention (Table 12).

5.9. Comparison of Environment Domain Scores of WHOQOL of Participants in Clinic Group across Baseline, Second, Fourth, and Sixth Week of Intervention. The mean environment domain scores of WHOQoL of participants in clinic group (CG) were not significantly different across baseline, second week, fourth week, and sixth week of intervention (Table 13).

5.10. Between-Group Comparison of Participants' Physical Health Domain of WHOQoL at Baseline, Second, Fourth, and Sixth Week of Intervention. The mean physical health domain scores of WHOQoL of the participants in the two groups (clinic group versus telephysiotherapy group) were not significantly different at baseline, second, fourth, and sixth week of intervention (Table 14). This is also represented on bar charts (Figure 1).

5.11. Between-Group Comparison of Participants' Psychological Domain of WHOQoL at Baseline, Second, Fourth, and Sixth

TABLE 12: Comparison of environment domain scores of WHOQoL of participants in telephysiotherapy group across baseline, second, fourth, and sixth week of intervention.

Time point	N	ED Mean ± SD	F	P value
Baseline	25	64.52 ± 7.76		
Second week	25	65.08 ± 7.16	1.570	0.20
Fourth week	25	67.76 ± 8.11		
Sixth week	25	68.48 ± 8.09		

ED: environment domain; WHOQoL: World Health Organization Quality of Life scale.
*Significant level is at 0.05.

TABLE 13: Comparison of environment domain scores of WHOQoL of participants in clinic group across baseline, second, fourth, and sixth week of intervention.

Time point	N	ED Mean ± SD	F	P value
Baseline	25	59.08 ± 8.01		
Second week	25	59.76 ± 8.58	1.750	0.16
Fourth week	25	62.24 ± 8.48		
Sixth week	25	63.76 ± 7.80		

*Significant level is at 0.05.

TABLE 14: Between-group comparison of participants' physical health domain of WHOQoL at baseline, second, fourth, and sixth week of intervention.

Time point	Group	N	PHD Mean ± SD	t	P value
Baseline	CG	25	51.48 ± 15.61	−0.579	0.57
	TG	25	53.72 ± 11.40		
Second week	CG	25	55.68 ± 14.00	−0.482	0.63
	TG	25	57.32 ± 9.70		
Fourth week	CG	25	64.08 ± 13.05	0.000	1.00
	TG	25	64.08 ± 9.28		
Sixth week	CG	25	71.16 ± 12.00	0.579	0.57
	TG	25	69.28 ± 10.94		

*Significant level is at 0.05.

Week of Intervention. The mean psychological domain scores of WHOQoL of the participants in the two groups (clinic group versus telephysiotherapy group) were not significantly different at baseline, second, fourth, and sixth week of intervention (Table 15). This is also represented on bar charts (Figure 2).

5.12. Between-Group Comparison of Participants' Social Relationships Domain of WHOQoL at Baseline, Second, Fourth, and Sixth Week of Intervention. The mean social relationships domain scores of WHOQoL of the participants in the two groups (clinic group versus telephysiotherapy group) were not significantly different at baseline, second, fourth, and sixth week of intervention (Table 16). This is represented on bar charts (Figure 3).

TABLE 15: Between-group comparison of participants' psychological domain of WHOQoL at baseline, second, fourth, and sixth week of intervention.

Time point	Group	N	PD Mean ± SD	t	P value
Baseline	CG	25	61.04 ± 10.45	−1.187	0.24
	TG	25	64.48 ± 10.03		
Second week	CG	25	66.60 ± 10.74	−0.156	0.88
	TG	25	67.04 ± 9.10		
Fourth week	CG	25	69.64 ± 9.45	−0.032	0.97
	TG	25	69.72 ± 7.97		
Sixth week	CG	25	71.40 ± 8.26	0.025	0.80
	TG	25	71.96 ± 7.55		

*Significant level is at 0.05.

TABLE 16: Between-group comparison of participants' social relationships domain of WHOQoL at baseline, second, fourth, and sixth week of intervention.

Time point	Group	N	SRD Mean ± SD	t	P value
Baseline	CG	25	65.76 ± 12.37	0.315	0.75
	TG	25	64.80 ± 8.92		
Second week	CG	25	67.04 ± 11.62	0.843	0.40
	TG	25	64.52 ± 9.41		
Fourth week	CG	25	67.00 ± 11.22	0.072	0.94
	TG	25	66.80 ± 8.29		
Sixth week	CG	25	69.04 ± 10.58	0.739	0.46
	TG	25	67.04 ± 8.44		

*Significant level is at 0.05.

TABLE 17: Between-group comparison of participants' environment domain of WHOQoL at baseline, second, fourth, and sixth week of intervention.

Time point	Group	N	ED Mean ± SD	t	P value
Baseline	CG	25	59.08 ± 8.01	−2.439	0.02*
	TG	25	64.52 ± 7.76		
Second week	CG	25	59.76 ± 8.58	−2.379	0.02*
	TG	25	65.08 ± 7.16		
Fourth week	CG	25	62.24 ± 8.48	−2.353	0.02*
	TG	25	67.76 ± 8.11		
Sixth week	CG	25	63.76 ± 7.80	−2.099	0.04*
	TG	25	68.48 ± 8.09		

*Significant level is at 0.05.

5.13. Between-Group Comparison of Participants' Environment Domain of WHOQoL at Baseline, Second, Fourth, and Sixth Week of Intervention. The mean environment domain scores of WHOQoL of the participants in the two groups (clinic group versus telephysiotherapy group) were significantly different at baseline, second, fourth, and sixth week of intervention (Table 17). This is represented on bar charts (Figure 4).

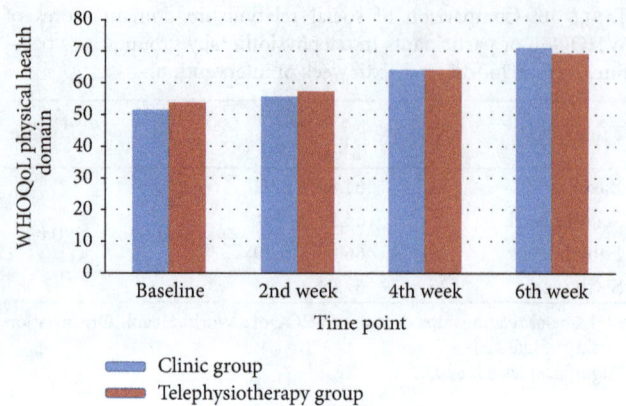

FIGURE 1: Bar chart showing between-group comparisons of participants' physical health domain of WHOQoL following six weeks of intervention.

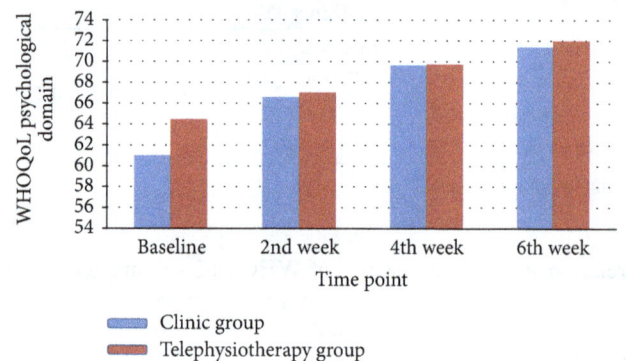

FIGURE 2: Bar chart showing between-group comparisons of participants' psychological domain of WHOQoL following six weeks of intervention.

6. Discussion

This study has scientifically investigated the effect of a 6-week telephysiotherapy programme on quality of life of patients with osteoarthritis of the knee. Fifty patients (26 males and 24 females) with osteoarthritis of the knee participated in the study. 96% of the participants are between the age range of 40–69 years and this is in line with the age prevalence of knee OA as documented in several studies [6, 29].

Sophisticated telecommunication means such as real-time video conferencing and satellite which are widely used in developed countries are not widely available for general use in developing countries like Nigeria, basically because they are expensive for average Nigerians. Thus, this research employed the use of mobile telephone which is an affordable and widely used telecommunication means in Nigeria. This medium (mobile telephoning) has been documented to be an acceptable form of telehealth/telemonitoring system [22, 23]. It appears there are no documented studies on the effect of telephysiotherapy among individuals with knee osteoarthritis in Nigeria. Therefore, the findings from this research would be compared with related works from other parts of the world and studies in different patients' population.

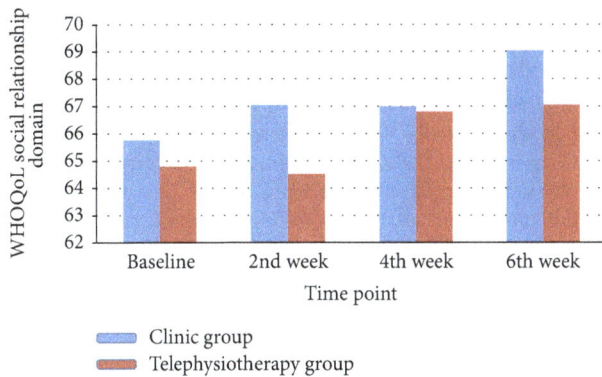

FIGURE 3: Bar chart showing between-group comparisons of participants' social relationship domain of WHOQoL following six weeks of intervention.

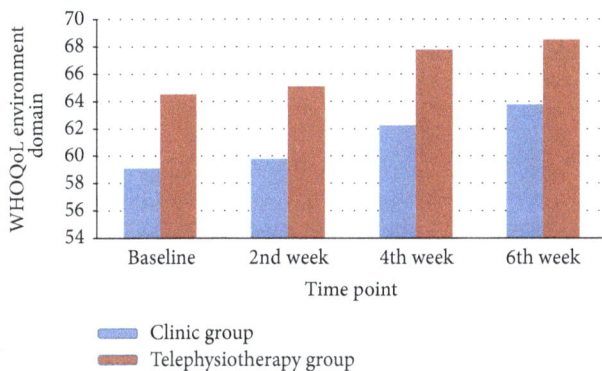

FIGURE 4: Bar chart showing between-group comparisons of participants' environment domain of WHOQoL following six weeks of intervention.

Dar et al. [30] reported no significant difference in typical elderly population of heart failure patients between those in usual care group and telemonitoring group in overall health-related quality of life as measured through the generic Euroqol (EQ5D) over the 6-month follow-up period and quality of life measured through the disease specific Minnesota living with heart failure questionnaire (MLwHF) ($P = 0.5$ for EQ5D and $P = 0.6$ for MLwHF).

Also, Russell [21] documented that the achieved outcomes following six weeks of either traditional outpatient rehabilitation services or internet-based outpatient rehabilitation (telerehab group) in 65 patients who underwent total knee replacement (TKR) are similar. The patients were randomized to receive six weeks of either traditional outpatient rehabilitation services or telerehabilitation exercises. Patients in the telerehab group received rehabilitation exercises (open and closed kinetic loop active exercises) through real-time (live video and audio) interaction with a physical therapist via an internet-based system and therapy sessions were limited to 45 minutes.

The above reports are similar to our research findings which showed no significant difference ($P > 0.05$) in physical,

psychological, and social relationship domains of quality of life between patients with knee osteoarthritis (OA) in telephysiotherapy group and clinic based group at baseline, second, fourth, and sixth week of intervention.

Furthermore, the efficacy of telephysiotherapy as shown in our findings where significant differences were noted in quality of life of patients in telephysiotherapy group between weeks 0–4, 0–6, 2–4, and 2–6 in physical health domain and weeks 0–4, 0–6, and 2–6 in psychological domain of WHOQoL is similar to the outcomes of two recent studies discussed below.

Keerthi et al. [31] assessed the efficacy of telerehabilitation via videoconferencing when compared to telephonic consultation for home based treatment of patients with knee OA using exercise. The results of this study showed percentage difference in pain, stiffness, and physical function in both groups, that is, patients in telerehabilitation via videoconferencing and patients in telephonic consultation group. The percentage difference in the former is a better home based exercise program in osteoarthritis of the knee though. The significant improvements in outcomes of pain, stiffness, and physical function documented in the telephonic consultation group are similar to the significant improvements in physical health and psychological domains of WHOQoL that were recorded in patients with knee OA in telephysiotherapy group during six weeks of intervention in our research.

Likewise, Margolis [32] reported that patients receiving telemonitoring along with high blood pressure management support from a pharmacist were more likely to lower their blood pressure than those not receiving extra support. They studied 450 patients with uncontrolled high blood pressure. Approximately half (222) of the patients were assigned to traditional care through their primary care providers while the remaining 228 patients in the intervention group saw a primary care provider and received additional telemonitoring support from a pharmacist. The latter measured their blood pressure at home and sent the readings electronically to a secure website. Participating pharmacists accessed the information and consulted the patients every two to four weeks by phone. The researchers found that blood pressure decreased more in the telemonitoring group. At the start of the study, patients' blood pressures averaged 148/85 mmHg while at six months the average was 126/76 mmHg in the telemonitoring intervention and 138/82 mmHg in the traditional care group. This result is also similar to the significant improvements in physical health and psychological domains of WHOQoL we recorded in patients with knee OA in telephysiotherapy group during six weeks of intervention in our research. However, the results of Keerthi et al. [31] and Margolis [32] discussed above are contrary to our findings in social relationship and environment domains of WHOQoL where no significant differences were noted during 6 weeks of telephysiotherapy intervention.

Summarily, our study showed that the outcome of quality of life in patients with osteoarthritis of the knee under telephysiotherapy treatment is comparable to those in clinic based group following six weeks of intervention. Besides, there were significant improvements in physical and psychological domains of quality of life in patients with osteoarthritis of the knee following 6 weeks of telephysiotherapy intervention. The effectiveness and usability of telephysiotherapy in the management of patients with knee osteoarthritis have been demonstrated in this study. This mode of therapeutic intervention in patients with knee OA would undoubtedly reduce clinic visits, clinic waiting time, and cost incurred on transportation to the clinic, especially for patients living at distant places from physiotherapy clinics.

7. Conclusion

Telephone-based physiotherapy intervention is effective in management of patients with knee osteoarthritis and it produces a similar outcome in terms of quality of life to conventional clinic based physiotherapy as documented in this research. Thus, this mode of treatment may be considered in the management of patients with osteoarthritis of the knee and more research should be carried out on the usability and effectiveness of telephysiotherapy in the management of other conditions amenable to physiotherapy.

References

[1] C. S. O'Reilly and M. Doherty, "Signs, symptoms and laboratory test," in *Osteoarthritis*, K. D. Brandt, M. Doherty, and L. S. Lohmander, Eds., pp. 197–210, Oxford University Press, New York, NY, USA, 2nd edition, 2003.

[2] J. Warner, Obesity, knee osteoarthritis hurt seniors' life expectancy, Quality of life also reduced by knee OA and obesity, researchers say, Osteoarthritis Health Center, 2011, http://www.webmd.com/osteoarthritis.

[3] Arthritis Foundation of Australia, "The prevalence, cost and disease burden of arthritis in Australia," 2001, http://www.boneandjointdecade.org/.

[4] Y. Zhang and J. M. Jordan, "Epidemiology of osteoarthritis," *Clinics in Geriatric Medicine*, vol. 26, no. 3, pp. 355–369, 2010.

[5] H. Bliddal and R. Christensen, "The treatment and prevention of knee osteoarthritis: a tool for clinical decision-making," *Expert Opinion on Pharmacotherapy*, vol. 10, no. 11, pp. 1793–1804, 2009.

[6] T. Molly, "Epidemiology of knee osteoarthritis," in *Management of Osteoarthritis of the Knee: An International Consensus*, H. Freddie and D. Bruce, Eds., American Academy of Orthopaedic Surgeons, 2003.

[7] A. O. Akinpelu, T. O. Alonge, B. A. Adekanla, and A. C. Odole, "Prevalence and pattern of symptomatic knee osteoarthritis in Nigeria: a community-based study," *Internet Journal of Allied Health Sciences and Practice*, vol. 7, no. 3, 2009.

[8] S. O. Ogunlade, T. O. Alonge, A. B. Omololu, and O. S. Adekolujo, "Clinical spectrum of large joint osteoarthritis in Ibadan, Nigeria," *European Journal of Science and Research*, vol. 11, pp. 116–122, 2005.

[9] D. J. Hunter and D. T. Felson, "Osteoarthritis: effective pain management for patients with arthritis," *British Medical Journal*, vol. 332, no. 7542, pp. 639–642, 2006.

[10] D. Gregory, R. Johnston, G. Pratt, and S. Whatmore, *Quality of Life*, Dictionary of Human Geography, 2009.

[11] G. Jamtvedt, K. T. Dahm, I. Holm, and S. Flottorp, "Measuring physiotherapy performance in patients with osteoarthritis of the knee: a prospective study," *BMC Health Services Research*, vol. 8, article 145, 2008.

[12] B. T. Maurer, A. G. Stern, B. Kinossian, K. D. Cook, and H. R. Schumacher, "Osteoarthritis: isokinetic quadriceps exercise versus an educational intervention," *Archives of Physical Medicine and Rehabilitation*, vol. 24, pp. 455–445, 1999.

[13] World Health Organisation, *Adherence to Long Term Therapies—Evidence for Action*, 2003.

[14] B. W. Nelson, E. O'Reilly, M. Miller, M. Hogan, J. A. Wegner, and C. Kelly, "The clinical effects of intensive, specific exercise on chronic low back pain: a controlled study of 895 consecutive patients with 1-year follow up," *Orthopedics*, vol. 18, no. 10, pp. 971–981, 1995.

[15] M.-M. Bernard, F. Janson, P. K. Flora, G. E. J. Faulkner, L. Meunier-Norman, and M. Fruhwirth, "Videoconference-based physiotherapy and tele-assessment for homebound older adults: a pilot study," *Activities, Adaptation and Aging*, vol. 33, no. 1, pp. 39–48, 2009.

[16] V. F. S. Fook, S. Z. Hao, A. A. P. Wai et al., "Innovative platform for tele-physiotherapy," in *Proceedings of the 10th International Conference on e-Health Networking, Applications and Service (HEALTHCOM '08)*, pp. 59–65, July 2008.

[17] C. Harper, "What is telemonitoring, Wisegeek conjecture corporation," 2012, http://www.wisegeek.com.

[18] P. Kittipanya-ngam, X. Yu, and H.-L. Eng, "Computer vision technologies for monitoring system in tele-physiotherapy," in *Proceedings of the 3rd International Convention on Rehabilitation Engineering and Assistive Technology (ICREATE '09)*, April 2009.

[19] H. Zhou, H. Hu, and N. Harris, "Wearable Inertial Sensors for arm motion tracking in home-based rehabilitation," in *Proceedings of the 9th International Conference on Intelligent Autonomous Systems (IAS-9 '06)*, pp. 930–937, 2006.

[20] H. Zheng, R. J. Davies, and N. D. Black, "Web-based monitoring system for home-based rehabilitation with stroke patients," in *Proceedings of the 18th IEEE Symposium on Computer-Based Medical Systems*, pp. 419–424, June 2005.

[21] T. Russell, "Tele-rehabilitation as successful as out-patient physiotherapy post total knee replacement," *Journal of Bone and Joint Surgery*, vol. 93, pp. 113–120, 2011.

[22] American Telemedicine Assocation, "Telemedicine frequently asked questions (FAQs)," 2013, http://www.americantelemed.org/learn/what-is-telemedicine/faqs.

[23] Rhiggs, "What is Telemedicine?" 2010, http://www.icucare.com/PageFiles/Telemedicine.pdf.

[24] World Health Organisation Quality of Life Group, "WHOQOL-bref. Introduction, administration, scoring and generic version of the assessment. The WHOQOL Group Programme on Mental Health," 1996, http://www.who.int/mental_health/media/en/76.

[25] World Health Organisation Quality of Life Group, "Development of the World Health Organization WHOQOL-BREF quality of life assessment," *Psychological Medicine*, vol. 28, no. 3, pp. 551–558, 1998.

[26] S. M. Skevington, M. Lotfy, and K. A. O'Connell, "WHO centre for the study of quality of life," *Quality of Life Research*, vol. 13, no. 2, pp. 299–310, 2004.

[27] A. O. Akinpelu, F. A. Maruf, and B. O. Adegoke, "Validation of a Yoruba translation of the World Health Organization's quality of life scale—short form among stroke survivors in Southwest Nigeria," *African Journal of Medicine and Medical Sciences*, vol. 35, no. 4, pp. 417–424, 2006.

[28] D. Zelman, "Exercises for OA of the knee," 2013, http://www.webmd.com/osteoarthritisjoint-/injections-13/slideshow-knee-exercises.

[29] Centers for Disease Control and Prevention, "Osteoarthritis," 2009, http://www.cdc.gov/arthritis/.

[30] O. Dar, J. Riley, C. Chapman et al., "A randomized trial of home telemonitoring in a typical elderly heart failure population in North West London: results of the home-HF study," *European Journal of Heart Failure*, vol. 11, no. 3, pp. 319–325, 2009.

[31] R. Keerthi, I. Chandra, and A. Deepak, "Can telerehabilitation add a new dimension in the treatment of osteoarthritis knee?" *Journal of Pain and Relief*, vol. 2, no. 1, 2013.

[32] K. Margolis, "Telemonitoring helps to lower blood pressure rates," 2012, http://www.fiercehealthit.com/story.

Feasibility of Telerehabilitation Implementation as a Novel Experience in Rehabilitation Academic Centers and Affiliated Clinics in Tehran: Assessment of Rehabilitation Professionals' Attitudes

Sara Movahedazarhouligh,[1] Roshanak Vameghi,[2] Nikta Hatamizadeh,[3] Enayatollah Bakhshi,[4] and Seyed Muhammad Moosavy Khatat[5]

[1] Department of Rehabilitation Management, University of Social Welfare and Rehabilitation Sciences, Tehran, Iran
[2] Pediatric Neurorehabilitation Research Center, University of Social Welfare and Rehabilitation Sciences, Tehran, Iran
[3] Department of Rehabilitation Management, Pediatric Neurorehabilitation Research Center,
 University of Social Welfare and Rehabilitation Sciences, Tehran, Iran
[4] Department of Biostatistics, University of Social Welfare and Rehabilitation Sciences, Tehran, Iran
[5] Department of Social Welfare, University of Social Welfare and Rehabilitation Sciences, Tehran, Iran

Correspondence should be addressed to Roshanak Vameghi; r_vameghi@yahoo.com

Academic Editor: Fei Hu

Introduction. This study aimed to assess rehabilitation professionals' attitude toward implementation and application of telerehabilitation technology as a novel study in rehabilitation academic centers and affiliated clinics in Tehran. *Methods.* It was a descriptive cross-sectional study. To collect data, a researcher-designed questionnaire was developed. 141 rehabilitation experts participated in the study. *Results.* A majority of faculty members (78%) and clinicians (89.7%) either were in "definite agreement" or "somewhat agreed" with implementation and application of this technology, which demonstrates an overall positive attitude. *Discussion.* Based on the positive attitudes of the majority of participants toward implementation and application of this technology and their preferences in offering different telerehabilitation services, it seems that there is an appropriate and desirable acceptance and administrative culture to implement this technology among rehabilitation experts in Tehran. It is thus expected that implementation and application of this technology will be a promising experience in rehabilitation academic centers and affiliate clinics in Tehran.

1. Introduction

Today, new technologies have come into existence in different occupations and work areas, one of which is information and communication technology [1]. Due to rapid advances in information technology many aspects of work environments worldwide have been faced with fundamental changes. The field of healthcare has not been exempt from these effects [2] as technological aspects of patient care are constantly undergoing changes [3]. Rapid development of technology and health informatics has encouraged healthcare organizations to provide advanced services with better quality [4].

Today, healthcare organizations are faced with a new technology called telehealth. Telehealth is the use of information and communication technologies to provide remote healthcare services [5]. The World Health Organization, citing its many benefits, has stated that telehealth should be one of the main parts of healthcare strategic plans to change health systems in the 21st century [6]. Telehealth covers other specialized areas such as e-health, telemedicine, telematics, and telerehabilitation. Telerehabilitation delivers remote rehabilitation services via information and communication technologies [7].

Telerehabilitation is a relatively new area which was first defined by the National Institute of Disability and Rehabilitation in the United Sates in 1997 [8]. It encompasses a considerable range of rehabilitation services which are offered in different formats including teleassessment, teletreatment, telemonitoring, teleconsultation, telesupport, teleconferencing, teleeducation, teletherapy, telecoaching, and teleplay [9]. Telerehabilitation includes application of different technologies which can be categorized into three main modes. (1) The first mode is the store-and-forward (asynchronous) mode, in which information is recorded and stored and used when needed. As an example, in a rural community telerehabilitation site, a patient X-ray of a fracture in the knee is scanned and captured as an electronic file. This file, including accompanying medical notes, is sent electronically to the rehabilitation expert in the tertiary care telerehabilitation site. The rehabilitation professional in the tertiary care site opens the file and reviews the X-rays and notes in order to get to know about the patient's medical history and determine a general therapeutic plan. The file and accompanying notes are then returned to the rural telerehabilitation site. The patient is informed of the therapeutic plan without having to meet the physical therapist. (2) The second mode is real-time (synchronous) interactions, in which live interactive interventions take place between the service provider and receiver. As an example for the same knee fracture, here the patient and the physical therapist can arrange a video conferencing meeting in the chatroom of the rural community of the telerehabilitation site and using live interaction consultation, the therapist can instruct the patient how to do some specific exercises. (3) The third mode is the hybrid mode, which is a combination of the two mentioned modes [10]. The technologies that are used are categorized as follows: (1) textual-based technologies like e-mails, (2) audio-based (voice/sound) technologies like phones, audio recorders, and telephone answering machines, (3) vision-based technologies like video conferencing, (4) virtual reality like computer games and avatars, (5) web-based technologies like real-time chatrooms and discussion boards, (6) wireless technologies like PDAs (Personal Digital Assistants) and GPS (Global Positioning Systems), and (7) integrated systems like robots [11].

Telerehabilitation has the potential to benefit both the consumers and providers of rehabilitation services by lessening the inconvenience and/or cost of patient transfers and reducing unnecessary travel time [12]. The many benefits of this technology include elimination of distance barriers, improvement of access to healthcare services and information both for the users and for the providers in particular remote access in Iran, lessening of the inconvenience and/or cost of patient transfers and reduction of unnecessary travel time for rehabilitation professionals, and playing of an invaluable role in situations where moving a patient may be undesirable or not feasible [13]. In our country, Iran, principles of e-health have already been taken into consideration in recent years and efforts have been made to implement related systems and software [14]. It seems that factors such as rehabilitation experts' tendency to live in larger cities and, thus, lack of easy access to experts and services in smaller towns,

geographical broadness, vast distribution of the population, and the existence of somewhat optimal telecommunication infrastructures in Iran can be considered as incentives for implementation of this technology in the country [15]. However, other factors can also play important roles and should not be overlooked. For example, implementation of an effective telerehabilitation system in any community requires awareness, motivation [16], and positive attitude of the people involved, in particular end-users and therapists.

Attitude plays an important role in our lives, thoughts, and our individual and social behaviors. In fact our views on various issues determine our actions and reactions and justify our motivation or reluctance to show certain behaviors [17]. Attitude toward technology is not an exception [18]. The techniques that are used for measuring attitudes, beliefs, and perceptions have gone beyond using questionnaires or having people interviewed and this is probably due to the importance of attitude studies [19]. Normally, to assess attitudes different scales such as Likert and Thurston and interview methods are used. Today, the most common way to measure attitude is grading scales among which Likert rating is the most popular [20].

In the past few years in Iran, there have been feasibility or review studies which have addressed different aspects of telemedicine and e-health including telelaparoscopy [5], telepsychiatry [21], telenursing [22], telesurgery [23], and e-health [24] but no study has ever been conducted on telerehabilitation yet. Telerehabilitation, specifically, does not even exist in the country, either in urban or in rural areas. No study has been ever conducted on telerehabilitation in the country and this research is a pioneer in this regard, both in the academic sense and in the clinical sense.

Due to the very newness of this technology in our country and considering the importance and advantages of this technology, this study aims to assess rehabilitation professionals' attitude towards implementation and application of telerehabilitation technology in rehabilitation academic centers in the city of Tehran. In the present study, attitude toward telerehabilitation implementation was defined as the respondents' views on the efficacy and the potential benefits of application of this technology in therapy and therapeutic systems.

Since rehabilitation professionals working in academic environments are expected to have more realistic attitudes towards this issue based on their more update knowledge in the rehabilitation domain and the fact that they are the most familiar ones with the current position and status of rehabilitation in the country, thus they were considered as a desirable population for conducting this study.

2. Method and Materials

This was a descriptive cross-sectional study conducted on faculty members of four universities and clinicians of affiliated rehabilitation centers in Tehran. A preliminary draft of an attitude questionnaire was developed by integration and cultural adaptation of different tools collected in the field of telehealth implementation. The face and content validity of the questionnaire was evaluated by a panel of rehabilitation faculty members in the University of Social Welfare and Rehabilitation Sciences using Lawshe's method and the reliability was assessed by test-retest correlation and Cronbach's alpha determinations. Finally, a researcher-designed questionnaire with favorable validity and reliability was obtained.

The designed questionnaire consisted of 51 questions scored by a Likert scale of 5, ranging from "definitely agree" with a score of 5 to "definitely disagree" with a score of 1. The higher the score, the more positive the attitude it reflected. By using 4 cut-off points for the total attainable score, 5 levels of total attitude were defined.

The questions in the questionnaire were categorized in 4 different groups, including questions that dealt with the possible positive or negative impacts of telerehabilitation implementation on (1) the experts' own work domain, (2) the work domain of colleagues, (3) the quality of therapeutic procedures and service delivery for the clients, and (4) the national health and ICT system. Overall, the questions were meant to determine what attitude the experts expressed regarding each of the suggested positive or negative outcomes or impacts of telerehabilitation implementation and application. Some examples of the questionnaire's content are stated in Table 1.

The study received an approval from the IRB and Ethical Committee of the University of Social Welfare and Rehabilitation Sciences. The study population included rehabilitation experts (faculty members and clinicians) in the University of Social Welfare and Rehabilitation Sciences and Tehran, Iran, and Shahid Beheshti Universities of Medical Sciences. Stratified sampling was used. The universities were considered as the main classes and the experts' positions as a faculty member or a clinician constituted the subclasses. The samples from each class and subclass were selected by simple random sampling. The questionnaire then was distributed manually by the researcher and participants were asked to complete the questionnaire in a few days, after which the researcher returned to collect them. Totally, 150 rehabilitation experts were recruited of which 141 participated by completing them.

3. Results

Table 2 shows the demographic characteristics of the participants. The results are presented in terms of two main categories: faculty members and clinicians.

Table 3 shows the distribution of the rehabilitation experts' overall attitude towards implementation and application of telerehabilitation, in terms of their groups of faculty members and clinicians. As can be seen a majority of faculty members (78%) and clinicians (89.7%) were either in "definite agreement" or "somewhat agreed" with implementation and application of this technology, which demonstrates an overall positive attitude. If "overall positive attitude" be defined as the sum of the total percentage of "definite agreement" and the total percentage of "somewhat agreement", then according to Table 4 which shows the distribution of the rehabilitation experts' attitude in terms of their age, Table 5 which shows the distribution of the rehabilitation experts' attitude in terms

TABLE 1

Category	Questions
Possible impacts of telerehabilitation implementation on the experts' own work domain	(i) Benefits of telerehabilitation application in enhancing professional contacts (ii) Challenges of telerehabilitation application (iii) Benefits of different modes of telerehabilitation in different rehabilitation specialties
Possible impacts of telerehabilitation implementation on their colleagues' work domain	(i) Benefits of telerehabilitation application in professional responsibilities of colleagues (ii) Ethical challenges of telerehabilitation application by colleagues (iii) Rehabilitation professionals' resistance toward telerehabilitation application
Possible impacts of telerehabilitation implementation on the treatment procedure and service delivery for the client	(i) Efficacy of telerehabilitation in different rehabilitation specialties (ii) Efficacy of telerehabilitation in different stages of therapy
Possible impacts of telerehabilitation implementation on the national supportive system	(i) Economical advantages and challenges of telerehabilitation application (ii) Reimbursement issues of telerehabilitation application (iii) Required IT infrastructures of telerehabilitation implementation

of their sex, Table 6 which shows the distribution of the rehabilitation experts' attitude in terms of their educational status, Table 7 which shows the distribution of the rehabilitation experts' attitude in terms of their university of employment and Table 8 which shows the distribution of the rehabilitation experts' attitude in terms of their working experience, the highest percent of overall positive attitude was observed in participants with >30 years of age, female participants, participants with a PhD degree, participants who were employed in the Tehran University of Medical Sciences and in participants with more than 20 years of experience.

Table 9 shows the distribution of the respondents' total attitudes towards the implementation and application of telerehabilitation technology according to their specialty. As

TABLE 2: Demographic characteristics of the participants.

Demographic characteristics	Participants	
	Faculty members	Clinicians
	%	%
Age		
<30	0	15.4
30–40	20.7	53.8
40–50	34.9	20.5
>50	44.4	10.3
Total	**100**	**100**
Sex		
Male	58.7	35.9
Female	41.3	64.1
Total	**100**	**100**
Educational status		
B.A.	0	30.8
M.A.	27	51.3
Ph.D./doctorate	73	17.9
Total	**100**	**100**
University of employment		
University of Social Welfare and Rehabilitation Sciences	55.6	74.4
Tehran University of Medical Sciences	4.7	13.8
Shahid Beheshti University of Medical Sciences	14.3	6.5
Iran University of Medical Sciences	25.4	5.3
Total	**100**	**100**
Working experience (years)		
<5	0	3.8
5–10	11.1	55.1
10–15	30.2	29.5
15–20	38.1	10.3
>20	20.6	1.3
Total	**100**	**100**

the results show speech therapy and occupational therapy were the only specialties in which some "definite agreement" overall was detected (13.3% and 2.9%, resp.). The lowest level of attitude belonged to the orthotists, 37.5% of whom had "no idea" regarding the issue and none were in "definite agreement" with it.

Table 10 shows the distribution of respondents' positive attitudes towards the implementation and use of various telerehabilitation services, in terms of their specialty. According to this table, teleconferences were the only remote service with which all respondents of all different specialties showed definite positive attitude (100% definite agreement). Other more popular telerehabilitation services included tele-experts consultation, tele-patient consultation, and tele-patient referrals. Teleevaluation seemed to be the least popular.

4. Discussion

Regarding the implementation and application of telerehabilitation technology, as the results show both faculty members and clinicians expressed a high percentage of positive attitude toward the implementation of telerehabilitation technology. This finding is somewhat in concordance with studies conducted by Mirhosseini et al. in the Kerman University of Medical Sciences [25] and Alizadeh in the Mazandaran University of Medical Sciences [26], both of whom demonstrated a positive attitude among medical experts to implement and apply telemedicine.

In our study clinicians surpassed the faculty members in their positive attitude toward this technology. It may be that since the majority of clinicians practice in clinical centers and are thus more familiar with the present obstacles of patient treatment they have a better understanding of the possible advantages of this technology. On the other hand, probably because faculty members in this study had higher seniority and thus more experience (see Table 2), they are more aware of the possible challenges and problems of implementation of this technology in the present situation and have a more realistic look into the matter and so tend to express a more cautious attitude.

Based on the results, with increasing age a predominantly decreasing trend of definite positive attitude has emerged. It seems that since people less than 30 years of age have more interest in and are in more contact with a variety of modern technologies they thus have a more positive view towards implementation of this modern technology. Also, our results showed that the percentage of "definite agreement" in participants with 40 to 50 years and above 50 years of age was 0%. It seems that aging has a considerable impact on the participants' cautious views, since older participants may have a better and deeper understanding about the possible challenges of implementation of this technology in our current situation, based on their higher experience. However, in a study conducted on medical students' points of view toward establishment of telemedicine in Mazandaran University of Medical Sciences, no significant correlation was found between age and attitude [26]. Evidently, in the Mazandaran study all participants were medical students whose age range was not as wide as that of the present study. Additional studies may clarify the role of age in this issue.

If "overall positive attitude" is defined as the sum of the total percentage of "definite agreement" and the total percentage of persons who responded with "somewhat agree," our results showed that participants with a Ph.D. degree expressed more positive attitude than other degree holders.

TABLE 3: The distribution of the rehabilitation experts' attitude in terms of their groups.

	Attitude					
	Definitely agree %	Somewhat agree %	Have no idea %	Somewhat disagree %	Definitely disagree %	Total %
Groups						
Faculty members	0	77.8	22.2	0	0	100
Clinicians	3.8	85.9	10.3	0	0	100

TABLE 4: The distribution of the rehabilitation experts' attitude in terms of their age.

	Attitude					
	Definitely agree %	Somewhat agree %	Have no idea %	Somewhat disagree %	Definitely disagree %	Total %
Age (years)						
<30	8.3	83.3	8.4	0	0	100
30–40	3.6	81.9	14.5	0	0	100
40–50	0	84.2	15.8	0	0	100
>50	0	80.6	19.4	0	0	100

TABLE 5: The distribution of the rehabilitation experts' attitude in terms of their sex.

	Attitude					
	Definitely agree %	Somewhat agree %	Have no idea %	Somewhat disagree %	Definitely disagree %	Total
Sex						
Male	1.5	80	18.5	0	0	100
Female	2.6	84.2	15.6	0	0	100

TABLE 6: The distribution of the rehabilitation experts' attitude in terms of their educational status.

	Attitude					
	Definitely agree %	Somewhat agree %	Have no idea %	Somewhat disagree %	Definitely disagree %	Total %
Educational status (degree)						
B.A.	4.2	79.2	16.6	0	0	100
M.A.	3.5	84.2	12.3	0	0	100
Ph.D./doctorate	0	88.4	11.6	0	0	100

TABLE 7: The distribution of the rehabilitation experts' attitude in terms of their university of employment.

	Attitude					
	Definitely agree %	Somewhat agree %	Have no idea %	Somewhat disagree %	Definitely disagree %	Total %
University of employment						
USWR*	3.2	80.8	16	0	0	100
TUMS**	0	92.3	7.7	0	0	100
Sh.B UMS***	0	78.6	21.4	0	0	100
IUMS****	0	85	15	0	0	100

*University Of Social Welfare and Rehabilitation Sciences.
**Tehran University of Medical Sciences.
***Shahid Beheshti University of Medical Sciences.
****Iran University of Medical Sciences.

TABLE 8: The distribution of the rehabilitation experts' attitude in terms of their working experiences.

	Attitude					
	Definitely agree	Somewhat agree	Have no idea	Somewhat disagree	Definitely disagree	Total
	%	%	%	%	%	%
Working experience (years)						
<5	0	66.7	33.3	0	0	100
5–10	4	80	16	0	0	100
10–15	2.4	82.9	14.7	0	0	100
15–20	0	84.4	15.6	0	0	100
>20	0	85.7	14.3	0	0	100

TABLE 9: Distribution of the respondents' total attitude towards the implementation and application of telerehabilitation technology in terms of specialty.

	Attitude					
	Definitely agree	Somewhat agree	Have no idea	Somewhat disagree	Definitely disagree	Total
	%	%	%	%	%	
Specialty						
Physical therapist	0	91.7	8.3	0	0	100
Occupational therapist	2.9	79.5	17.6	0	0	100
Audiometer	0	90.9	9.1	0	0	100
Optometrist	0	100	0	0	0	100
Speech therapist	13.4	53.3	33.3	0	0	100
Rehabilitation consultant	0	83.3	16.7	0	0	100
Ergonomist	0	100	0	0	0	100
Orthotists	0	62.5	37.5	0	0	100
Nurse	0	100	0	0	0	100
Other specialties	2.1	91.65	6.25	0	0	100

However, participants with a Ph.D. degree were the only group among whom no "definite agreement" was obtained. The findings of a study which was conducted by Alizadeh et al. showed that in Mazandaran University of Medical Sciences medical students with more years of education had more positive attitude than those with lower levels of education toward telemedicine [26].

The findings show that the University of Social Welfare and Rehabilitation Sciences was the only university in which some participants showed "definite agreement" with implementation of telerehabilitation. This may be due to the fact that this university is the only specialized university in the field of rehabilitation in Iran, with exclusive focus on welfare and rehabilitation sciences. However, if "overall positive attitude" is defined as the sum of the total percentage of "definite agreement" and the total percentage of persons who responded with "somewhat agree," it is noteworthy that the highest percent of positive attitude belonged to the Tehran University of Medical Sciences and the lowest belonged to the Shahid Beheshti University of Medical Sciences.

As the findings show teleconferences were the most popular telerehabilitation service, followed by tele-experts consultation and tele-patient consultation, in all of which it is possible to establish a live connection between the therapist and his colleague or patient and it is also possible to benefit from both sound and image in interactions.

5. Conclusion

Overall, based on the results of the present study it can be anticipated that, in case of implementation of this technology in the field of rehabilitation, an overall positive trend in its acceptance and application by experts can be expected.

One of the limitations the authors faced was that to their knowledge, no study of any kind had ever been conducted before regarding telerehabilitation in Iran or even in other countries of the region. All similar studies including feasibility studies or review articles, have been conducted on different domains of telemedicine, e- helath and tele-health implementation. Thus we have been faced with lack of adequate national or regional research benefits from similar experiences in this field for further comparison and discussion of the results. It seems that further feasibility studies are required in this field in Iran and similar developing countries to enhance rehabilitation service quality by implementing telerehabilitation technology.

Ethical Approval

All ethical issues (such as informed consent, conflict of interests, plagiarism, misconduct, coauthorship, and double submission) have been considered. Also, it should be mentioned that this study received an approval from the IRB and

TABLE 10: Distribution of respondents' positive attitude towards implementation of different telerehabilitation services in terms of specialty.

Telerehabilitation service	Physical therapist (%)	Occupational therapist (%)	Audiologist (%)	Optometrist (%)	Speech therapist (%)	Rehabilitation consultant (%)	Ergonomist (%)	Orthotists (%)	Nurse (%)	Other specialties (%)
Tele-expert consultations	100	24.1	90.1	100	100	100	100	100	100	100
Teleconferences	100	100	100	100	100	100	100	100	100	100
Tele-follow-ups	75	73.2	72.7	62	60	83.4	100	25	80	79.1
Tele-patient referrals	95.7	91.1	7.8	100	93.4	100	100	87.5	100	100
Tele-patient assessment	58.3	52.9	45.5	50	46.6	66.7	100	12.5	60	80
Telemonitoring	66.7	64.7	63.6	62.5	16.6	66.7	100	12.5	80	80
Teleevaluation	45.8	60	45.5	50	40.7	33.3	50	12.5	60	47.9
Tele-patient consultation	100	91.2	100	100	100	100	100	100	100	100

Ethical Committee of the University of Social Welfare and Rehabilitation Sciences.

Acknowledgment

The authors acknowledge and appreciate the cooperation of the rehabilitation experts who participated in this study.

References

[1] T. Cornford and E. Klecun, "The organizing vision of tele-health," in *Proceedings of the 10th European Conference on Information Systems, Information Systems and the Future of the Digital Economy (ECIS '02)*, Gdańsk, Poland, June 2002, http://eprints.lse.ac.uk/id/eprint/27120.

[2] M. B. Buntin, M. F. Burke, M. C. Hoaglin, and D. Blumenthal, "The benefits of health information technology: a review of the recent literature shows predominantly positive results," *Health Affairs*, vol. 30, no. 3, pp. 464–471, 2011.

[3] J. K. H. Tan, *E-Health Care Information Systems: An Introduction for Students and Professionals*, Jossey-Bass, San Francisco, Calif, USA, 2005.

[4] H. M. Judi, A. A. Razak, N. Sha'ari, and H. Mohamed, "Feasibility and critical success factors in implementing telemedicine," *Information Technology Journal*, vol. 8, no. 3, pp. 326–332, 2009.

[5] M. Najafi Semnani, N. Simforush, M. Bahlgerdi, M. Ghazizadeh, and H. Hosseipour, "Real-time point to point wireless intranet connection: first implication for surgical demonstration, decision making and telementoring in laparoscopy in Iran," *Journal of Birjand University of Medical Sciences*, vol. 14, no. 1, pp. 60–66, 2007.

[6] Ministry of Health and Medical Education, *Health in Iran in the Fifth Economic, Development, Social Program*, 2009, http://hamahangi.behdasht.gov.ir.

[7] British Colombia Ministry of Health Services, "Telehealth Contacts. A practical guide," 2001, http://www.health.gov.bc.ca/cpa/publications/practicalguide.pdf.

[8] American Telemedicine Association, Commmittee members. A blue print for telerehabilitation guideline, 2010, http://www.americantelemed.org/.

[9] J. Cason, "Telerehabilitation: an adjunct service delivery model for early intervention services," *International Journal of Telerehabilitation*, vol. 3, no. 1, 2011, http://telerehab.pitt.edu/ojs/index.php/Telerehab/article/view/6071.

[10] M. Pramuka and L. van Roosmalen, "Telerehabilitation technologies: accessibility and usability," *International Journal of Telerehabilitation*, vol. 1, no. 1, pp. 85–98, 2009.

[11] M. R. Schmeler, R. M. Schein, M. McCue, and K. Betz, "Telerehabilitation clinical and vocational applications for assistive technology: research, opportunities, and challenges," *International Journal of Telerehabilitation*, vol. 1, no. 1, pp. 59–72, 2009.

[12] K. Feyzi and R. Pourdehzad, "E-health system in Iran (obstacles and challenges)," Tehran, Iran, 2007, http://www.civilica.com/Paper-ICTM04-ICTM04_024.html.

[13] J. L. Schutte, S. Gales, A. Filipponi, A. Saptono, P. Bambang, and M. McCue, "Evaluation of a telerehabilitation system for community-based rehabilitation," *International Journal of Telerehabilitation*, vol. 4, no. 1, pp. 25–32, 2012.

[14] M. Heyvi Haghighi, H. Alipour, Z. Mastaneh, and L. Mouseli, "Feasibility of telemedicine implementation in the Medical University of Hormozgan," *Medical Journal of Hormozgan University*, vol. 15, no. 2, pp. 128–137, 2011.

[15] R. E. Scott, "e-Records in health—preserving our future," *International Journal of Medical Informatics*, vol. 76, no. 5-6, pp. 427–431, 2007.

[16] P. M. Schlag, K. T. Moesta, S. Rakovsky, and G. Graschew, "Telemedicine: the new must for surgery," *Archives of Surgery*, vol. 134, no. 11, pp. 1216–1221, 1999.

[17] D. M. Brennan and L. M. Barker, "Human factors in the development and implementation of telerehabilitation systems," *Journal of Telemedicine and Telecare*, vol. 14, no. 2, pp. 55–58, 2008.

[18] T. Teo and J. Noyes, "An assessment of the influence of perceived enjoyment and attitude on the intention to use technology among pre-service teachers: a structural equation modeling approach," *Computers and Education*, vol. 57, no. 2, pp. 1645–1653, 2011.

[19] J. Behner and M. Vanak, *Attitude and Changes*, Junghel Publishing Group, Tehran, Iran, 2006.

[20] M. Henreson, *Attitude Assessment*, Farhang Maktub, Tehran, Iran, 1381.

[21] S. Mazhari and K. Bahaedinbeighi, "Telepsychiatry applications in Iran," *Iranian Journal of Psychiatry and Clinical Psychology*, vol. 17, no. 4, pp. 336–338, 2012.

[22] E. Maserat, M. Samadi, N. Mehrnoosh, R. Mohammadi, and M. Zali, "Telenursing, a novel method for patients education," *Journal of Health and Care*, vol. 13, no. 3, 2012.

[23] A. Hosseini, H. Moghaddasi, F. Asadi, and M. Karimi, "Feasibility study of implementing of telesurgery in hospitals affiliated to Tehran Universities of Medical Sciences, Iran," *Health Information Management*, vol. 9, no. 1, article 74, 2012.

[24] A. Najafipour, R. Najafbeighi, and M. Rahmani, "A study on effective factors on E-health in Iran," *Scientific Journal of Teemedicine*, vol. 12, no. 6, 2010.

[25] M. Mirhosseini, D. Ziyadlu, N. Nasiri, and A. Saberiniya, "An assessment on knowledge and attitudes of staff of Kerman University of Medical Sciences towards telemedicine technology," 2014, http://journals.tums.ac.ir/.

[26] A. Alizadeh, A. Mohammadi, A. Khademlu, and H. Hosseini, "An assessment on the medical students' point of view toward development of telemedicine in the Mazandaran University of Medical Sciences," *Journal of Medical Education Development Center*, vol. 2, no. 10, pp. 129–141, 1392.

4

A Framework for Sustainable Implementation of E-Medicine in Transitioning Countries

Stephen Robert Isabalija,[1] Victor Mbarika,[2] and Geoffrey Mayoka Kituyi[3]

[1] Department of Business Administration, Makerere University Business School, 1337 Kampala, Uganda
[2] International Center for Information Technology and Development, Southern University and A and M College, P.O. Box 9723, Baton Rouge, LA 70813-9723, USA
[3] Department of Business Computing, Makerere University Business School, 1337 Kampala, Uganda

Correspondence should be addressed to Geoffrey Mayoka Kituyi; kimayoka@gmail.com

Academic Editor: Ron A. Winkens

Organizations in developed countries such as the United States of America and Canada face difficulties and challenges in technology transfer from one organization to another; the complexity of problems easily compounds when such transfers are attempted from developed to developing countries due to differing socioeconomic and cultural environments. There is a gap in the formation of research and education programs to address technology transfer issues that go beyond just transferring the technologies to sustaining such transfers for longer periods. This study examined telemedicine transfer challenges in three Sub-Sahara African countries and developed a framework for sustainable implementation of e-medicine. Both quantitative and qualitative research methods were used. The study findings indicate that e-medicine sustainability in Sub-Saharan Africa is affected by institutional factors such as institutional environment and knowledge management practices; technical factors such as the technological environment and technology transfer project environment; social environmental factors such as social environment and donor involvement. These factors were used to model the proposed framework.

1. Introduction

Healthcare is unarguably one of the most fundamental needs for Sub-Saharan Africa (SSA), considering the region's multiple medical problems. The health statistics of SSA are deplorable. The academic and practitioner literature report many medical problems of SSA. Yet SSA is the most vulnerable to disease, given the prevalent social, economic, and environmental factors. For instance, the World Health Organization (WHO) reports that by the end of year 2009, over 32.9 million people worldwide were living with HIV/AIDS. Out of these, 22 million (approximately 68%) live in SSA [1]. By the end of year 2009, the percentages of people living with HIV/AIDS in Botswana, Central African Republic, and Swaziland were still the highest in the world [1, 2].

Further to the above, out of the estimated 9.7 million number of children under the age of five who die every year due to lack of access to medical facilities worldwide, 41% live in SSA. Research shows that malaria is responsible for as many as half the deaths of African children under the age of five. This disease kills more than one million children (2,800 per day) each year in Africa alone. In regions of intense transmission, 40% of toddlers may die of acute malaria. In most malaria cases, however, there is a good chance of survival if timely and appropriate medical attention is provided. Other diseases that plague the continent and lead to the loss of millions of lives every year in Africa include dysentery, cholera, typhoid, yellow fever, and diarrhea [1].

One notable challenge in SSA is the shortage of medical personnel and facilities. Many developing countries have an acute shortage of doctors, particularly specialists. SSA has, on average, fewer than 10 doctors per 100,000 people, and 14 countries do not have a single radiologist [3, 4]. The specialists and services that are available are concentrated in large urban cities.

In the healthcare sector, rising costs and new types of health problems result in increasing pressure on the healthcare system and stimulate new approaches for improving access and reducing the cost of healthcare [5, 6]. Telemedicine initiatives represent potential solutions to improve healthcare accessibility and quality. Modern day healthcare is offering more and more treatment alternatives on the Internet, called e-medicine also sometimes generally referred to as telemedicine [7].

E-medicine is one of the most powerful initiatives for enabling access to health services in rural areas which are in most cases hard-to-reach. E-medicine is the use electronic means to transfer medical data from one place to another. At advanced levels, e-medicine may involve conducting clinical practices using telecommunication facilities such as teleconferencing. Simple applications of e-medicine may be manifested in medical record keeping, data processing, and information sharing. At a lower level e-medicine may also involve teleconsultation, whereby health workers can offer consultancy services to peers and/or patients [1]. In this study, our emphasis was placed on the use of health information systems, teleconferencing facilities, and medical data processing application in the hospitals. Studies by [8, 9] and [3] show that these are the most commonly used e-medicine systems in SSA.

The high penetration of mobile devices and networks globally implies that mobile technologies can be used very effectively in the field of healthcare in order to compensate for the scarcity of resources, particularly in developing countries [10]. In general, e-medicine has advantages where there is relatively inadequate or nonexistent access to healthcare resources, uneven geographical distribution of expertise, and continuing increases in the cost of healthcare services. In these circumstances, e-medicine improves access to healthcare, reducing the cost. Also, by improving communication between health centers (peripheral) and secondary or tertiary hospitals, e-medicine has been shown to speed up the referral process, reduce unnecessary referrals, and improve quality of care [3, 9, 11]. In some cases, e-medicine may be cheaper than the conventional practice [9].

The advent of e-medicine has presented numerous opportunities for countries without adequate human resources to benefit from global manpower that resides in the developed world. However, many telemedicine projects initiated in Sub-Saharan Africa have always failed without tangible benefits. One of the causes of failure is because there are inappropriate telemedicine implementation frameworks [9]. Scholars [12] argue that there should be telemedicine implementation and sustainability frameworks tailored to the local needs of countries in SSA. The purpose of the study therefore was to develop a framework which can facilitate the development, implementation, and sustainability of e-medicine in SSA employing a mixed research approach.

2. Materials

This section presents a brief review relevant literature that was consulted to enrich and ground the study on theory. The section presents the contextual analysis of Sub-Saharan Africa and examines the sustainability network theory, the technological environment, and the social environment factors that influence the sustainability of e-medicine outcomes in transitioning countries, especially Sub-Saharan Africa.

2.1. Overview of Sub-Saharan Africa. Sub-Saharan Africa is the part of the African continent that stretches out from Senegal, Niger, Mali, Chad, Djibouti, and Ethiopia, coming southwards to South Africa. It is sometimes referred to as the Black Africa because most of its inhabitants are black. The majority of people in SSA form part of the world's poorest people, whereby over 60% live below the poverty line of $1 per day. In addition, the region is characterized by high birth and death rates with low life expectancy (between 45 and 55 years) in different countries. For example, the United Nations study puts birth rates from years 2005 to 2010 for SSA at 5.1 per woman [13]. Further, [13] estimates that the population for SSA region will shoot from 0.86 billion people in year 2010 to 1.96 billion people in year 2050. This means that there is greater need for efficiency in healthcare service delivery, which requires e-medicine. Moreover, studies on the uptake of e-medicine and telemedicine in this region have revealed appalling findings as most projects do not live even for a year [3, 8, 9].

2.2. Sustainability Network Theory. According to [14], sustainability networks concern properties that arise in systems of many objects linked together and displaying both static and dynamic complexity. From a static perspective, networks are characterized by a number of key concepts such as connectivity (nodes, links, and flows), criticality, loops and cycles, dynamics, modularity, trees, and hierarchies. But it is the dynamics of industrial systems that are particularly challenging, and it is here that the need for sustainability network theory (SNT) [14] becomes apparent, because many of the behaviors of such systems arise not from the substantive factors that are the usual focus of analysis but from their underlying networks structure and dynamics. Thus, tightly coupled networks are more resistant to change than loosely coupled networks. This is a characteristic of complex systems that explains why changes to pollution control equipment regulations are more easily accomplished than changes to product design or manufacturing process regulations. In the former case, the technology is only loosely coupled to underlying product and manufacturing networks and thus can be changed with only minimal implications for other aspects of the product and manufacturing networks.

2.3. The Technological Environment. The technological environment largely involves the current state of ICT infrastructure in a country [15]. This factor impacts transfer of e-medicine to developing countries in terms of the basic ICT infrastructures, such as levels of basic telephone penetration (teledensity—the number of land telephone lines per capita). A country needs a solid ICT infrastructure for telemedicine to be possible. Due to various socioeconomic and political problems, SSA has the lowest levels of ICT-related infrastructures in the world [12]. SSA countries share a common set of problems regarding ICT, among which are a huge gap between supply and demand, a strong distribution imbalance favoring urban over rural areas, poor quality of service, long waiting times for new services, and peak traffic demands that exceed network capacity [12]. These problems result in extremely low levels of basic telephone penetration, which remain the base framework for both voice and data communications.

Overall, current models of ICT transfer within developed countries assume an existing ICT infrastructure on which applications such as telemedicine can be built. This is far from reality in SSA continues and remains a major bottleneck to e-medicine transfer within the region. Although some telemedicine projects have succeeded in SSA, these projects have been less sophisticated such as in teleradiology that does not require real-time transmission of X-ray images. The region is therefore limited to store-and-forward telemedicine practices as opposed to more sophisticated and needed practices such as telesurgery, which requires real-time transmission. Yet less sophistication or complexity is a viable approach to the current problem in the short run; however, for long-term solutions, SSA countries must expend efforts to improve on their underlying technology infrastructure so that they can enjoy more state-of-the-art telemedicine technologies.

2.4. Social Environment.
Social environment encompasses the factors that influence the uptake of technologies emanating from the community where the technology is implemented. Social environment model is a traditional ICT transfer model that theorizes that, in general, three general classes of precursors are required for successful transfer: the existence of the specific ICTs that need to be transferred; a basic ICT infrastructure to support the new technology; and appropriate implementation of the transfer project [16]. As in any project, it is imperative that the underlying processes be optimized before initiating ICTs. For regions such as SSA, this means revamping current healthcare practices and system from their present glut of bureaucracy, corruption, and social stigmas to a coordinated flow of materials and information. For example, in anticipation of violence, ostracism, and even murder, many people in SSA fear to reveal their ailments. In cases where conditions are diagnosed, rampant bureaucracy and corruption result in gross delays in delivery of solutions.

While it is generally taken for granted that traditional healthcare is in a functional state in most developed countries (relative to developing nations), the effectiveness of the system in developing countries as those in SSA is an important consideration in the potential effectiveness of telemedicine. In a study of developed countries, the prior state and effectiveness of the national healthcare industry—encompassing, for example, hospitals and clinics, health professionals, effectiveness, and efficiency of health administrations—would never be tested for, but this must be explicit in a model of the effects of telemedicine in SSA. ICT transfer models created in developed countries assume that the transfer domain is already healthy and just needs to be wired (or unwired) with ICTs to make it even better. However, when the base domain is in poor condition, as in many developing countries, successful transfer is jeopardized by this fact alone. Thus,

we contend that telemedicine projects supported by a more robust national healthcare system are likely to produce more favorable outcomes compared to telemedicine projects that lack support of a robust healthcare system.

2.5. Sustainability of E-Medicine Outcomes in Transitioning Countries.
The challenges faced by developing nations are complex, cutting across all sectors of society, and they can be addressed effectively only by implementation of transformative and sustainable change. Prerequisites for such change include a long-term commitment to system reform and resource development. Partnerships focused on capacity building can serve as important resources for the needed change [17]. Sustainability is the capacity of programs to continuously respond to community issues and maintenance of focus on set goals. Achieving sustainability has become a central issue of program implementation. The challenges of how we can become sustainable continue to simmer over basic issues such as what it even means to be sustainable and what new knowledge is required to become sustainable [18]. We look at sustainability in terms of how programs contract and others expand. Whereas some programs maintain original program activities, some become aligned with other organizations and established institutions, and still others maintain their independence. The key element of sustainability is providing continued benefits, regardless of particular activities delivered or the format (institutionalization versus independence) in which they are delivered. Thus, it is more important to sustain benefits to communities than to sustain program activities per se.

The emerging field of sustainability science provides a fresh perspective on learning because of its focus on several major learning challenges in policy and sustainable development [19]. Scholars in this community generally agree that learning is a critical hinge for sustainability [20], but how we get there is another problem. So far there has been no systematic treatment of learning for sustainability. Despite some attempts to outline a comprehensive research program, for example, [20], the development of strategies to promote learning for sustainability remains an elusive goal. Many scholars recognize the need for institutions that promote learning in the face of complex and uncertain problems.

A growing literature on "collaborative policy," for example, argues that networks spanning otherwise fragmented groups of stakeholders promote an effective exchange of information and the learning of common worldviews. However, there is sparse evidence that those collaborative institutions and the social networks they produce actually promote learning and improve outcomes. This underscores a central problem with the literature on institutional design to promote sustainability. The process of learning is often treated as a black box, and the design of strategies to promote learning is thus based primarily on anecdotal evidence rather than on lessons from theoretically grounded and empirically based models. A better understanding of how and why agents learn, including a detailed map of the parameters that influence this process, is a prerequisite for thinking about the types of institutions that are needed to promote

TABLE 1: Comparison of traditional and constructivist criteria.

Traditional criteria	Trustworthiness criteria	Measurement of criteria
Internal validity	Credibility	(i) Extended engagement in the field (ii) Variety of data types (iii) Peer debriefing
External validity	Transferability	(i) Purposive and theoretical sampling (ii) Detailed description
Objectivity	Conformability	Meticulous data management and recording
Reliability	Dependability	(i) Snow balling (ii) Accurate records maintained (iii) Participants confidentiality protected

learning. Understanding which types of actors are most likely to engage in constructive discussion, for example, will inform decisions regarding whom to invite to participate in a shared learning space, such as a scientific assessment process or a collaborative planning effort. These decisions must be based on a stronger theoretical and empirical understanding of how and why learning occurs. In order to accomplish this, however, we need an integrative framework that resolves the confusions and contradictions that often surround the study of learning.

One idea is that the most basic framework for understanding sustainability does not rely on understanding the interrelationship between its principal values (ecosystem health, social justice, and human needs); rather, the most basic framework for understanding sustainability may be the interrelationship between its technical and philosophical dimensions. These dimensions were dubbed by [21] as the substantive and no substantive aspects of sustainability, respectively. By this assessment, the technical dimension seems valuable for its ability to define problems precisely and to be usefully applied to many specific cases that differ greatly in circumstance (e.g., achieving a sustainable harvest of some particular population or achieving sustainable water use in some local community). This value is clearly demonstrated by the framework that supports sustainability science [22].

For sustainability of e-medicine outcomes, we note that standard knowledge hierarchy of data, information, and knowledge—in which data or simple facts become information when they are interpreted and become meaningful, and information becomes knowledge when it is put into a larger context—has been challenged by the construction of a reversed knowledge hierarchy that argues that data and information emerge only after knowledge is already available. But when the knowledge creation process is seen as a temporal sequence, sustainability is questioned [23]. These views can be combined without contradiction that previous knowledge is required to organize methodologically the production of new data or information and to interpret data and information for sustainability.

We examine seven major elements of sustainability: leadership competence, effective collaboration, understanding the community, demonstrating program results, strategic funding, staff involvement and integration, and program responsivity. These elements are mainly within the control of program leaders and stakeholders, but a program may have limited life because of factors outside the control of the program, such as state or local budget shortfalls or the emergence of other programs and organizations [24].

3. Methods

3.1. A Mixed Research Approach. A combination of methods and the sequence of the methods chosen in any particular study are critical decisions that were informed not just by the research question but also by the researchers' epistemological commitment and ontological views. Based on existing different epistemological assumptions, information system and social sciences research utilizes both quantitative and qualitative methods [25, 26]. Quantitative research methods were preferred because the research findings will apply to more than one population, thereby increasing the possibility of generalizing the research findings.

For purposes of this study, the research questions required systematically a variety of methods and techniques. Multiple methods were used in obtaining the findings [27, 28] in this case, the sustainability of e-medicine in SSA which links well with the guiding theoretical framework of this research. The focus was on studying the impacts of key factors within specific policy implementation, infrastructural, and knowledge management, with an overall goal of constructing a model that captures the synergistic relationships among key domain factors influencing sustainable e-medicine outcomes.

3.2. Methods Used to Improve Trustworthiness Criteria in Qualitative Methods. Research within a natural inquiry approach is guided by specific criteria to establish its validity (traditional criteria) or trustworthiness [29, 30]. The study examined four levels in trustworthiness: credibility (internal validity), transferability (external validity), conformability (objectivity), and dependability (reliability). This is summarized in Table 1.

In establishing the true value of findings, credibility was established through using two sources and cross-checking data. Transferability was considered by making certain claims that were limited by sample characteristics and providing a thick description of concepts and categories. Conformability, which requires that findings would emerge again if the study were conducted with similar situations, was maintained with

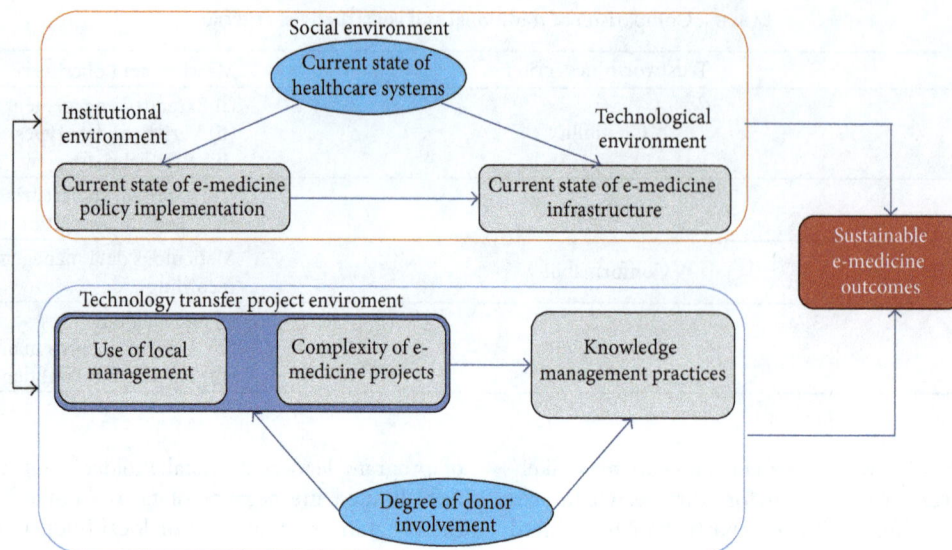

FIGURE 1: Hypothetical structural model for e-medicine sustainability.

careful management of data. All interviews were transcribed verbatim and clearly labeled as per respondent. To warrant that the findings reflect the interpretation of the participants, dependability was ensured through clear record of the study which was recorded and stored supported with snowballing.

3.3. Sample Size. A sample of 416 was chosen purposively from Uganda (sample = 135), Ethiopia (sample = 131), and Nigeria (sampler = 150) to participate in this study. These included hospital administrative and ICT staff.

In Uganda, the sample distribution included 25 doctors (10 from Nsambya hospital and 10 from Mulago hospital), 58 nurses (32 from Nsambya hospital and 26 from Mulago hospital), 38 hospital administrators (20 from Nsambya hospital and 18 from Mulago hospital), and 27 information technology/information systems employees (15 from Nsambya hospital and 12 from Mulago hospital).

In Nigeria, 70 respondents came from Pan-African Telemedicine, University of Ibadan teaching hospital, whereas 80 came from Lagos hospital. In Pan-African Telemedicine, University of Ibadan teaching hospital, the sample was distributed as follows: 18 medical doctors, 25 nurses, 12 hospital administrators, and 15 information technology/information systems employees. In Lagos hospital, the sample was distributed as follows: 20 medical doctors, 30 nurses, 15 hospital administrators, and 15 information technology/information systems employees, while in Ethiopia, the sample 130 came from Bethel teaching hospital and was distributed as follows: 15 medical doctors, 50 nurses, 45 hospital administrators and 26 information technology/information systems employees.

The above sample was selected using purposive sampling method, which is nonprobability sampling method. There are sound theoretical reasons why most qualitative research uses non-probability sampling techniques and good practical reasons why qualitative researchers deal with small numbers of instances to be researched.

The sample size is unlikely to be known with precision or certainty at the start of the study. Second, the sample size will generally be very small. Both points can be unnerving. They go against the grain as far as conventional survey approaches are concerned and open up the prospect of accusations of sloppy and biased research design. The researcher is quite explicit about the use of non-probability sampling [31, 32]. Another point is that phenomenology is well suited to purposeful sampling. This type of sampling permits the selection of interviewees whose qualities or experiences permit an understanding of the phenomenon in question and are therefore valuable. This is the strength of snowballing.

It is purely for this reason that the researcher decided to interview 10 participants with special qualifications for the study per country site from the medical organizations, that is, medical personnel, hospital administrators, IT personnel, nurses, and telemedicine center managers. This small sample size is quite good in keeping with the nature of qualitative data. Findings by [33] reveal that results based on a small sample (under 10) tend to be unstable so for this reason a sample of 10 respondents was chosen. The researcher focused on individuals' interpretations of their environment and behavior (self and others), and the presentation of data lies in understanding the participants and their terms [34].The main purpose of qualitative research is to study a social reality [34]. In this case study, the focus will be on telemedicine projects selected from five SSA countries. The study focuses on how the firm works in relation to key success factors for sustainable outcomes of e-medicine.

3.4. Empirical Models and Method of Data Analysis

3.4.1. Structural Equation Model. In addition to qualitative analysis, in this study through a survey, respondents were asked to evaluate different statements on all the postulated domains in Figure 1. The respondents were asked to indicate their degree of agreement with the statements, using a seven-point Likert scale. Important to note is that the seven domains in Figure 1 (i.e., social environment; institutional environment; technological environment; degree of donor involvement; technological transfer environment; knowledge management environment; and e-medicine outcomes or e-medicine sustainability) are latent variables. Based on the responses, each item or statement for each domain can be analyzed separately or summed to create a score for a group of items or a summative scale. However, analyzing single-item responses pertaining to a latent variable (e.g., sustainability of e-medicine) is not reliable.

Generally, it is not advisable to make inferences based upon the analysis of single-item responses that are used in measuring a scaled latent variable. For this study, the format of the statements or responses can be either treated as ordinal or interval-level measurements. Responses to a single Likert item are normally treated as ordinal data because not all responses are equidistant. Such ordinal data can show how high the scores are from each other but may not indicate how much higher they are. When responses to several items are summed to measure a latent variable such as sustainability of e-medicine, all statements in a survey instrument use the same Likert scale; the responses are treated as interval data. This means that the interval between two points and the differences between each response are equal in distance.

The relationship of responses to statements or items and latent variables can be estimated using different procedures. Structural equation modeling was however adopted for this study. Structural equation model (SEM) allows both confirmatory and exploratory modeling, which is suited to both theory testing and theory development. Confirmatory modeling usually starts out with a hypothesis that gets represented in a causal model. The concepts used in the model must then be operationalized to allow testing of the relationships between the concepts in the model. The model is tested against the obtained measurement data to determine how well the model fits the data. The causal assumptions embedded in the model often have falsifiable implications which can be tested against the data [35]. With an initial theory, SEM can be used inductively by specifying a corresponding model and using data to estimate the values of free parameters. Often the initial hypothesis requires adjustment in light of model evidence.

The SEM was adopted due to the ability to construct variables, which are not measured directly but are estimated in the model from several measured variables, each of which is predicted to "tap into" the latent variables [36]. This allows the modeler to explicitly capture the unreliability of measurement in the model, which in theory allows the structural relations between latent variables to be accurately estimated.

In general, SEM is a combination of factor analysis and multiple regressions. The variables in SEM are measured (observed or manifested) variables (indicators or items in the survey instrument) and factors (latent variables) represented as seven domains in Figure 1. Variables and factors in SEM may be classified into endogenous/dependent variables or independent exogenous variables.

3.4.2. Model Specifications. SEM is used as a confirmatory technique; researchers [35] suggest that when building the correct model, the researcher uses two different kinds of variables, namely, exogenous and endogenous variables. The distinction between these two types of variables is whether the variable regresses on another variable or not [37]. In SEM, other variables regress on exogenous variables. Exogenous variables can be recognized in a graphical version of the model, as the variables sending out arrowheads, denoting which variable it is predicting. A variable that regresses on a variable is always an endogenous variable, even if this same variable is also used as a variable to be regressed on. Endogenous variables are recognized as the receivers of an arrowhead in the model. In this study, we have institutional environment (IE), technical environment (TE), technology transfer project environment (TTE), knowledge management practices (KM), social environment (SE), and donor involvement (DI) as exogenous variables or independent variables, while sustainable e-outcome (ST) is the dependent variable (DV).

The measured variables are within rectangles and the names of factors or latent variables are ellipses. Rectangles and ellipses are connected with lines having an arrowhead on one end (unidirectional causation) or two (implying no specification of direction on causality). Dependent variables are those which have one-way arrows pointing to them and independent variables are those which do not. Dependent variables have residuals (denoted as e). The residual is not perfectly related to the other variables in the model and is indicated by arrow pointing to measured or latent variables. Therefore, a line with an arrow at both ends indicates a covariance between the two variables, with no implied direction of effect. An arrow pointing to each measured variable implies that the factor does not predict the measured variable perfectly. There is variance (residual) in the measured variable that is not accounted for by the factor. The structural model is illustrated below.

3.4.3. Interpretation of Model and Discussion. All model constructs were estimated by R package Lavaan. The R package Lavaan is a free, open-source R package for latent variable analysis. You can use Lavaan to estimate a large variety of multivariate statistical models, including path analysis, confirmatory factor analysis, structural equation modeling, and growth curve models. According to the author [38], the Lavaan package was developed to provide users with a free, open-source but commercial-quality package for latent variable modeling. The long-term goal of Lavaan is to implement all the state-of-the-art capabilities that are currently available in commercial packages.

Two confirmatory data analysis models were estimated for each country. As explained before, the first model was for testing institutional, technical, and social environmental variables relationships. The second model was testing donor involvement, technology transfer project environment, and knowledge management practices relationship. Each model was estimated as a stack of system of equations and used the "GROUP" option in Lavaan to get the estimate of the model at the country level.

We used four different measures to test the model fit. The comparative fit index (CFI) assesses fit relative to other models and uses an approach based on the noncentral parameters distribution with noncentrality parameter distribution. The larger the value CFI is, the better the model fit is. The CFI values greater than .9 often are indicative of good fitting models. The RMSEA estimates the lack of fit in a model compared to a perfect or saturated model. Essentially, RMSEA is a measure of noncentrality relative to sample size and degrees of freedom. For a given noncentrality, large numbers of observations and degrees of freedom imply a better fitting model, that is, a smaller RMSEA. Values of .06 or less indicate a close-fitting model. Values larger than .10 are indicative of poor-fitting models. However, the index is less preferable with small samples. Other test statistics used in the study were Chi-square and the likelihood ratio test.

4. Results and Discussion

4.1. Confirmatory Analysis for the Model. The fit test statistics for the model are as follows: CFI (0.91), RMSEA (0.1) with a 90% confidence interval of 0.086 and 0.113, the standardized root mean square residual was 0.076, and the Chi-square and log of likelihood that test the null hypothesis that all parameters are equal to zero was significant to the 1% level. The hypothesized model appears to be a good fit to the data. There was no need to conduct post hoc modifications of the model because of the good fit of the data to the model.

Tables 2–4 show the estimated coefficients for Ethiopia, Uganda, and Nigeria confirmatory factor analysis as related to institutional environment, technological environment, and social environment. In the tables, estimates are estimated parameters, Std.err is standard error, and std.lv and Std., respectively, represent estimates of the model when items are standardized and the latent variables are not standardized and when both variables are standardized. The latter is often called the completely standardized solution.

In the first column of Tables 2–4, parameters of items are unstandardized, and the first item in each domain is fixed to 1 to allow model identification. The associated, therefore, values and probabilities are not estimated. The estimated values are equivalent to factor loading for each item. If the unstandardized parameter estimates are divided by their respective standard errors, a Z score is obtained for each estimated parameter. The Z score is used because the standard errors are adjusted for nonnormality. The probability values generated using the Z-score are used to test the null hypothesis that the unstandardized regression coefficients are equal to zero.

Apart from factor loadings, covariances between latent variables and variances (residual variances) are also reported. Loadings show the effect of latent variable on the measure; if a measure loads on only one factor, the standardized loading is the measure's correlation with the latent variables and can be interpreted at the square root of the measure's reliability. In the tables, the variance (or the residual variance) in the measure is not explained by the latent variable; error variance does not imply that the variance is random or not meaningful, just that it is unexplained by the latent variables. To estimate the standardized models, the factor variance is set equal to one and all the loadings are free to vary. For unstandardized models, as mentioned before, one of the loadings is set to one (called the marker variable), the others are free, and the factor variance is free. Covariances between latent variables measure how much two latent variables change together. However, standardized covariances are easy to understand, as they are based on the same distribution and scale.

Results of the model for Ethiopia (Table 2) indicate that all item loadings were statistically significant (P value < 0.01). Therefore, we reject the null hypothesis and accept the alternative that all items included in the model influence the respective latent variables. Likewise, the residual variances are statistically significant at (P value < 0.01), rejecting the null hypothesis that the items are measured without errors. It can also be seen that there is a statistically significant positive covariation (P value < 0.05) between institutional environment and technological environment. This means that the two latent variables influence each other. There was a positive covariation between Institutional Environment involvement and Social Environment and Technological environment; however, it was not statistically significant. The results showing a positive covariance between technological environment and social environment were not statistically significant.

Based on these results, the standardized loadings (last column) indicate the importance of each item at loading on the respective latent variables. For example, IE1 with a loading factor of 0.947 was more important than IE3 with a loading factor of 0.922. The item IE5 was the least important, with a loading factor of 0.361.

During our interviews with key stakeholders, technological environment was echoed as an important factor in institutional environment for e-medicine sustainability. A doctor in Uganda argued, "We use computers for different reasons citing the pharmacy and laboratories, the doctor said they don't have a strategy; everything is done on a piece-meal basis, with IT technicians only helping in trouble shooting."

The model results for Uganda (Table 3) also reveal that all item loadings were statistically significant (P value < 0.01). Therefore, we reject the null hypothesis and accept the alternative that all items included in the model influence the respective latent variables. The results also show that, except for TE3, all residual variances were statistically significant at P value < 0.01. The null hypothesis that the items are measured without errors is therefore rejected. It can also be seen that there was a statistically significant positive covariation (P value < 0.05) between institutional environment and technological environment. This means that the two latent variables influence each other. There was positive nonstatistical significant covariation between institutional environment and social environment.

Based on these results, the standardized loadings (last column) indicate the importance of each item at loading on the respective latent variables. For example, Uganda SE2 with a loading factor of 0.714 was more important than SE3 with

TABLE 2: Confirmatory factor analysis results for Ethiopia on institutional, technical, and social environmental variables relationship.

Variable	Estimate	Std.err	Z value	P (>|z|)	Std.lv	Std.all
Institutional environment						
IE1	1.000				1.456	0.946
IE2	0.946	0.046	20.548	0.000	1.377	0.951
IE3	0.696	0.074	9.348	0.000	1.013	0.661
IE4	0.706	0.067	10.591	0.000	1.028	0.712
IE5	0.567	0.078	7.254	0.000	0.826	0.556
Technological environment						
TE1	1.000				0.613	0.473
TE2	1.658	0.304	5.45	0.000	1.016	0.758
TE3	2.224	0.435	5.116	0.000	1.362	0.978
Social environment						
SE1	1.000				0.998	0.81
SE2	0.985	0.096	10.31	0.000	0.983	0.872
SE3	0.792	0.102	7.771	0.000	0.791	0.664
SE4	0.823	0.096	8.546	0.000	0.821	0.72
Covariance among latent variables						
Institutional environment to						
technical environment	0.33	0.107	3.081	0.002	0.37	0.37
social environment	0.57	0.153	3.729	0.000	0.392	0.392
Technical environment to						
social environment	0.206	0.074	2.793	0.005	0.336	0.336
Variances						
IE1	0.248	0.066	3.746	0.000	0.248	0.105
IE2	0.199	0.058	3.434	0.001	0.199	0.095
IE3	1.32	0.17	7.783	0.000	1.32	0.563
IE4	1.025	0.133	7.68	0.000	1.025	0.493
IE5	1.522	0.192	7.916	0.000	1.522	0.691
TE1	1.305	0.167	7.815	0.000	1.305	0.777
TE2	0.766	0.146	5.233	0.000	0.766	0.426
TE3	0.086	0.2	0.43	0.668	0.086	0.044
SE1	0.524	0.092	5.698	0.000	2.524	0.345
SE2	0.304	0.071	4.268	0.000	0.304	0.239
SE3	0.791	0.11	7.166	0.000	0.791	0.558
SE4	0.627	0.092	6.811	0.000	0.627	0.482
IE	2.119	0.297	7.141	0.000	1	1
TE	0.375	0.138	2.723	0.006	1	1
SE	0.996	0.188	5.3	0.000	1	1

loading factor of 0.578. The item SE1 was the least important, with a loading factor of 0.407.

The model results for Nigeria (Table 4) also reveal that all item loadings were statistically significant (P-value < 0.01). Therefore, we reject the null hypothesis and accept the alternative that all items included in the model influence the respective latent variables. The results also indicate that most of the residual variances were statistically significance at P-value < 0.01 apart from SE 2 (P-value < 0.01 = 0.064). We therefore reject the null hypothesis that the items are measured without errors. It can also be seen that there was a statistically significant positive covariation (P-value < 0.05) between institutional environment, technological environment, and social environment. This means that the two latent variables influence each other. There was a positive institutional environment and social environment relationship between and statistically significant.

Based on these results, the standardized loadings (last column) indicate the importance of each item at loading on the respective latent variables. For example, in Nigeria, SE2 with a loading factor of 0.967 was more important than SE1 with a loading factor of 0.895. The item SE3 was the least important with a loading factor of 0.450.

4.2. Discussion and Framework Development. As mentioned earlier in the study, applying e-medicine concepts in SAA has been a pressing issue [8, 39]. This study sought to

TABLE 3: Confirmatory factor analysis for Uganda on the institutional, technical, and social environmental variables relationship.

Variable	Estimate	Std.err	Z value	P (>|z|)	Std.lv	Std.all
Institutional environment						
IE1	1.000				1.488	0.947
IE2	0.506	0.071	7.135	0.000	0.753	0.556
IE3	0.987	0.066	14.910	0.000	1.468	0.922
IE4	0.383	0.085	4.532	0.000	0.570	0.381
IE5	0.390	0.091	4.273	0.000	0.581	0.361
Technological environment						
TE1	1.000				0.553	0.415
TE2	1.540	0.496	3.104	0.002	0.851	0.679
TE3	0.868	0.309	2.807	0.005	0.480	0.414
Social environment						
SE1	1.000				0.669	0.407
SE2	1.284	0.362	3.546	0.000	0.859	0.714
SE3	1.101	0.319	3.448	0.001	0.736	0.578
SE4	1.098	0.338	3.248	0.001	0.734	0.495
Covariance among latent variables						
Institutional environment to						
technical environment	0.388	0.143	2.706	0.007	0.472	0.472
social environment	0.299	0.132	2.271	0.023	0.300	0.300
Technical environment to						
social environment	0.189	0.085	2.222	0.026	0.511	0.511
Variances						
IE1	0.248	0.066	3.746	0.000	0.248	0.105
IE2	0.199	0.058	3.434	0.001	0.199	0.095
IE3	1.320	0.170	7.783	0.000	1.320	0.563
IE4	1.025	0.133	7.680	0.000	1.025	0.493
IE5	1.522	0.192	7.916	0.000	1.522	0.691
TE1	1.305	0.167	7.815	0.000	1.305	0.777
TE2	0.766	0.146	5.233	0.000	0.766	0.426
TE3	0.086	0.200	0.430	0.667	0.086	0.044
SE1	0.524	0.092	5.698	0.000	0.524	0.345
SE2	0.304	0.071	4.268	0.000	0.304	0.239
SE3	0.791	0.110	7.166	0.000	0.791	0.558
SE4	0.627	0.092	6.811	0.000	0.627	0.482
IE	2.119	0.297	7.141	0.000	1.000	1.000
TE	0.375	0.138	2.723	0.006	1.000	1.000
SE	0.996	0.188	5.300	0.000	1.000	1.000

develop a framework which would facilitate the development, implementation, and sustainability of e-medicine in Sub-Sahara Africa. The results presented in the study not only show how technological, institutional social environmental, technology transfer environment, and donor involvement factors have impacted on sustainable e-medicine transfer but also the impacts of knowledge management on sustainable e-medicine transfer outcomes.

4.2.1. Social Environment. The revamping of contemporary healthcare practices and system from their present glut of bureaucracy, corruption, and social stigmas to a coordinated flow of materials and information has been a major problem

in SSA. However, the potential effectiveness of telemedicine can no longer be taken for granted. This is, as the results of the study indicate, a healthy technology transfer domain and telemedicine projects supported by a more robust national healthcare system are likely to produce more favorable outcomes compared to telemedicine projects that lack support of a robust healthcare system.

The results of this study showed that the social environment strongly influenced the level of institutional and technological environments on sustainable e-medicine outcomes.

The social environment as far as technology transfer is concerned has been supported by many scholars. For instance, [8] argue that although general ICT policies have little effect on the success of e-medicine in SSA, policies

TABLE 4: Confirmatory factor analysis results for Nigeria on the institutional, technical, and social environmental variables relationship.

Variable	Estimate	Std.err	Z value	P (>|z|)	Std.lv	Std.all
Institutional environment						
IE1	1.000				1.399	0.907
IE2	1.029	0.063	16.435	0.000	1.440	0.955
IE3	0.452	0.086	5.275	0.000	0.632	0.414
IE4	0.608	0.067	9.114	0.000	0.851	0.639
IE5	0.476	0.077	6.170	0.000	0.666	0.473
Technical environment						
TE1	1.000				0.775	0.704
TE2	1.125	0.114	9.834	0.000	0.873	0.866
TE3	1.259	0.127	9.920	0.000	0.976	0.930
Social environment						
SE1	1.000				1.171	0.895
SE2	1.020	0.059	17.335	0.000	1.195	0.967
SE3	0.575	0.099	5.827	0.000	0.674	0.450
SE4	0.701	0.059	11.953	0.000	0.821	0.759
Covariance among latent variables						
Institutional environment to						
technological environment	0.278	0.102	2.735	0.006	0.256	0.256
social environment	0.281	0.144	1.950	0.051	0.172	0.172
Technical environment to						
social environment	0.265	0.086	3.074	0.002	0.292	0.292
Variances						
IE1	0.422	0.096	4.411	0.000	0.422	0.177
IE2	0.199	0.090	2.223	0.026	0.199	0.088
IE3	1.930	0.226	8.547	0.000	1.930	0.828
IE4	1.052	0.127	8.258	0.000	1.052	0.592
IE5	1.538	0.181	8.501	0.000	1.538	0.776
TE1	0.610	0.079	7.727	0.000	0.610	0.504
TE2	0.254	0.052	4.850	0.000	0.254	0.250
TE3	0.149	0.057	2.630	0.009	0.149	0.135
SE1	0.342	0.064	5.366	0.000	0.342	0.200
SE2	0.098	0.053	1.853	0.064	0.098	0.064
SE3	1.790	0.210	8.545	0.000	1.790	0.798
SE4	0.495	0.063	7.879	0.000	0.495	0.424
IE	1.957	0.283	6.924	0.000	1.000	1.000
TE	0.601	0.126	4.771	0.000	1.000	1.000
SE	1.372	0.200	6.849	0.000	1.000	1.000

that are specifically targeted at e-medicine were necessary if telemedicine has to provide meaningful results. Also, while looking at technology adoption at the individual level of analysis, [40] tested a comprehensive model of the moderating effects of national cultural dimensions on technology transfer and found that all dimensions of culture [41] had effects on decisions to use technology. In their studies, Straub and others found that both cultural subconstructs have a mediating effect on IT implementation [42, 43]. In other words, beliefs, values, and culturation affect the effectiveness of IT implementation, in addition to their direct effects on IT outcomes.

The purpose of the study was to develop a framework which will facilitate the development, implementation, and sustainability of e-medicine in Sub-Saharan Africa; the study therefore presents the tested model as per results of the study as illustrated in Figure 2.

5. Conclusion

5.1. Policy Contributions and Implications of the Study. This study contributes to the methodological discourse in information science and social sciences and on action research. We identify vital, yet underdeveloped, quality criteria for action

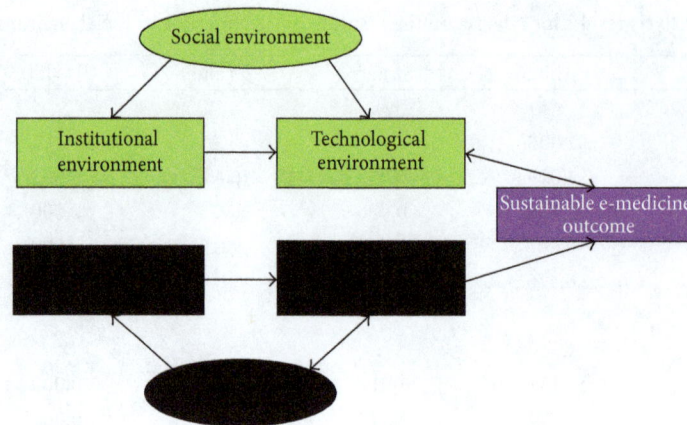

FIGURE 2: Framework for e-medicine sustainability.

research in information science and social science model for the sustainability of interventions. The researcher was against the notion of action research projects that end up with changes that last only as long as the attention of action researchers remains or, similarly, end up with a prototype but never routinely used systems. The study postulates a model for sustainability of e-medicine that is much needed in sub-Saharan Africa.

Our findings suggest a roadmap for being deliberate about sustainability efforts by virtue of the development and implementation of a sustainability plan in e-medicine. Intention is particularly important in light of research that discusses how early sustainability planning is an important step toward actually sustaining programs and that calls for the need to be ethically responsible for continuing programs once begun, particularly for those in the neediest communities.

The study recommends program teams to develop, implement, and monitor a sustainability plan which was not found consistent in the organizations where the study was done. Training should be a major component for sustainability, and continuous assessment of e-medicine programs in the country sites should be embraced both at the individual level and at the organizational level. Sustaining initiatives is a process that benefits from continual monitoring and adaptation to meet individual, family, program, and community needs. The sustainability conceptual model developed will help in providing e-medicine professionals with grounded, reliable, and valid information on which to build their sustainability efforts in an intentional, cohesive, comprehensive, and efficient way.

The central contribution of this work is a call to IS researchers and telemedicine practitioners to extend the sustainability of information systems to the developing world as a part of our communal research agenda. The study highlighted this need specifically by outlining a research framework for telemedicine sustainability in Sub-Saharan Africa; the perspectives offered are by no means limited to the specific region but are applicable for the developing world with a fragile healthcare system. This research will set a stage for IS researchers to continue in this vein by developing and augmenting IS theories to examine the sustainability interplay of ICTs in societies. The study proposes an inductive

ICT transfer framework that researchers can institute to investigate myriad factors that lead to and influence ICT transfers in the developing world. The development of this theoretical framework is a step towards creating a new reference frame of social development: one that is parallel to the mature phenomenon of organizational development.

References

[1] WHO, *Global Summary of the HIV/AIDS Epidemic*, United Nations, 2006, http://www.unaids.org/.

[2] M. E. Rutherford, K. Mulholland, and P. C. Hill, "How access to health care relates to under-five mortality in sub-Saharan Africa: systematic review," *Tropical Medicine and International Health*, vol. 15, no. 5, pp. 508–519, 2010.

[3] M. V. Kifle, V. Mbarika, and F. Payton, "Testing integrative technology (telemedicine) acceptance models among ethiopian physicians," in *Proceedings of the Southeast Decision Sciences Institute Conference (DSI '05)*, Raleigh, NC, USA, 2005.

[4] H. S. F. Fraser and S. J. D. McGrath, "Information technology and telemedicine in sub-Saharan Africa," *The British Medical Journal*, vol. 321, no. 7259, pp. 465–466, 2000.

[5] K. Subrahmanyam and N. Mariyam, "Evaluation of critical success factors for telemedicine implementation," *International Journal of Computer Applications*, vol. 12, no. 10, pp. 29–36, 2011.

[6] S. Sudhahar, D. Vatsalan, D. Wijethilake et al., "Enhancing rural healthcare in emerging countries through an eHealth solution," in *Proceedings of the 2nd International Conference on eHealth, Telemedicine, and Social Medicine (eTELEMED '10)*, pp. 23–28, St. Maarten, Antilles, February 2010.

[7] A. H. M. van Limburg and J. van Gemert-Pijnen, "Towards innovative business modeling for sustainable eHealth applications," in *Proceedings of the 2nd International Conference on eHealth, Telemedicine, and Social Medicine (eTELEMED '10)*, pp. 11–16, St. Maarten, Antilles, February 2010.

[8] B. Aynu, C. Okoli, and V. Mbarika, "IT training in sub-saharan Africa: a moderator of IT transfer for sustainable development," in *Proceedings of the 4th Annual Global Information Technology Management*, 2003.

[9] G. M. Kituyi, A. Rwashana, V. Mbarika, and R. Isabalija, "A framework for designing sustainable telemedicine information systems in developing countries," *Emerald Journal of Systems and Information Technology*, vol. 14, no. 3, pp. 200–219, 2012.

[10] D. Vatsalan, S. Arunatileka, K. Chapman et al., "Mobile technologies for enhancing eHealth solutions in developing countries," in *Proceedings of the 2nd International Conference on eHealth, Telemedicine, and Social Medicine (eTELEMED '10)*, pp. 84–89, St. Maarten, Antilles, February 2010.

[11] T. L. Huston and J. L. Huston, "Is telemedicine a practical reality?" *Communications of the ACM*, vol. 43, no. 6, pp. 91–95, 2000.

[12] V. Mbarika, *Africa's Least Developed Countries' Teledensity Problems and Strategies*, ME & AGWECAMS Publishers, Yaoundé, Cameroon, 2001.

[13] United Nations, *World Population Prospects: The 2010 Revision*, Department of Social Affairs, Population Division, United Nations, New York, NY, USA, 2011.

[14] J. B. Kim and A. Xu, *Sustainability Network Theory and Industrial Systems*, Center for Sustainable Engineering, 2007.

[15] P. Wolcott, L. Press, W. McHenry, S. E. Goodman, and W. Foster, "A framework for assessing the global diffusion of the Internet," *Journal of the Association for Information Systems*, vol. 2, article 6, 2001.

[16] E. M. Rogers, *Diffusion of Innovations*, Free Press, New York, NY, USA, 1995.

[17] D. L. Powell, C. L. Gilliss, H. H. Hewitt, and E. P. Flint, "Application of a partnership model for transformative and sustainable international development," *Public Health Nursing*, vol. 27, no. 1, pp. 54–70, 2010.

[18] J. A. Vucetich and M. P. Nelson, "Sustainability: virtuous or vulgar?" *BioScience*, vol. 60, no. 7, pp. 539–544, 2010.

[19] W. C. Clark, "Sustainability science: a room of its own," *Proceedings of the National Academy of Sciences of the United States of America*, vol. 104, no. 6, pp. 1737–1738, 2007.

[20] E. A. Parson and W. C. Clark, "Sustainable development as social learning: theoretical perspectives and practical challenges for the design of a research program," in *Barriers and Bridges to the Renewal of Ecosystems and Institutions*, L. H. Gunderson, C. S. Holling, and S. S. Light, Eds., Columbia University Press, New York, NY, USA, 1995.

[21] P. B. Thompson, "Agricultural sustainability: what it is and what it is not," *International Journal of Agricultural Sustainability*, vol. 5, pp. 5–16, 2007.

[22] Y. Kajikawa, "Research core and framework of sustainability science," *Sustainability Science*, vol. 3, no. 2, pp. 215–239, 2008.

[23] K. Bruckmeier and H. Tovey, "Knowledge in sustainable rural development: from forms of knowledge to knowledge processes," *Sociologia Ruralis*, vol. 48, no. 3, pp. 313–329, 2008.

[24] J. A. Mancini and L. I. Marek, "Sustaining community-based programs for families: conceptualization and measurement," *Family Relations*, vol. 53, no. 4, pp. 339–347, 2004.

[25] G. Goldkuhl and C. Stefan, "Adding theoretical Grounding to grounded theory: toward multi-grounded theory," *International Journal of Qualitative Methods*, vol. 9, no. 2, pp. 187–205, 2010.

[26] S. E. Myers, *Factors Affecting the Technology Readiness of Health Professionals*, Walden University Press, 2011.

[27] L. E. Suter, "Multiple methods: research methods in education projects at NSF," *International Journal of Research and Method in Education*, vol. 28, no. 2, pp. 171–181, 2005.

[28] T. D. Cook and D. T. Campbell, *Quasi Experimentation: Design and Analytical Issues for Field Settings*, Rand McNally, Chicago, Ill, USA, 1979.

[29] E. G. Guba and Y. S. Lincoln, "Paradigmatic controversies, contradictions, and emerging influences," in *The Sage Handbook of Qualitative Research*, N. K. Denzin and Y. S. Lincoln, Eds., pp. 191–215, 3rd edition, 2005.

[30] Y. Lincoln and E. G. Guba, *Naturalist Inquiry*, Sage, Newbury Park, Calif, USA, 1985.

[31] M. Miles and A. Huberman, *Qualitative Data Analysis*, Sage, Thousand Oaks, Calif, USA, 1994.

[32] C. Mills, "Phenomenological," *Surgical Nurse*, pp. 27–29, 1994.

[33] G. LoBiondo-Wood and J. Haber, *Nursing Research—Methods, Critical Appraisal and Utilization*, Mosby, St. Louis, Mo, USA, 4th edition, 1998.

[34] N. Nakkeeran, "Knowledge, truth, and social reality: an introductory note on qualitative research," *Indian Journal of Community Medicine*, vol. 35, no. 3, pp. 379–381, 2010.

[35] K. A. Bollen and S. J. Long, *Testing Structural Equation Models*, vol. 154, SAGE Focus Edition, 1993.

[36] R. C. MacCallum and J. T. Austin, "Applications of structural equation modeling in psychological research," *Annual Review of Psychology*, vol. 51, pp. 201–226, 2000.

[37] R. B. Kline, *Principles and Practice of Structural Equation Modeling*, Guilford Press, New York, NY, USA, 3rd edition, 2010.

[38] Y. Rosseel, "Lavaan: latent variable analysis," R package version 0.4-3, 2010.

[39] D. Maher, L. Smeeth, and J. Sekajugo, "Health transition in Africa: practical policy proposals for primary care," *Bulletin of the World Health Organization*, vol. 88, no. 12, pp. 943–948, 2010.

[40] S. McCoy, *The effect of national culture dimensions on the acceptance of information technology: a trait based approach [dissertation]*, University of Pittsburgh, Pittsburgh, Pa, USA, 2002.

[41] G. Hofstede, *Culture's Consequences: International Differences in Work-Related Values*, Sage, Beverly Hills, Calif, USA, 1980.

[42] R. M. Checchi, G. R. Sevcik, K. D. Loch, and D. Straub, "An instrumentation process for measuring ICT Policies and culture," in *Proceedings of the International Conference on Information Technology, Communications, and Development*, Kathmandu, Nepal, December 2002.

[43] D. W. Straub, K. D. Loch, R. Evaristo, E. Karahanna, and M. Srite, "Toward a theory-based measurement of culture," *Journal of Global Information Management*, vol. 10, no. 1, pp. 13–23, 2002.

5

Effect of Wireless Channels on Detection and Classification of Asthma Attacks in Wireless Remote Health Monitoring Systems

Orobah Al-Momani and Khaled M. Gharaibeh

Yarmouk University, Irbid 21163, Jordan

Correspondence should be addressed to Khaled M. Gharaibeh; kmgharai@yu.edu.jo

Academic Editor: Velio Macellari

This paper aims to study the performance of support vector machine (SVM) classification in detecting asthma attacks in a wireless remote monitoring scenario. The effect of wireless channels on decision making of the SVM classifier is studied in order to determine the channel conditions under which transmission is not recommended from a clinical point of view. The simulation results show that the performance of the SVM classification algorithm in detecting asthma attacks is highly influenced by the mobility of the user where Doppler effects are manifested. The results also show that SVM classifiers outperform other methods used for classification of cough signals such as the hidden markov model (HMM) based classifier specially when wireless channel impairments are considered.

1. Introduction

The application of wireless telemedicine in monitoring patients is seen as a useful and potentially powerful tool to help patients seek medical treatment [1, 2]. In remote monitoring systems of asthmatic patients, cough signals (as well as other body vital signs) are collected by sensors attached to the patient and sent to a PC located in a hospital using wireless technology [3–7]. A classification algorithm is then applied to the received signals in order to decide the state of the patient. Doctor intervention can then be done by calling the patient to take precautions, take a certain medication, or to go to a health care centre for proper treatment.

One of the main purposes of such systems is to help patients take precautions in the case of asthma attacks [4]. An asthma attack is a sudden worsening of asthma symptoms caused by an exposure to allergens or irritants such as inhaling dry and cold air and certain allergens such as pets, pollen, dust, and smoke. The symptoms of asthma attack may vary in severity and duration from person to person. The main symptom that indicates an asthma attack is coughing which has different frequency and strength from regular coughing [4]. Other signs of Asthma attack include headache,

blue colour in skin, difficulty in talking, and difficulty in breathing. When these signs of asthma attack are noticed, a patient should immediately seek medical treatment in order to prevent severe asthma attacks which may cause death [5].

With wireless transmission, channel impairments such as amplitude variations, time dispersion, and Doppler effects result in degradation of the receiver ability to recover the transmitted signal. This means that the classification accuracy of medical signals transmitted over wireless channels will be deteriorated as a result of errors in the received data. Unlike voice data, medical signals are more influenced by channel impairments because these signals have low bandwidths and are very sensitive to channel impairments [8]. Therefore, it is important to relate the classification accuracy and hence diagnosability of body signs to channel parameters in order to identify the channel conditions under which transmission is not recommended from a clinical point of view.

This problem has been investigated in the literature where the objective was to determine the transmission conditions where diagnosability of received signals is possible [8–11]. For example, it was shown in [8] that successful transmission of ECG is highly influenced by the mobility of the transmitter where it was shown that the receiver BER exceeds the acceptable limit required for correct classification and diagnosability of ECG signals at speeds above 50 Km/Hr. In [9], a wireless telemedicine system for transmission of photoplethysmography (PPG) signals was analyzed where it was shown that successful transmission of medical data over the tested channels requires a receiver bit error rate of less than 10^{-7}.

In this paper, support vector machines (SVM's) are used for classification of cough signals transmitted through a wireless channel in order to make decision about the occurrence of asthma attacks of asthmatic patients who are free to move. SVM classifiers have extensively been used in classification of speech-like signals and were shown to provide higher classification capability for classification of cough than other techniques [12, 13].

The performance of the SVM classification algorithm in detection of asthma attacks is evaluated by computing the probability of correct classification at different channel conditions (channel models) and is compared to the performance of hidden markov model (HMM) classifier [14]. The classification accuracy is related to the channel SNR in order to determine the channel conditions under which the classifier produces acceptable results for detection of asthma attacks.

2. Wireless Remote Health Monitoring System for Asthma Patients

Figure 1 shows a system model for a wireless remote health monitoring system which can be used for detection of asthma attacks of patients who are free to move. In this system, cough data are captured by a microphone and then transmitted through a wireless channel. At the receiver side, the received signal is demodulated and then entered into a feature extraction block. Extracted features of the received signal are used by the classification algorithm which makes a decision about the existence of an asthma attack.

One of the main challenges in the design of wireless remote health monitoring system is the reliability of the communication channel [13]. Communication channels introduce impairments to the transmitted signal which result in the inability of the receiver to recover the original signal correctly. Hence, errors introduced by the wireless channel impact signal classification and result in wrong interpretation of medical data.

There are two main types of signal degradation introduced by wireless channels: the first is attenuation and random variation of signal amplitude, and the second is distortion of the signal spectrum. Signal attenuation results from the degradation of the signal power level over distance while random variation of signal amplitude results from channel noise and multipath fading effects. Noise effects are modelled by additive white Gaussian noise (AWGN) with a power spectral density that depends on the channel signal-to-noise ratio (SNR).

With AWGN channel model, white Gaussian noise is added to the transmitted signal based on a specified SNR; therefore, the received signal can be expressed as

$$r(t) = s(t) + n(t), \qquad (1)$$

where $s(t)$ is transmitted signal and $n(t)$ is a noise signal. The noise signal is assumed to be statistically independent of $s(t)$, stationary Gaussian noise process with zero mean and two-sided PSD of $N_0/2$ Watts/Hz. The AWGN model is particularly simple to use in the detection of signals and in the design of optimum receiver in most communication systems.

Random variations of signal amplitude due to multipath fading effects are usually modelled by the Rayleigh channel model [14, 15]. In a Rayleigh channel model, signals from different paths having different phases and similar signal strengths are received to produce a Rayleigh distributed signal amplitude. The received signal from a Rayleigh fading channel is modelled as [13, 15]

$$r(t) = h(t) s(t) + n(t), \qquad (2)$$

where $h(t)$ is the fading amplitude which has a Rayleigh probability density function (PDF) given by

$$f_h(h) = \frac{h}{\sigma^2} e^{-h^2/2\sigma^2}, \quad h \geq 0, \qquad (3)$$

where σ^2 is the average received power and h is the signal magnitude.

Distortion of signal spectrum is usually attributed to two main phenomena: the first is multipath delay and the second is the Doppler effects. Multipath delay results from multipath phenomena in wireless channels where the received signal consists of multiple reflected signal components which have different delays. Delay distortion results in intersymbol interference (ISI) where successive symbols interfere and have significant effects on transmitted signals when their bandwidth is larger than the coherence bandwidth of the fading channel (frequency selective channels) [16]. The Doppler spread is a measure a spectral broadening caused by time varying nature of the channel. Doppler spread is usually related to the mobility of either the receiver or the transmitter and is defined as the frequency range in which the frequency of the received signal changes due to Doppler effects. Doppler shift leads to signal distortion which causes errors in the received signal. The Doppler power spectrum for a narrowband fast fading channel is modelled as [16]

$$S(f) = \frac{1}{\pi f_D \sqrt{1 - (f/f_D)^2}}, \quad |f| \leq f_D, \qquad (4)$$

where f_D is the maximum Doppler shift introduced by the channel which is linearly related to the speed of either the transmitter or the receiver. The Doppler spectrum specifies the frequency spectrum of the Rayleigh fading signal and hence its autocorrelation function.

Since medical signals usually have smaller bandwidths than the channel coherence bandwidth, the delay spread can be neglected. On the other hand, small variations in signal spectrum due to Doppler spread can cause significant distortion to the transmitted signal when the signal bandwidth is small. Therefore, in the simulations that will follow, delay spread will be neglected and the performance of the classification system will be tested under different values of the Doppler spread.

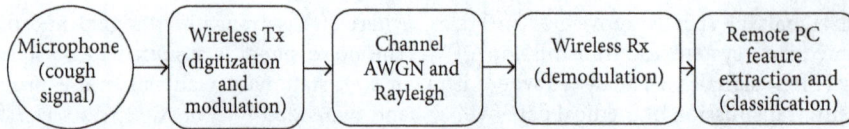

FIGURE 1: Block diagram of a wireless monitoring system for asthma attack detection.

3. Support Vector Machine (SVM) Classification

SVM classifiers have extensively been used in classification of speech-like signals and were shown to provide higher classification capability for classification of cough than other techniques [12].

SVM is a classification algorithm that performs a classification task by constructing a hyperplane in a multidimensional space that separates data into two different categories. An SVM classifier consists of L training points, where each input $\mathbf{x}_i$ has D dimensions and belongs to one of two classes H_1 and H_2 which correspond to $y_i = -1$ or $+1$, where y_i denotes the classifier output. Training data can be represented in the form $\{\mathbf{x}_i, y_i\}$ where $i = 1, 2, \ldots, L$ and $\mathbf{x} \in R^D$ [17]. If the data is linearly separable, then classification of a data point $\mathbf{x}$ is done by maximizing the margin separating the two hyperplanes, which results in a decision rule of the form [18]:

$$\text{Decide Class 1 if } \text{sign}\left(\sum_{i=1}^{L} \alpha_i \mathbf{x}_i y_i \cdot \mathbf{x} + b\right) = 1,$$

$$\text{Decide Class 2 if } \text{sign}\left(\sum_{i=1}^{L} \alpha_i \mathbf{x}_i y_i \cdot \mathbf{x} + b\right) = -1, \tag{5}$$

where sign($\cdot$) is the sign function and α_i are Lagrange multipliers and are referred to as the support vectors (SV) [18].

When data is not linearly inseparable, a kernel function is used to map data to higher dimension such that the resulting data is linearly separable [18]. The original formulation of the SVM classifier remains the same except that every dot product in (5) is replaced by a nonlinear kernel function. Therefore, with using a kernel function, the decision rule in (5) is reformulated as [18]

$$\text{Decide Class 1 if } \text{sign}\left(\sum_{i=1}^{L} \alpha_i y_i K(\mathbf{x}_i, \mathbf{x}) + b\right) = 1,$$

$$\text{Decide Class 2 if } \text{sign}\left(\sum_{i=1}^{L} \alpha_i y_i K(\mathbf{x}_i, \mathbf{x}) + b\right) = -1, \tag{6}$$

where $K(\mathbf{x}_i, \mathbf{x})$ is the kernel function which has different forms depending on the application. The most common kernel functions are the polynomial, the radial basis function (RBF), and the sigmoid kernel functions [19].

The parameters of the SVM classification algorithm (including the parameters of the kernel function) can be found using cross-validation of the available training data where the parameters that give the best classification accuracy are selected [17].

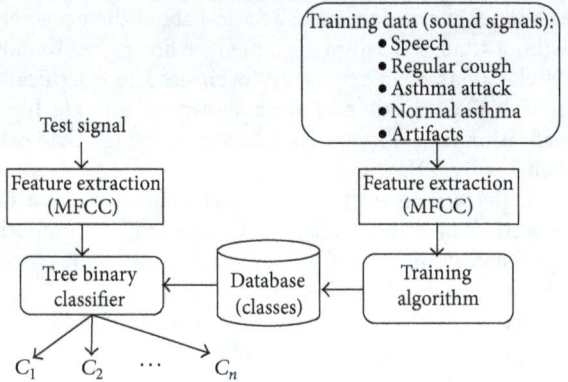

FIGURE 2: Classifier model.

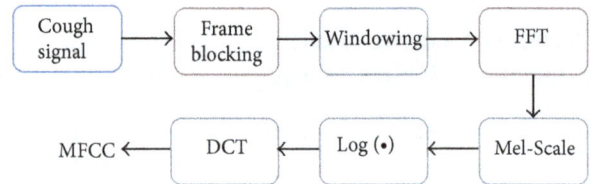

FIGURE 3: Block diagram of feature extraction process using MFCC [20].

4. Asthma Attack Detection Using SVM Classification

Figure 3 shows the SVM classification model used in this paper for detection of asthma attacks. The classification process involves extraction of features, generation of a classifier data base from a training set, and decision making for a given test signal.

4.1. Feature Extraction. In the classification model in Figure 2, features of cough signals are extracted and then used by the classification algorithm in order to reduce the dimensionality of the classification problem. Feature extraction can be done using different methods, such as Fourier transform and Wavelet transform-based methods [21].

One of the common Fourier transform-based methods is the Mel Frequency Cepstral Coefficient (MFCC) technique which has been used extensively in feature extraction of speech-like signals [22]. MFCC is a type of parametric representation of speech-like signals and has been extensively used in speech recognition because of its ability to capture relevant information of human speech [20]. MFCC feature extraction process is known for its robustness against time varying nature of speech signals which is a desired feature when processing cough data from asthmatic patients.

MFCCs are the coefficients that represent the short-term power spectrum of a signal obtained from linear cosine transform of the log power spectrum on a nonlinear "Mel" scale of frequency [22]. The process of calculating MFCCs is illustrated in Figure 3. Digitized cough data is first processed by the framing block which performs segmentation of the cough signal samples into N frames. Windowing is applied to the resulting frames before being spectrally analyzed using the fast Fourier transform (FFT). The power spectrum is mapped onto the Mel scale using the approximation [20]:

$$f_m = 2595 \log_{10}\left(1 + \frac{f}{700}\right), \qquad (7)$$

where f (Hz) is the normal frequency and f_m is the Mel frequency. MFCCs are calculated from the discrete cosine transform (DCT) of the log of the signal spectrum which is equivalent to passing the Mel scaled log spectrum through a bank of triangular shaped bandpass filters, distributed along a Mel scaled frequency band of interest [14].

4.2. MultiClass Classification of Cough Signals. The initial form of SVM classifier is binary as clear from (1) and (2) where the output of the learned function is either positive or negative. Asthma attack detection requires classification of cough signals into five classes: normal cough, cough related to asthma attack, cough related to a regular asthma episode, speech, and artefacts (sounds from patient daily activity including drinking, laughing, clearing through, and crying). To generate multiclass SVMs from binary SVMs, a number of methods have been proposed in the literature [23–25]. One of the most popular methods is the binary tree support vector machine (BTSVM) which combines SVM and binary trees. BTSVM decomposes an N-class problem into N–1 subproblem, each separating a pair of classes with SVM classifier. BTSVM has a number of characteristics such as lower number of binary classifiers and faster decision speed [23].

Figure 5 shows a tree-based classification process of cough signals. The classifier uses four stages of classification for classifying a sound signal into the five classes mentioned above. The training set for the tree classifier is generated by dividing the database into two disjoint groups at each classification stage.

4.3. Kernel Function Selection. Given the diversity of the sound signals incorporated in the training set of the classifier, training data constitutes a linearly inseparable database. Therefore, an RBF kernel function is used as in (2). The RBF kernel has less hyperparameters and less numerical complexity than other kernel functions [17]. The RBF kernel function is described by [18]

$$K\left(\mathbf{x}_i, \mathbf{x}_j\right) = e^{(-|\mathbf{x}_i - \mathbf{x}_j|^2 / 2\sigma^2)}. \qquad (8)$$

The parameter σ determines the area of influence of the support vector (SV) over the data space. Large value of σ will

TABLE 1: MFCC parameters used in feature extraction of cough signals.

Parameter	Value
Number of MFCC coefficient	20
Window	Hamming: $w(n) = 0.54 - 0.46 \cos(2n/(N-1))$
Window length (N)	256
Frame size	25 ms
FFT size	256
Feature vector dimension	69

allow a SV to have a strong influence over a large area and reduces the SV, but reducing the SV results in increased error [17].

5. Simulation and Verification

In the model shown in Figure 6, test signals are transmitted through the wireless channel after performing analogue to digital (A/D) conversion and digital modulation. At the receiver, the signal is converted back to the analogue domain after digital demodulation and then applied to the classifier to make a decision about the existence of asthma attacks.

The performance of the classification system under wireless channel impairments is quantified by computing the probability of correct classification (P_c) (the classification rate). The probability of correct classification (P_c) is defined as the ratio of the number of correctly classified samples and the total number of the samples [19]:

$$P_c\,(\%) = \frac{\text{Numbr of correctly classified samples}}{\text{Total number of samples}} \times 100. \qquad (9)$$

5.1. Data Collection. The classification system was tested using recordings of cough signals from real asthmatic patients. The recordings were obtained from 18 patients at the King Abdullah University Hospital (KAUH) in Jordan in order to develop the training set of the classifier (Data was obtained after getting the consent of patients through the hospital procedure and policies). The causes of cough in these patients were as follows: 10 patients had cough caused by asthma and 8 patients had cough caused by an asthma attack. All recording were sampled at frequency 11025 Hz and were divided into samples where each patient produces at least 5 samples or 6 samples. On the other hand, 144 samples from normal subjects including normal cough, speech, and artefacts (drink, laughter, clearing through, and crying) were obtained from http://www.freesound.org/ [26]. Table 3 shows the five types of sound signals used for training the classifiers. The recordings were digitized at a frequency of 11025 samples/second and encoded at 16 bits per sample.

Table 1 shows the parameters used for feature extraction of cough signals using MFCC as discussed in the previous

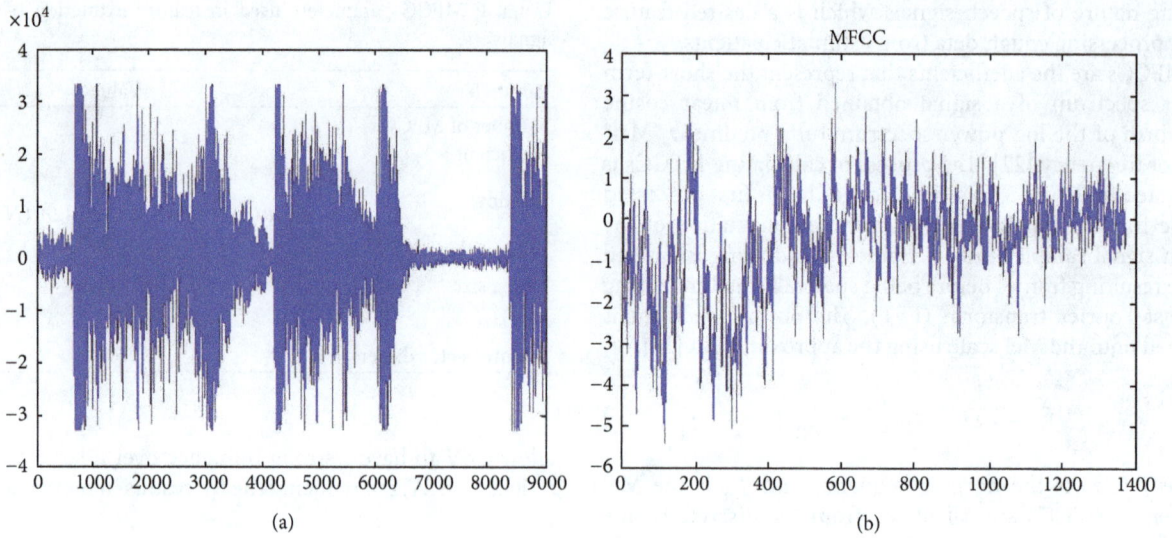

FIGURE 4: (a) A cough signal of an asthmatic patient and (b) its MFCC.

TABLE 2: Fading channel parameters.

Modulation order M	8
Fading sequence length (N)	180019
φ_n, θ_n	Uniformly distributed random variables $\varphi_n = \theta_n = 2 * \text{pi} * \text{rand}\,(1, N) - \text{pi};$
Doppler shift	0, 10, 100 Hz
SNR	0–35 dB

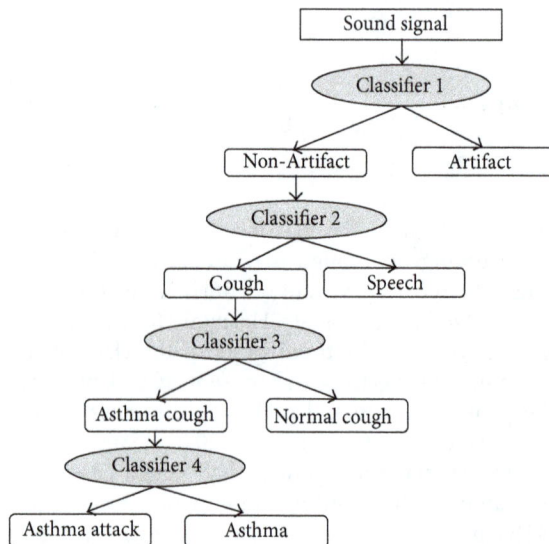

FIGURE 5: Tree SVM classifier for detection of asthma attacks.

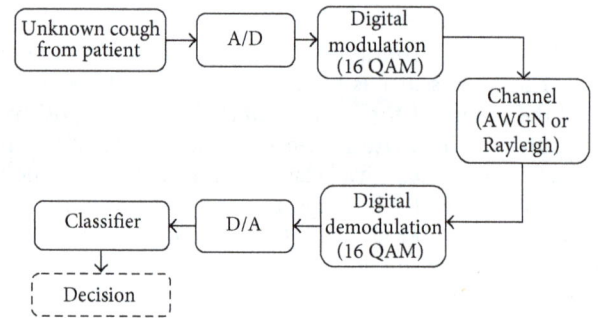

FIGURE 6: Block diagram of simulation model.

channel model. With AWGN channel, noise is simply added to the transmitted signal using the Matlab function "awgn" function where SNR can be specified. A Rayleigh fading channel model is generated using the sum-of-sinusoids method in which complex Gaussian noise with a power spectral density (PSD) that is equal to the Doppler power spectrum in (8) is approximated by a finite sum of weighted sinusoids as [27]:

$$h(t) = \sqrt{\frac{2}{M}} \sum_{n=1}^{M} \cos\left(\omega_d t \cos \alpha_n + \varphi_n\right)$$
$$+ j\sqrt{\frac{2}{M}} \sum_{n=1}^{M} \cos\left(\omega_d t \sin \alpha_n + \varphi_n\right), \quad (10)$$

where $\alpha_n = (2\pi n - \pi - \theta_n)/4M$, $n = 1, 2, \ldots, M$, ω_d is the maximum angular Doppler frequency, φ_n and θ_n are independent random variables uniformly distributed on $[-\pi, \pi]$ for all n. With this formulation, the fading amplitude ($|h(t)|$) approximates a Rayleigh random variable with a PDF as in (7). The parameters of the channel model in (10) used in the simulations which will follow are shown in Table 2.

section. Figures 4(a) and 4(b) show a cough signal and its MFCC features.

5.2. *Wireless Channel Models.* Two channel models are considered: an AWGN channel model and a Rayleigh fading

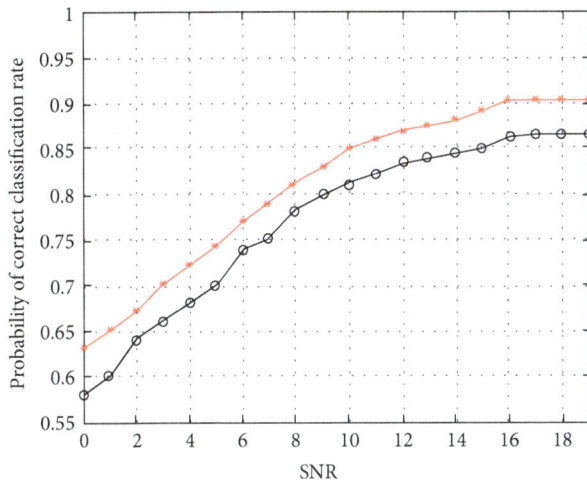

FIGURE 7: Probability of correct classification in AWGN channel versus SNR; *SVM and °HMM.

TABLE 3: Sound signals used in generating the training set of the classifier.

Class	Number of samples
Artefacts	48
Speech	48
Normal cough	48
Asthma cough	48
Asthma attack	48
Total	**240**

In the simulation model shown in Figure 6, test signals are transmitted through both channel models at different SNRs and Doppler shifts and the number of correctly classified samples is counted. The minimum SNR required for an acceptable P_c is determined for both channel models. Furthermore, in the case of Rayleigh fading channel, the maximum Doppler frequency that results in acceptable classification rate is determined at a given SNR.

5.3. Simulation Results. Using the AWGN channel model, the average classification rate of the SVM classifier was computed at different SNRs and compared to the classification rate obtained from using the hidden markov models approach in [14]. Figure 7 shows P_c versus SNR for the SVM classifier and compared to that of an HMM classifier.

Under a Rayleigh channel model, P_c is calculated at different SNRs and different values of the Doppler shift of the channel. Figures 8(a)–8(c) show P_c versus SNR at Doppler shifts of 0, 10, and 100 Hz of the SVM classifier and compared to the HMM-based classifier.

5.4. Discussion. In the case of AWGN channel, the simulation results show that a maximum P_c of 90% is obtained for the SVM classifier at SNR = 16 dB and 86% for the HMM-based classifier at SNR = 17 dB. The results show that the SVM classifier outperforms the HMM classifier at all SNRs.

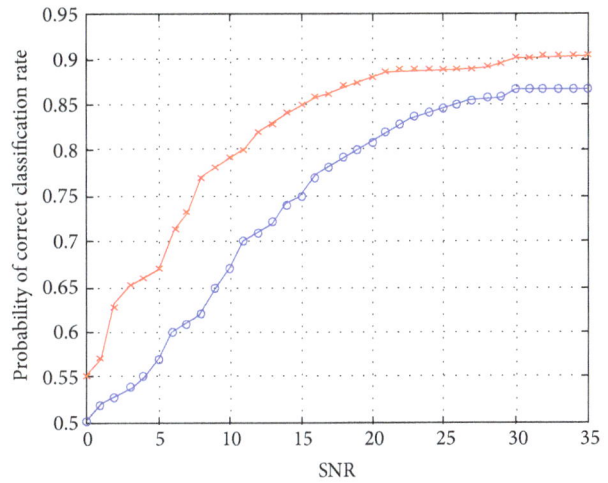

(a)

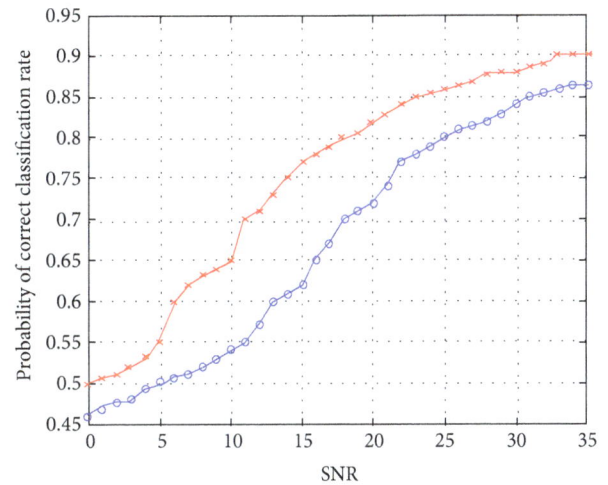

(b)

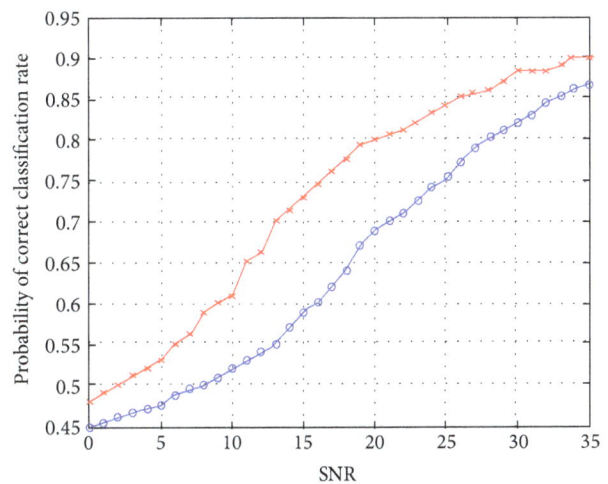

(c)

FIGURE 8: Probability of correct classification in Rayleigh fading channel versus SNR (a) $f_D = 0$ Hz, (b) $f_D = 10$ Hz, and (c) $f_D = 100$ Hz; *SVM and °HMM.

In Rayleigh fading channel, the simulation results show that the SVM classifier outperforms the HMM classifier at all Doppler frequency shifts. From Figures 8(a)–8(c), the maximum P_c of both classifiers is obtained at SNRs above 33 dB which is about 14 dB higher than the case of using an AWGN channel. This means that SNR needs to be increased in order to overcome the loss in P_c due to the mobility of the transmitter. In general, the simulation results show that the SVM classifier outperforms the HMM classifier when channel impairments are considered. The maximum difference in P_c between the two classifiers is about 17% at $f_D = 100$ Hz and SNR = 15 dB.

6. Conclusion

In this paper, classification of cough signals in a wireless remote health monitoring scenario using SVM classification algorithm has been analyzed. The reliability of the classification system has been tested under different wireless channel models (AWGN and Rayleigh fading) where it has been shown that channel impairments have a significant effect on the accuracy of the classification system. The simulation results show that SVM classification is capable of detecting asthma attacks from cough signals transmitted through a wireless communication channel provided that the channel SNR is increased to overcome the channel impairments caused by noise, amplitude variations due to fading, and the mobility of the wireless transmitter at the patient's side. The simulation results also show that SVM classifier provides better classification accuracy than the HMM-based classifier under the same channel conditions. The results presented in this paper can be used in the design of remote health monitoring systems for asthmatic patients where system parameters can be designed considering the minimum requirements for channel SNR required for achieving the desired classification accuracy.

Acknowledgments

The authors would like to thank Dr. Nedal Shawagfeh and Dr. Alaa Ayasra from King Abdullah University Hospital (KAUH) for their help in providing the cough data.

References

[1] B. Woodward, R. Istepanian, and C. Richards, "Design of a telemedicine system using a mobile telephone," *IEEE Transactions on Information Technology in Biomedicine*, vol. 5, no. 1, pp. 13–15, 2001.

[2] A. Abidoye, N. Azeez, A. Adesina, and K. Agbele, "Using Wearable Sensors for Remote Healthcare Monitoring System," *Journal of Sensor Technology*, vol. 1, pp. 22–28, 2011.

[3] J. Finkelstein and R. H. Friedman, "Home asthma tele-monitoring system," in *Proceedings of IEEE Annual Northeast Bioengineering Conference*, pp. 103–104, Storrs, Conn, USA, 2000.

[4] J. Finkelstein and R. Friedman, "Telemedicine system to support asthma self-management," in *Proceedings of the IEEE EMBS International Conference on Information Technology Applications in Biomedicine*, pp. 164–167, Arlington, Va, USA, 2000.

[5] H. Chu, C. Chang, Z. Hui, and J. Tsai, "A ubiquitous warning system for asthma-inducement," in *Proceedings of the IEEE International Conference on Sensor Networks, Ubiquitous, and Trustworthy Computing*, pp. 186–191, Taichung, Taiwan, 2006.

[6] M. Okubo, Y. Imai, T. Ishikawa, T. Hayasaka, and S. Ueno, "Respiration monitoring for home-care patients of respiratory diseases with therapeutic aids," in *Proceedings of the of the 4th European Conference of the International Federation for Medical and Biological Engineering*, vol. 22, pp. 1117–1120, Antwerp, Belgium, November 2008.

[7] A. Bumatay, R. Chan, K. Lauher et al., "Coupled mobile phone platform with peak flow meter enables real-time lung function assessment," *IEEE Sensors Journal*, vol. 12, no. 3, pp. 685–691, 2012.

[8] R. Habib, "Modeling of GSM mobile telemedical system," in *Proceedings of the IEEE Annual Engineering in Medicine and Biology Society Conference*, pp. 926–930, Hong Kong, 1998.

[9] R. Istepanian and M. Brien, "Modeling of photo plethysmography mobile telemedicine system," in *Proceedings of the IEEE International Conference EMBS*, pp. 987–990, Chicago, Ill, USA, 1997.

[10] J. R. Gállego, Á. Hernández-Solana, M. Canales, J. Lafuente, A. Valdovinos, and J. Fernández-Navajas, "Performance analysis of multiplexed medical data transmission for mobile emergency care over the UMTS channel," *IEEE Transactions on Information Technology in Biomedicine*, vol. 9, no. 1, pp. 13–22, 2005.

[11] http://www.webmd.com.

[12] J.-C. Wang, J.-F. Wang, C.-B. Lin, K.-T. Jian, and W. Kuok, "Content-based audio classification using support vector machines and independent component analysis," in *Proceedings of the IEEE International Conference on Pattern Recognition (ICPR '06)*, pp. 157–160, Hong Kong, August 2006.

[13] J. Chol and M. Zhou, "Recent advances in wireless sensor networks for health monitoring," *International Journal of Intelligent Control and Systems*, vol. 15, pp. 49–58, 2010.

[14] M. Sergio, S. S. Birring, I. D. Pavord, and D. H. Evans, "Detection of cough signals in continuous audio recordings using hidden Markov models," *IEEE Transactions on Biomedical Engineering*, vol. 53, no. 6, pp. 1078–1083, 2006.

[15] B. Sklar, "Rayleigh fading channels in mobile digital communication systems," *IEEE Communications Magazine*, vol. 35, no. 7, pp. 90–100, 1997.

[16] S. Popa, N. Draghiciu, and R. Reiz, "Fading types in wireless communications systems," *Journal of Electrical and Electronics Engineering*, vol. 1, no. 1, pp. 233–237, 2008.

[17] C. Burges, *A Tutorial on Support Vector Machines For Pattern Recognition*, Kluwer Academic Publishers, Boston, Mass, USA, 1998.

[18] D. Srivstain and L. Bhambu, "Data classification using support vector machine," *Journal of Theoretical and Applied Information Technology*, vol. 12, no. 1, pp. 1960–1971, 2009.

[19] C. Hsu, C. Chang, and C. Lin, "A Practical Guide to Support Vector Classification," http://www.csie.ntu.edu.tw/.

[20] A. Bala, A. Kumber, and N. Birla, "Voice command recognition system based on MFCC and DWT," *International Journal of Engineering Science and Technology*, vol. 2, pp. 7335–7342, 2010.

[21] H. Chatrzarrin, A. Arcelus, R. Goubran, and F. Knoefel, "Feature extraction for the differentiation of dry and wet cough sounds," in *Proceedings of the IEEE International Symposium on Medical Measurements and Applications (MeMeA '11)*, pp. 162–166, Bari, Italy, May 2011.

[22] R. Hasan, M. Jamil, and G. Rabbain, "Speaker identification using Mel frequency cepstral coefficients," in *Proceedings of the 3rd International Conference on Electrical & Computer Engineering (ICECE '04)*, pp. 565–568, Dhaka, Bangladesh, 2004.

[23] H. Hoa, T. An, and T. Dat, "Semi-supervised tree support vector machine for online cough recognition," in *Proceedings of the International Speech Communication Association (ISCA '11)*, pp. 1637–1640, Florence, Italy, 2011.

[24] G. Sun, Z. Wang, and M. Wang, "A new multi-classification method based on binary tree support vector machine," in *Proceedings of the IEEE International Conference on Innovative Computing Information and Control*, Liaoning, China, June 2008.

[25] M. Pal, "Multiclass approaches for support vector machine based land cover classification," in *Proceedings of the 8th Annual International Conference, Map India*, 2005, http://arxiv.org/ftp/arxiv/papers/0802/0802.2411.pdf.

[26] http://www.freesound.org/.

[27] N. Kostov, "Mobile radio channels modelling in MATLAB," *Radio Engineering*, vol. 12, pp. 12–16, 2003.

6

Online Medicine for Pregnant Women

Sharon Davidesko,[1] David Segal,[2,3] and Roni Peleg[1,4]

[1] Ben-Gurion University of the Negev, P.O. Box 653, 84105 Beer-Sheva, Israel
[2] Division of Obstetrics and Gynecology, Soroka Medical Center, P.O. Box 151, 84101 Beer-Sheva, Israel
[3] Women Health Center, Clalit Health Services, Southern District, Henrietta Szold 1, 89428 Beer-Sheva, Israel
[4] The Department of Family Medicine and Siaal Research Center for Family Practice and Primary Care,
  Division of Community Health, Faculty of Health Sciences, Ben-Gurion University of the Negev,
  P.O. Box 653, 84105 Beer-Sheva, Israel

Correspondence should be addressed to Roni Peleg; pelegr@bgu.ac.il

Academic Editor: Carlos De Las Cuevas

Objective. To assess the use of cell phones and email as means of communication between pregnant women and their gynecologists and family physicians. *Study Design*. A cross-sectional study of pregnant women at routine followup. One hundred and twenty women participated in the study. *Results*. The mean age was 27.4 ± 3.4 years. One hundred nineteen women owned a cell phone and 114 (95%) had an email address. Seventy-two women (60%) had their gynecologist's cell phone number and 50 women (42%) had their family physician's cell phone number. More women contacted their gynecologist via cell phone or email during pregnancy compared to their family physician ($P = 0.005$ and 0.009, resp.). Most preferred to communicate with their physician via cell phone at predetermined times, but by email at any time during the day ($P < 0.0001$). They would use cell phones for emergencies or unusual problems but preferred email for other matters ($P < 0.0001$). *Conclusions*. Pregnant women in the Negev region do not have a preference between the use of cell phones or email for medical consultation with their gynecologist or family physician. The provision of the physician's cell phone numbers or email address together with the provision of guidelines and resources could improve healthcare services.

1. Introduction

Israel passed a Health Insurance law in 1995 that mandates healthcare services by healthcare funds (HMOs) for the entire population. There is competition among the funds to improve efficiency and provide optimal care to the satisfaction of their patients, while still meeting budgetary constraints. One of the ways to achieve these goals is the use of advanced means of communication such as provision of physicians' cell phone numbers and email addresses to patients for those cases in which this form of communication can make patient-physician communication more efficient. The use of cell phones and email to reduce the work burden of clinic physicians and to improve patient-physician communication has been shown to be effective [1]. Experience has shown that cell phone consultations are more effective than in-person consultations in the clinic [2, 3] especially for the ongoing

treatment of chronic diseases [4, 5]. Educated use of this form of consultation enables patients to get counsel when they require it. Cell phone consultations can save travel time as well as waiting time in the clinic [6].

Patients often contact their physicians by cell phone [7]. One study showed that 83.1% of the patients that contacted their physician by cell phone solved their problem and did not have to come to the clinic. In addition, in 52.8% of the cases it was possible to monitor the patients by phone [8]. In another study most of the family physicians surveyed thought that cell phone consultation was of equal value to a face-to-face appointment [9].

Electronic communication is a revolutionary development in healthcare services [10]. The results of a survey, which assessed communication between patients and physicians, showed that patients were satisfied with the option of electronic communication with their physicians.

The investigators found that email was a convenient, useful way for physicians to achieve their objectives without any reported problems [11].

In order to evaluate this development in the field of patient-physician communication one should assess the advantages and disadvantages of its use. Proper use of email can improve communication and serve as a primary instrument for consulting in the healthcare system [12]. A study that investigated the use of email for communication with patients found that the main reasons for choosing this mode of communication, among physicians who were satisfied with its use, was that it saved time (33%) and helped provide better care (20%). Among physicians who were not happy with this mode of communication the major reason for its use was that patients requested it (80%) [13]. In another study of communication with patients by email the physicians reported a high degree of satisfaction with this mode of communication [14]. Physicians should be aware of the advantages and disadvantages of electronic communication with patients so as to make the best possible use of it.

Although provision of cell phone numbers [15] or email addresses [13] to patients is simple and can make patient-physician communication easier, it can also increase the physician's work load and have a negative effect on the physician's work environment and even on their free time [16].

Pregnant women comprise a unique population that needs monitoring over the course of pregnancy. Pregnancy entails potential condition-related complications on the one hand while necessitating increased monitoring of chronic diseases that are unrelated to gender or pregnancy on the other. This unique situation requires the professional skills of the gynecologist together with the ongoing care of the family physician. The latter knows the patients and their medical and biopsychosocial circumstances and information that is very important for the decision-making process. The mode of communication with the gynecologist and the family physician is important as well as its availability at times of need under these unique medical circumstances. Over the course of pregnancy women often feel a need to contact their physician about their pregnancy, per se, as well as any causes of concern that may arise or new and troublesome symptoms. To our knowledge no paper has been published to date on patient-physician communication among pregnant women.

1.1. Setting. In Israel the treatment and followup of pregnant women are carried out by family physicians as well as obstetricians and gynecologists. Deliveries are performed by obstetricians and midwifes, but not by family physicians. In the current study family physicians serve as a reference group for comparison with obstetricians. In Israel there is a combined residency program for obstetrics and gynecology, so for convenience we use the term gynecologist when referring to either gynecologists or obstetricians.

2. Materials and Methods

The primary aim of the study was to evaluate the use of cell phones or email by pregnant women to consult with their gynecologist or family physician and their use of the Internet to search for information on their pregnancy.

The secondary aims of the study were as follows:

(i) to assess whether pregnant patients have the cell phone number or the email address of their gynecologist or family physician,

(ii) to compare how pregnant women consult with their gynecologist and family physician,

(iii) to evaluate the advantages and disadvantages of these modes of communication,

(iv) to assess the effect of patient age, educational level, and other sociodemographic variables on the preferred mode of communication,

(v) to assess use of Internet searches to obtain information on pregnancy-related issues,

(vi) to improve our understanding of this new mode of healthcare service.

This was a cross-sectional study. Personal interviews were conducted with Hebrew-speaking pregnant women of 18 years of age or older who came to the Women's Health Center of the Clalit Healthcare Services in Beer-Sheva for a routine pregnancy checkup and agreed to participate in the study. Women with cognitive problems and those who were unable to answer the questionnaire items were not included in the study.

The study instrument was a questionnaire completed by personal interview. The first part covered patient attitudes towards getting their physicians' cell phone number and email address for medical consultations during pregnancy and use of the Internet to obtain medical information. The second part included patient sociodemographic data. The questionnaire was tested in a pilot study with 10 participants and was revised in light of their comments.

Statistical analyses were conducted with the SPSS software package; version 19.0. Statistical tests were used for differences between the two primary study groups. In univariate analyses the Chi-square test was used for categorical variables and t-tests for continuous variables. Statistical significance was set at $P < 0.05$.

The Helsinki Committee of the Meir Medical Center approved the study (number 140/2012).

3. Results

One hundred and twenty women participated in the study. Their mean age was 27.4 ± 3.4. One hundred and five women (96%) were married and most lived in Beer-Sheva (59%). Ninety-eight women (82%) were born in Israel. The sociodemographic characteristics of the study population are shown in Table 1.

3.1. Attitudes towards the Use of Cell Phones for Consultations with Gynecologists and Family Physicians (Table 2). One hundred and nineteen of the 120 participants have cell phones. Most of the participants were very interested in receiving

TABLE 1: Sociodemographic and health characteristics of the study population ($N = 120$).

Variable	Result
Age in years	
Mean ± SD	27.4 ± 4.3
Range	18–38
Family status [N (%)]	
Single	5 (4)
Married	115 (96)
Place of residence [N (%)]	
Beer-Sheva	71 (59)
Nearby city	20 (17)
Agricultural settlement	11 (9)
Bedouin sector	18 (15)
Country of birth [N (%)]	
Israel	98 (82)
Former USSR	12 (10)
Europe	5 (4)
USA/Canada	3 (3)
Africa/Asia	2 (2)
Years of education	
Mean ± SD	11.8 ± 0.7
Range	9–14
Present work status [N (%)]	
Employed	82 (68)
Student	16 (13)
Unemployed	22 (18)
Income	
Low	63 (53)
Average	43 (36)
High	14 (12)
How would you rate your health condition? [N (%)]	
Excellent	81 (68)
Very good	25 (21)
Good	4 (3)
Reasonable	8 (7)
Poor	2 (2)
Do you suffer from a chronic disease? [N (%)]	
Yes	12 (10)
No	108 (90)
Population sector? [N (%)]	
Jewish	93 (78)
Bedouin	27 (23)
Number of children	
Mean ± SD	1.08 ± 1.31
Range	0–7
Week of pregnancy	
Mean ± SD	20.87 ± 8.05
Range	7–37

the cell phone number of their gynecologist and family physician (92.5% and 95%, resp.). Most of them felt that having their physician's cell phone number could improve the quality of their communication (4.53 for their gynecologist and 4.56 for their family physician on a scale from 1 to 5, with 5 representing strong agreement). The women also agreed that having their physician's cell phone number would increase their personal sense of security even if they did not actually contact the physician. The women agreed that calling the physician during work hours could impair the physician's work (4.0 for the gynecologist and 4.05 for the family physician).

In the majority of issues surveyed there were no statistically significant differences in the participants' responses between gynecologists and family physicians. The exceptions were that more women had their gynecologist's number than their family physician's number ($P = 0.004$) and more women actually contacted their gynecologist than their family physician by cell phone during pregnancy ($P = 0.005$).

3.2. Attitudes towards the Use of Email for Consultations with Gynecologists and Family Physicians (Table 3). One hundred and fourteen participants (95%) have email addresses. Most of the women were very interested in getting email addresses from their gynecologist (89.2%) and their family physician (88.3%). Most of them felt that having their physician's cell phone number could improve the quality of their communication (4.6 for their gynecologist and 4.58 for their family physician). Similarly, the women agreed that having their physician's cell phone number would increase their personal sense of security even if they did not actually contact the physician. They thought that having the cell phone number could help solve medical problems and reduce the number of visits to the clinic and emergency room. The women responded that calling the physician during work hours could impair the physician's work to a moderate degree (3.2 for both the gynecologist and the family physician).

The participants thought that there is greater risk of impaired communication through email with their family physician (4.03) than with their gynecologist (3.08) ($P < 0.0001$). More women had their gynecologist's email address (61%) than their family physician's email address (38%) ($P = 0.005$). More women contacted their gynecologist by means of email during pregnancy (34%) than their family physician (9%) ($P = 0.009$).

3.3. A Comparison of Attitudes towards Getting the Family Physician's Cell Phone Number or Email Address (Table 4). There was no statistically significant preference for getting a cell phone number or email address or as to which would be more likely to improve communication with the family physician, provide a greater sense of personal security, or reduce the number of clinic or emergency room visits. More women said that they would prefer to contact their family physician by cell phone at predetermined days or hours compared with any hour of the day by email ($P < 0.0001$). Similarly, women prefer the cell phone to email in unusual circumstances ($P < 0.001$).

3.4. A Comparison of Attitudes towards Getting the Gynecologist's Cell Phone Number or Email Address (Table 5). There was no statistically significant preference for getting a cell phone number or email address or as to which would be

TABLE 2: Attitudes towards medical consultation through cell phones.

Variable	Gynecologist	Family physician	P
How do you feel about getting your physician's cell phone number? [N (%)]			
Very interested	111 (92.5)	114 (95.0)	
Would not object	8 (6.7)	5 (4.2)	
Not interested	1 (0.8)	1 (0.8)	0.747
Do you agree with the following statements regarding getting your physician's cell phone number? (scale of 1–5)			
It could improve the relationship between us:			
Mean ± SD	4.53 ± 0.78	4.58 ± 0.71	
Range	2–5	2–5	0.678
It could improve my sense of security even if I do not use it:			
Mean ± SD	4.53 ± 0.78	4.57 ± 0.71	
Range	2–5	2–5	0.604
The cell phone is an effective mode of communication that could solve my problems:			
Mean ± SD	4.28 ± 0.74	4.37 ± 0.71	
Range	2–5	2–5	0.377
The cell phone can cut down on the number of clinic visits:			
Mean ± SD	4.28 ± 0.74	4.33 ± 0.73	
Range	2–5	2–5	0.598
The cell phone can reduce the number of emergency room visits:			
Mean ± SD	4.28 ± 0.74	4.33 ± 0.74	
Range	2–5	2–5	0.602
At what times would you call the physician? [N (%)]			
I do not intend to call	2 (2)	2 (2)	
Only at appointed hours	47 (39)	49 (41)	
Only during daytime hours (except Saturdays and holidays)	56 (47)	54 (45)	
At all hours including nights, Saturdays, and holidays	15 (13)	15 (13)	0.994
Under which circumstance would you call your physician? [N (%)]			
I do not intend to call	1 (1)	1 (1)	
Only in unusual circumstances	75 (63)	73 (61)	
For any questions that I think I require a medical consultation	44 (37)	46 (38)	0.945
The physician should not be called because it could interfere with their privacy when they are not working (scale of 1–5):			
Mean ± SD	3.94 ± 0.86	4.03 ± 0.98	
Range	2–5	1–5	0.450
The physician should not be called because there are telephone centers that are active after clinic hours (scale of 1–5):			
Mean ± SD	4.08 ± 0.89	4.20 ± 0.83	
Range	2–5	1–5	0.281

TABLE 2: Continued.

Variable	Gynecologist	Family physician	P
The physician should not be called because in emergencies one can call for an ambulance or go to the emergency room (scale of 1–5):			
Mean ± SD	4.31 ± 0.71	4.23 ± 0.83	0.423
Range	2–5	1–5	
The physician should not be called because medical errors can occur if a physical examination is not performed (scale of 1–5):			
Mean ± SD	3.67 ± 0.99	3.73 ± 1.03	0.646
Range	1–5	1–5	
The physician should not be called because there is a risk of miscommunication (scale of 1 to 5):			
Mean ± SD	3.92 ± 0.94	3.98 ± 0.97	0.627
Range	1–5	1–5	
The physician should not be called because it can interfere with their clinic work (scale of 1 to 5):			
Mean ± SD	4.00 ± 0.90	4.05 ± 1.00	0.684
Range	1–5	1–5	
Have you asked for your physician's cell phone number in the past? [N (%)]			
Yes	33 (28)	29 (24)	0.555
Do you have your physician's cell phone number? [N (%)]			
Yes	72 (60)	50 (42)	0.004
Have you contacted your physician by cell phone since you became pregnant? [N (%)]			
Yes	46 (38)	26 (22)	0.005

TABLE 3: Attitudes towards medical consultation through email.

Variable	Gynecologist	Family physician	P
How do you feel about getting your physician's email address? [N (%)]			
Very interested	107 (89.2)	106 (88.3)	
Would not object	4 (3.3)	5 (4.2)	0.944
Not interested	9 (7.5)	9 (7.5)	
Do you agree with the following statements regarding getting your physician's email address? (scale of 1–5)			
It could improve the relationship between us:			
Mean ± SD	4.6 ± 0.69	4.58 ± 0.71	0.412
Range	2–5	2–5	
It could improve my sense of security even if I do not use it:			
Mean ± SD	4.59 ± 0.69	4.58 ± 0.71	0.456
Range	2–5	2–5	
Email is an effective means of communication that could solve my problems:			
Mean ± SD	4.33 ± 0.73	4.34 ± 0.72	0.457
Range	2–5	2–5	
Email can cut down on the number of clinic visits:			
Mean ± SD	4.38 ± 0.71	4.34 ± 0.72	0.667
Range	2–5	2–5	
Email can reduce the number of emergency room visits:			
Mean ± SD	4.38 ± 0.71	4.32 ± 0.75	0.500
Range	2–5	2–5	
At what times would you email the physician? [N (%)]			
I do not intend to call	9 (8)	9 (8)	
Only at appointed hours	8 (7)	7 (6)	0.994
Only during daytime hours (except Saturdays and holidays)	50 (42)	50 (42)	
At all hours including nights, Saturdays, and holidays	53 (44)	54 (45)	
Under which circumstance would you email your physician? [N (%)]			
I do not intend to contact by email	9 (8)	9 (8)	
Only in unusual circumstances	44 (37)	38 (32)	0.706
For any question	67 (56)	73 (61)	
The physician should not be sent an email because it could interfere with their privacy when they are not working (scale of 1 to 5):			
Mean ± SD	3.34 ± 1.42	3.41 ± 1.36	0.697
Range	1–5	1–5	
The physician should not be sent an email because medical errors can occur if a physical examination is not performed (scale of 1 to 5):			
Mean ± SD	3.88 ± 0.93	3.81 ± 0.96	0.566
Range	2–5	2–5	
The physician should not be sent an email because there is a risk of miscommunication (scale of 1 to 5):			
Mean ± SD	3.08 ± 0.85	4.03 ± 0.87	<0.0001
Range	2–5	1–5	
The physician should not be sent an email because it can interfere with their clinic work (scale of 1 to 5):			
Mean ± SD	3.20 ± 1.46	3.20 ± 1.47	1.000
Range	1–5	1–5	

TABLE 3: Continued.

Variable	Gynecologist	Family physician	P
I see no reason why I should not get the physician's personal email address (scale of 1–5):			
Mean ± SD	4.16 ± 0.92	4.39 ± 0.93	0.055
Range	1–5	1–5	
Have you asked for your physician's email address in the past? [N (%)]			
Yes	27 (23)	20 (17)	0.255
Do you have your physician's email address? [N (%)]			
Yes	73 (61)	46 (38)	0.0005
Have you contacted your physician by email since you became pregnant? [N (%)]			
Yes	41 (34)	23 (19)	0.009

TABLE 4: A comparison of attitudes towards receiving the family physician's cell phone number or email address.

Variable	Cell phone number	Email address	P
How do you feel about getting your physician's cell phone number or email address? [N (%)]			
Very interested	114 (95.0)	106 (88.3)	
Would not object	5 (4.2)	5 (4.2)	0.035
Not interested	1 (0.8)	9 (7.5)	
Do you agree with the following statements regarding getting your physician's cell phone number or email address? (scale of 1 to 5)			
It could improve the relationship between us:			
Mean ± SD	4.57 ± 0.71	4.58 ± 0.71	0.913
Range	2–5	2–5	
It could improve my sense of security even if I do not use it:			
Mean ± SD	4.58 ± 0.71	4.58 ± 0.71	0.913
Range	2–5	2–5	
Calls and email are effective means of communication that could solve my problems:			
Agree			
Do not agree			
Mean ± SD	4.37 ± 0.71	4.34 ± 0.72	0.745
Range	2–5	2–5	
Calls and email can cut down on the number of clinic visits:			
Mean ± SD	4.33 ± 0.73	4.34 ± 0.72	0.915
Range	2–5	2–5	
Calls and email can reduce the number of emergency room visits:			
Mean ± SD	4.33 ± 0.74	4.32 ± 0.75	0.917
Range	2–5	2–5	
At what times would you call or email the physician? [N (%)]			
I do not intend to call or send an email	2 (2)	9 (8)	
Only at appointed hours	49 (41)	7 (6)	<0.0001
Only during daytime hours (except Saturdays and holidays)	54 (45)	50 (42)	
At all hours including nights, Saturdays, and holidays	15 (13)	54 (45)	
Under which circumstance would you call or email your physician? [N (%)]			
I do not intend to call or contact by email	1 (1)	9 (8)	
Only in unusual circumstances	73 (61)	38 (32)	<0.0001
For any question	46 (38)	73 (61)	
The physician should not be called or sent an email because it could interfere with their privacy when they are not working (scale of 1 to 5):			
Mean ± SD	4.03 ± 0.98	3.41 ± 1.36	0.0001
Range	1–5	1–5	
The physician should not be called or sent an email because medical errors can occur if a physical examination is not performed (scale of 1 to 5):			
Mean ± SD	3.73 ± 1.03	3.81 ± 0.96	0.876
Range	1–5	2–5	
The physician should not be called or sent an email because there is a risk of miscommunication (scale of to 5).			
Mean ± SD	3.98 ± 0.97	3.20 ± 1.47	<0.0001
Range	1–5	1–5	
The physician should not be called or sent an email because it can interfere with their clinic work (scale of 1 to 5):			
Mean ± SD	3.20 ± 1.46	3.20 ± 1.47	1.000
Range	1–5	1–5	

TABLE 4: Continued.

Variable	Cell phone number	Email address	P
The family physician cannot help because I am pregnant: (scale of 1 to 5)			
Mean ± SD	1.98 ± 0.68	2.06 ± 0.74	0.384
Range	1–4	1–5	
I see no reason why I should not get the physician's personal cell phone number or email address (scale of 1 to 5):			
Mean ± SD	3.73 ± 1.05	4.39 ± 0.93	<0.0001
Range	1–5	1–5	
Have you asked for your physician's cell phone number or email address in the past? [N (%)]			
Yes	29 (24)	20 (17)	0.149
Do you have your physician's cell phone number or email address? [N (%)]			
Yes	50 (42)	46 (38)	0.598
Have you contacted your physician by cell phone or email since you became pregnant? [N (%)]			
Yes	26 (22)	23 (19)	0.631

TABLE 5: A comparison of attitudes towards receiving the gynecologist's cell phone number or email address.

Variable	Cell phone number	Email address	P
How do you feel about getting your physician's cell phone number or email address? [N (%)]			
Very interested	111 (92.5)	107 (89.2)	
Would not object	8 (6.7)	4 (3.3)	0.02
Not interested	1 (0.8)	9 (7.5)	
Do you agree with the following statements regarding getting your physician's cell phone number or email address? (scale of 1 to 5)			
It could improve the relationship between us:			
Mean ± SD	4.53 ± 0.78	4.60 ± 0.69	0.462
Range	2–5	2–5	
It could improve my sense of security even if I don't use it:			
Mean ± SD	4.53 ± 0.78	4.59 ± 0.69	0.528
Range	2–5	2–5	
Cell phone calls and email are effective means of communication that could solve my problems:			
Agree			
Do not agree			
Mean ± SD	4.28 ± 0.74	4.33 ± 0.73	0.598
Range	2–5	2–5	
Cell phone calls and email can cut down on the number of clinic visits:			
Mean ± SD	4.28 ± 0.74	4.38 ± 0.71	0.286
Range	2–5	2–5	
Cell phone calls and email can reduce the number of emergency room visits:			
Mean ± SD	4.33 ± 0.74	4.38 ± 0.71	0.286
Range	2–5	2–5	
At what times would you call or email the physician? [N (%)]			
I do not intend to call	2 (2)	9 (8)	
Only at appointed hours	47 (39)	8 (7)	<0.0001
Only during daytime hours (except Saturdays and holidays)	56 (47)	50 (42)	
At all hours including nights, Saturdays, and holidays	15 (13)	53 (45)	
Under which circumstance would you call or email your physician? [N (%)]			
I do not intend to contact by email	1 (1)	9 (8)	
Only in unusual circumstances	75 (63)	44 (37)	<0.0001
For any question	44 (37)	67 (56)	
The physician should not be called or sent an email because it could interfere with their privacy when they are not working: (scale of 1 to 5)			
Mean ± SD	3.94 ± 0.86	3.41 ± 1.36	0.0001
Range	2–5	1–5	
The physician should not be called or sent an email because medical errors can occur if a physical examination is not performed: (scale of 1 to 5)			
Mean ± SD	3.67 ± 0.99	3.88 ± 0.93	0.091
Range	1–5	2–5	
The physician should not be called or sent an email because there is a risk of miscommunication: (scale of 1 to 5)			
Mean ± SD	3.92 ± 0.94	3.08 ± 0.85	<0.0001
Range	1–5	2–5	
The physician should not be called or sent an email because it can interfere with his clinic work: (scale of 1 to 5)			
Mean ± SD	4.00 ± 0.90	3.20 ± 1.47	<0.0001
Range	1–5	1–5	

TABLE 5: Continued.

Variable	Cell phone number	Email address	P
I see no reason why I should not get the physician's personal cell phone number or email address: (scale of 1 to 5)			
Mean ± SD	3.62 ± 1.05	4.16 ± 0.92	<0.0001
Range	1–5	1–5	
Have you asked for your physician's cell phone number or email address in the past? [N (%)]			
Yes	33 (28)	27 (23)	0.371
Do you have your physician's cell phone number or email address? [N (%)]			
Yes	72 (60)	73 (61)	0.895
Have you contacted your physician by cell phone or email since you became pregnant? [N (%)]			
Yes	46 (38)	41 (34)	0.502

more likely to improve communication with the gynecologist, provide a greater sense of personal security, or reduce the number of clinic or emergency room visits. More women said that they would prefer to contact their gynecologist by cell phone at predetermined days or hours compared with any hour of the day by email ($P < 0.0001$). Similarly, women prefer the cell phone to email in unusual circumstances ($P < 0.0001$).

3.5. Internet Searches for Information Related to Pregnancy (Table 6). Most of the women (60%) reported that they conduct Internet searches on pregnancy often but 76% never discussed the information obtained with their gynecologist and 81% never did so with their family physician. The mean age of women who conducted Internet searches on pregnancy was higher than those who did not ($P < 0.001$). Most of the women who live in Beer-Sheva ($N = 71$) conducted Internet searches, while most of those who did not conduct Internet searches live in Bedouin regions ($P < 0.001$) and define themselves as religious ($P < 0.001$). Women who conducted fewer Internet searches or did not conduct them at all have fewer years of education ($P < 0.001$) and are more likely to be unemployed ($P < 0.001$) and have lower mean incomes ($P = 0.002$).

4. Discussion

The results of the study show that the participants were interested in receiving the cell phone number or email address of both of their treating physicians without any preference for either modality.

We found that most of the women were very interested in getting the cell phone number and email address of their gynecologist (92.5% and 89.2%, resp.) or family physician (95% and 88.3%, resp.). These findings are in contradiction to the results of other studies conducted in the same geographic region among Jews [17] and Bedouins (personal communication), which found a clear preference for cell phone number over email address. The difference in results may stem from differences in the study populations. Pregnant women are younger on average than the general population so that they may have more experience, knowledge, and access to electronic means of communication. In addition, pregnant women comprise a unique population that requires specific monitoring to prevent complications and to control chronic diseases that are not related to the pregnancy and because the group is composed solely of women. These circumstances necessitate the specific professional skills of gynecologists and the continuity of care and familiarity with patients over time in biopsychosocial terms that the family physician can provide. The mode of communication with patients practiced by gynecologists and family physicians as well as its availability and accessibility are of great importance.

More pregnant women had their gynecologists' cell phone number and/or email address and consulted with their gynecologist by electronic modes than with their family physician over the course of their pregnancy. A possible explanation for this finding is that pregnant women are

usually healthy and have little need in general for contact with healthcare services or family physicians, so they turn to gynecologists during pregnancy because they perceive them as the natural address for pregnancy-related issues.

Telephone calls interrupt the routine work of the physician in the clinic, while communication through email does not, because the physician can relate to the patient who sent an email message when they are not with another patient [17]. This is consistent with the findings of our study. Phone calls enable consultations in real time compared with email communication, which does not always elicit an immediate response. In the present study the women were asked about the circumstances under which they would consult with their physician by cell phone or email. The results show that women communicate by cell phone if the circumstances are urgent or unusual. On the other hand they use email for any question that arises. This finding highlights the possibility that patients are able to make reasonable use of varying communication modes for different healthcare needs. The women declared that they make contact with their gynecologist or family physician during all hours of the day by email, but only at predetermined times by cell phone. In another study conducted in a surgical medical center provision of cell phone numbers by the treating physician was interpreted as a sign of caring on the physician's part and patients made use of this service in an efficient manner when they needed it [18]. In general, patients are happier when they have the option of communicating with their physician by personal cell phone [9, 18].

Having the physician's cell phone number and/or email address can give patients a sense of personal security even if they do not actually use it. If used, it can lead to a reduction in clinic and emergency room visits and a decrease in the work burden of physicians in clinics and in the hospital. The results of another study showed that use of email for medical consultation led to a significant reduction in emergency room visits [6]. Even though there have been reports of email consultations from as long ago as a decade, the use of email has become popular later than the use of cell phones [19]. Most of the participants in the present study have email addresses (95%) compared to 85.5% and 22% in previous studies conducted in the same geographical region in Jewish [17] and Bedouin populations (personal communication), respectively. One possible explanation for these differences is that pregnant women are usually younger than patients in family medicine practices who made up the study populations in the earlier studies.

In the present study we found that all the women who did not perform pregnancy-related Internet searches were Bedouin women who defined themselves as religious. This indicates that there are significant differences between the Jewish and Bedouin sectors of the population in terms of use of the Internet and email. This may stem from lower availability and accessibility of computers and other means of electronic communication in the Bedouin sector compared to the Jewish sector.

TABLE 6: Characteristics related to conduct Internet searches on pregnancy.

Variable	Often	Sometimes	Never	P
Age in years				
Mean ± SD	27.99 ± 3.91	27.58 ± 4.38	21.13 ± 2.59	<0.001
Range	19–35	19–37	18–24	
Family status [N (%)]				
Single	4 (6)	1 (2.2)	0	0.517
Married	63 (94)	44 (97.8)	8 (100)	
Place of residence [N (%)]				
Beer-Sheva	50 (74.6)	21 (46.7)	0	
Nearby city	9 (13.4)	9 (20.0)	2 (25.0)	<0.001
Agricultural settlement	6 (9.0)	5 (11.1)	0	
Bedouin sector	2 (3.0)	10 (22.2)	6 (75.0)	
Country of birth [N (%)]				
Israel	52 (77.6)	38 (84.4)	8 (100)	0.251
Other	15 (22.4)	7 (15.6)	0	
Years of education				
Mean ± SD	12.8 ± 0.55	11.76 ± 0.609	11.13 ± 1.126	0.001
Range	9–14	10–12	9–12	
Present work status [N (%)]				
Employed	54 (80.6)	28 (62.2)	0	
Student	9 (13.4)	5 (11.1)	2 (25.0)	<0.001
Unemployed	4 (6.0)	2 (25.0)	6 (75.0)	
Income				
Low	25 (37.3)	30 (66.67)	8 (100)	
Average	31 (46.3)	12 (26.7)	0	0.002
High	11 (16.4)	3 (6.7)	0	
How would you rate your health condition? [N (%)]				
Excellent	47 (70.1)	27 (60.0)	7 (87.5)	
Very good	13 (19.4)	11 (24.4)	1 (12.5)	
Good	1 (1.5)	3 (6.7)	0	0.778
Reasonable	5 (7.5)	3 (6.7)	0	
Poor	1 (1.5)	1 (2.2)	0	
Do you suffer from a chronic disease? [N (%)]				
Yes	7 (10.4)	5 (11.1)	0	0.617
No	60 (89.6)	40 (88.9)	8 (100)	
Population sector? [N (%)]				
Jewish	64 (95.5)	29 (64.4)	0	<0.001
Bedouin	3 (4.5)	16 (35.6)	8 (100)	
Are you religious? [N (%)]				
Yes	17 (25.4)	22 (48.9)	8 (100)	<0.001
No	50 (74.6)	23 (51.1)	0	
Number of children				
Mean ± SD	0.81 ± 0.925	1.53 ± 1.673	0.88 ± 1.126	0.013
Range	0–4	0–7	0–3	
Week of pregnancy				
Mean ± SD	20.55 ± 7.83	21.89 ± 8.359	17.75 ± 8.013	0.366
Range	7–37	7–36	11–35	

In a previous study on the attitudes of physicians in the Negev to providing their email addresses to their patients, 65% expressed concern that the absence of a physical examination could lead to misdiagnosis and treatment, 58% stated that in the case of emergency they would recommend that their patients visit the emergency room, and 57% believed that communication through email could impair the quality of care and were concerned about medical negligence suits [20].

In a world in which an increasing number of people have access to the Internet and email and use them for many and varied needs, the provision of healthcare services through electronic communication could become, in the future, a central modality of medical consultation. However, there is a glaring lack of controlled studies supporting this means of communication for medical services or providing information on how to integrate these technologies into the daily work routine of the physician [11].

The use of email for patient-physician communication also raises an important ethical issue. Studies conducted in northern Europe found that medical confidentiality could not be guaranteed using these technologies and as a result hospitals developed computerized systems in which patients can contact their physicians in a secure manner [21, 22].

There are no clear regulations or guidelines in Israel regarding the use of cell phones, email, and social networks such as Facebook and Twitter for medical consultation and physicians use them as they see fit.

Although there are clear advantages to the use of cell phones and email for medical consultation, there are also disadvantages including invasion of the physician's free time beyond their defined and compensated work hours, interruption to the provision of medical care for other patients during clinic work hours, and the risk of mistakes in medical decision making [23]. All the participants in the present study agreed that gynecologists and family physicians should be reimbursed for healthcare provided through cell phones and email. The formulation of guidelines for the use of cell phones and email for medical consultations, such as setting aside dedicated time for this type of patient-physician communication, could improve physicians' willingness to use it [24]. Another possible means of improving medical service for pregnant women could be the inclusion of midwives who specialize in pregnancy monitoring in the team that provides consultation through cell phones and email. This could improve the service since it would reduce costs and improve availability.

This study has several limitations, including the relatively small study population of 120 pregnant women, which may have limited statistical power and led to a type II error. Since the vast majority in the study were very interested in getting the cell phone numbers and email addresses of their gynecologists and family physicians it was not possible to conduct a logistic regression analysis to look for characteristics of the participating women that would predict whether they preferred one modality over the other. This study was conducted in a specific geographical region in women's health clinic of the Negev region of Israel. Since there are significant differences relating to health and pregnancy in different classes and cultures, the results of this study cannot be generalized to all the populations of pregnant women in Israel and around the world. It is also possible that women who did not participate in the study, including women who do not come to the clinic for regular monitoring during pregnancy, could have different attitudes towards the study questions, thus leading to a potential bias.

5. Conclusions

Pregnant women in the Negev region do not have a preference between the use of cell phones or email for medical consultation with their gynecologist or family physician. The

provision of the physician's cell phone numbers or email address, together with provision of guidelines and resources, could improve healthcare services by reducing clinic and emergency room visits, providing a sense of personal security to patients, and improving the quality of the patient-physician relationship. Understanding the unique advantages and disadvantages of these modes of communication could lead to their effective use in different conditions, including treatment for pregnant women. To this end it is recommended to formulate ethical and legal guidelines relating to the use of cell phones and email for healthcare services.

We hope that the findings of this study will help further this understanding of the use of cell phones and email among pregnant women specifically and in healthcare services in general.

References

[1] J. Car and A. Sheikh, "Telephone consultations," *British Medical Journal*, vol. 326, pp. 966–969, 2003.

[2] J. Oldham, "Telephone use in primary care. Programme to shape demand has been started in several practices," *British Medical Journal*, vol. 325, article 547, 2002.

[3] M. Jiwa, N. Mathers, and M. Campbell, "The effect of GP telephone triage on numbers seeking same-day appointments," *The British Journal of General Practice*, vol. 52, no. 478, pp. 390–391, 2002.

[4] H. Pinnock, L. McKenzie, D. Price, and A. Sheikh, "Cost-effectiveness of telephone or surgery asthma reviews: economic analysis of a randomised controlled trial," *The British Journal of General Practice*, vol. 55, pp. 119–124, 2005.

[5] H. H. Fischer, S. L. Moore, D. Ginosar, A. J. Davidson, C. M. Rice-Peterson, and M. J. Durfee, "Care by cell phone: text messaging for chronic disease management," *American Journal of Managed Care*, vol. 18, pp. e42–e47, 2012.

[6] B. McKinstry, P. Watson, H. Pinnock, D. Heaney, and A. Sheikh, "Telephone consulting in primary care: a triangulated qualitative study of patients and providers," *The British Journal of General Practice*, vol. 59, pp. e209–e218, 2009.

[7] D. E. Hildebrandt, J. M. Westfall, R. A. Nicholas, P. C. Smith, and J. Stern, "Are frequent callers to family physicians high utilizers?" *The Annals of Family Medicine*, vol. 2, pp. 546–548, 2004.

[8] D. M. Elnicki, P. Ogden, M. Flannery, M. Hannis, and S. Cykert, "Telephone medicine for internists," *Journal of General Internal Medicine*, vol. 15, pp. 337–343, 2000.

[9] B. McKinstry, V. Hammersley, C. Burton et al., "The quality, safety and content of telephone and face-to-face consultations: a comparative study," *Quality & Safety in Health Care*, vol. 19, pp. 298–303, 2010.

[10] J. Car and A. Sheikh, "Email consultations in health care: 1—scope and effectiveness," *British Medical Journal*, vol. 329, pp. 435–438, 2004.

[11] M. Wallwiener, C. W. Wallwiener, J. K. Kansy, H. Seeger, and T. K. Rajab, "Impact of electronic messaging on the patient-physician interaction," *Journal of Telemedicine and Telecare*, vol. 15, pp. 243–250, 2009.

[12] J. Ye, G. Rust, Y. Fry-Johnson, and H. Strothers, "E-mail in patient-provider communication: a systematic review," *Patient Education and Counseling*, vol. 80, pp. 266–273, 2010.

[13] T. K. Houston, D. Z. Sands, B. R. Nash, and D. E. Ford, "Experiences of physicians who frequently use e-mail with patients," *Health Communication*, vol. 15, pp. 515–525, 2003.

[14] B. Gaster, C. L. Knight, D. E. DeWitt, J. V. Sheffield, N. P. Assefi, and D. Buchwald, "Physicians' use of and attitudes toward electronic mail for patient communication," *Journal of General Internal Medicine*, vol. 18, pp. 385–389, 2003.

[15] R. Peleg, "Off-the-cuff cellular phone consultations in a family practice," *Journal of the Royal Society of Medicine*, vol. 94, pp. 290–291, 2001.

[16] B. McKinstry, J. Walker, C. Campbell, D. Heaney, and S. Wyke, "Telephone consultations to manage requests for same-day appointments: a randomised controlled trial in two practices," *The British Journal of General Practice*, vol. 52, pp. 306–310, 2002.

[17] R. Peleg and E. Nazarenko, "Providing cell phone numbers and e-mail addresses to patients: the patient's perspective, a cross sectional study," *Israel Journal of Health Policy Research*, vol. 1, p. 32, 2012.

[18] K. R. Chin, S. B. Adams Jr., L. Khoury, and D. Zurakowski, "Patient behavior if given their surgeon's cellular telephone number," *Clinical Orthopaedics and Related Research*, vol. 439, pp. 260–268, 2005.

[19] G. R. Bergus, S. D. Sinift, C. S. Randall, and D. M. Rosenthal, "Use of an e-mail curbside consultation service by family physicians," *The Journal of family practice*, vol. 47, no. 5, pp. 357–360, 1998.

[20] R. Peleg, A. Avdalimov, and T. Freud, "Providing cell phone numbers and email addresses to patients: the physician's perspective," *BMC Research Notes*, vol. 4, article 76, 2011.

[21] H. van Os-Medendorp, C. van Veelen, M. Hover et al., "The digital eczema centre utrecht," *Journal of Telemedicine and Telecare*, vol. 16, pp. 12–14, 2010.

[22] V. van der Meer, W. B. van den Hout, M. J. Bakker, K. F. Rabe, P. J. Sterk, and W. J. Assendelft, "Cost-effectiveness of Internet-based self-management compared with usual care in asthma," *PLoS ONE*, vol. 6, Article ID e27108, 2011.

[23] H. W. Potts and J. C. Wyatt, "Survey of doctors'experience of patients using the Internet," *Journal of Medical Internet Research*, vol. 4, article e5, 2002.

[24] P. C. Tang, W. Black, and C. Y. Young, "Proposed criteria for reimbursing eVisits: content analysis of secure patient messages in a personal health record system," *AMIA Annual Symposium Proceedings*, pp. 764–768, 2006.

7

Evaluation of a Clinical Service Model for Dysphagia Assessment via Telerehabilitation

Elizabeth C. Ward,[1,2] **Clare L. Burns,**[3] **Deborah G. Theodoros,**[1] **and Trevor G. Russell**[1]

[1] *The University of Queensland, School of Health & Rehabilitation Sciences, St. Lucia, Brisbane, QLD 4072, Australia*
[2] *Centre for Functioning and Health Research, Queensland Health, Buranda, Brisbane, QLD 4102, Australia*
[3] *Speech Pathology Department, Royal Brisbane and Women's Hospital, Herston, Brisbane, QLD 4006, Australia*

Correspondence should be addressed to Elizabeth C. Ward; liz.ward@uq.edu.au

Academic Editor: Malcolm Clarke

Emerging research supports the feasibility and viability of conducting clinical swallow examinations (CSE) for patients with dysphagia via telerehabilitation. However, minimal data has been reported to date regarding the implementation of such services within the clinical setting or the user perceptions of this type of clinical service. A mixed methods study design was employed to examine the outcomes of a weekly dysphagia assessment clinic conducted via telerehabilitation and examine issues relating to service delivery and user perceptions. Data was collected across a total of 100 patient assessments. Information relating to primary patient outcomes, session statistics, patient perceptions, and clinician perceptions was examined. Results revealed that session durations averaged 45 minutes, there was minimal technical difficulty experienced, and clinical decisions made regarding primary patient outcomes were comparable between the online and face to face clinicians. Patient satisfaction was high and clinicians felt that they developed good rapport, found the system easy to use, and were satisfied with the service in over 90% of the assessments conducted. Key factors relating to screening patient suitability, having good general organization, and skilled staff were identified as facilitators for the service. This trial has highlighted important issues for consideration when planning or implementing a telerehabilitation service for dysphagia management.

1. Introduction

There is a small but emerging evidence base supporting the use of telerehabilitation to improve access to both clinical and instrumental dysphagia assessment services [1–8]. However, while the research conducted to date has focused on the evaluation of different types of system architecture [1, 4, 6], early feasibility data [1, 4, 7, 8], and the validity and reliability of online clinical decisions [2, 3, 5, 7, 8], no studies have examined the service characteristics (session durations, session complication rates, and equipment issues) associated with implementing a telerehabilitation clinical service. There is also limited information regarding potential facilitators and barriers to implementing a successful and time efficient telerehabilitation dysphagia service. Only one paper to date has discussed issues noted during the assessment of a small set of patients where certain patient factors (e.g., hearing

impairment, movement disorders) made the assessment process less efficient [9]. That paper highlighted important service considerations including the need for careful patient and clinician preparation prior to the session, having flexible system capabilities (e.g., multiple adjustable cameras, free field and lapel microphones, etc.) which allow for modifications/adjustments to assist the patient, and the importance of good support staff at the patient end to facilitate the session.

Integral to the evaluation of any new clinical service is also the examination of the consumer perspective. Without consumer support, from both the clinicians providing the services and the patients receiving them, new service models will not be adopted or sustained. Recent data from a cohort of 40 patients has shown that both clinician and patient satisfaction with dysphagia assessments provided via telerehabilitation were high [2]. However, although patient perceptions were positive, use of a pre- and postsession methodology revealed that a small proportion of patients had some presession reservations, stemming from a lack of awareness/understanding of what a telerehabilitation session would be like. Patient concerns about the "unknown" telerehabilitation service may have implications for the uptake of services.

Clinical service information is critical to inform the next step of telerehabilitation service planning and enable the incorporation of telerehabilitation services as a successful and viable service model for patients with dysphagia. The aim of the current research is to evaluate a short-term trial of a telerehabilitation service providing clinical assessments of dysphagia. By examining the service characteristics, barriers, facilitators, and the consumer perspective, the study aims to define the scope of the strengths and challenges involved with implementing this new service model.

2. Materials and Methods

A total of 100 patients being managed by the speech pathology department of the Royal Brisbane and Women's Hospital, QLD, Australia, were recruited to receive a clinical swallow examination via a weekly telerehabilitation dysphagia assessment clinic. Participants were recruited across a range of dysphagia severity levels (normal, mild, moderate, and severe) ensuring diversity within the sample. For recruitment, dysphagia severity was determined from a Clinical Swallow Examination (CSE) conducted by a clinician independent of this research, at a time no greater than 24 hours prior to the online clinic assessment. From the findings of that CSE, dysphagia severity was classified using the 7-level Dysphagia Outcome and Severity Scale [10] (nondysphagic: level 6-7; mild: level 5; moderate: level 3-4, severe: level 1-2). For inclusion, participants had to be deemed suitable for assessment by their treating medical officer and capable of remaining in a semiupright or upright position for the duration of the assessment. They were not required to have any knowledge or skills associated with computers or technology.

The participant group recruited was 54% male with a mean age of 67.08 years (SD = 16.99, range 21–112). One-quarter had a medically diagnosed cognitive deficit. Participants were from a range of aetiological groups (51% acute/degenerative disorder; 31% cancer care; 18% other) and presented with nil to severe dysphagia (25 nondysphagic; 25 mild, 25 moderate, and 25 severe). Consent was obtained for all participants. The study was granted ethical clearance from the Human Research Ethics Committees of both Queensland Health and The University of Queensland.

2.1. The Telerehabilitation Clinic.
The administrative, clinical, and technical guidelines for telerehabilitation practice [11] were used to establish the clinic and its processes. The trial clinic ran for 4 hours on a weekday morning with a maximum of 4 patients scheduled into any clinic. Clinic staff on any day included an online speech pathologist (O-SP) who arranged and led all assessments and an allied health assistant located at the patient end who was responsible for arranging inpatient transport to the telerehabilitation clinic,

setting up the system, positioning and preparing the patient, and assisting with physical tasks (e.g., feeding the patient during the food and fluid trials) under the direction of the O-SP. A second face to face speech pathologist (FTF-SP) was also involved in each clinic and was located in the room with the patient. The role of the FTF-SP was to conduct a simultaneous CSE (with the O-SP) in the FTF environment for each patient. This allowed later comparison of the online and FTF assessment results to calculate clinical agreement. The two SPs involved in any session (online or FTF) came from a pool of four clinicians, each with >5 years of experience in managing dysphagia in the acute care setting. For research purposes, distance was simulated, with the O-SP located in one room of the clinical setting and the patient, assistant, and FTF-SP located in a separate room within the same facility.

2.2. The Telerehabilitation System.
The telerehabilitation system used in this study has been described in detail elsewhere [1–3]. It consisted of notebook computers at the patient and clinician ends that incorporated custom video conferencing software audio and video compression technology for real-time videoconferencing. Audio was enabled using a free-field combined echo cancelling microphone and web-conference speaker, while the patient also wore a lapel microphone. Fixed and free standing cameras (with zoom capacity) were incorporated and remotely controlled by the O-SP. The system enabled the capture of audio and video (640 × 480 pixels) at the client end of the consultation for store-and-forward recordings of the sessions. An ad hoc 802.11 g wireless network with a throttled bandwidth of 128 Kbit/s was used for communication. This low bandwidth was purposefully chosen as it is the minimum bandwidth available across Australia's public health network.

2.3. Clinical Swallow Examination (CSE).
The CSE procedure has been reported in detail previously [1–3]. Prior to the session, both the online and FTF clinicians received a summary of the patient's relevant medical history. Each assessment was then led by the O-SP who based their clinical judgments on their online observations and/or on later review of the store and forward videos. The CSE followed a structured pro forma of 65 test items divided into four main sections including (1) general orientation and alertness, (2) oromotor and laryngeal function assessment, (3) performance during food and fluid trials, and (4) clinical decisions and recommendations.

2.4. Data Collection.
The study employed a mix methods design to examine patient outcomes, session statistics, and patient and clinician perceptions. Patient outcome data was collected from the simultaneous CSEs conducted by both the O-SP and FTF-SPs during the clinic sessions. For this study, data from only 3 key patient outcome parameters collected as part of the "Clinical Decisions and Recommendations" component of the CSE were examined: (a) decision regarding safety for oral/nonoral feeding (binary decision), (b) recommended safe fluid intake (4-level categorical data), and (c) recommended safe food intake (4-level categorical data). In addition, data regarding the patients need for review/ongoing

care was collated. For this study, this data was coded into 4 categories: review needed within 1 week; review within >1 week and <1 month; review in 3 months; or, patient can be discharged. Details of the levels of agreement for the full range of CSE items have been outlined elsewhere [3].

Session statistics were calculated from the session logs recorded by the videoconferencing system software. The system recorded the number of dropped connections/reconnections during any session. It also recorded the total time (in minutes) of the online session. The timing data related only to the duration of the online assessment and did not include time spent by the assistant preparing the room/patient or the time spent by the clinician reading the medical history or writing their report. Comments pertaining to any equipment failure or visual or auditory difficulties were collected through postsession reports completed by the O-SP.

Patient perceptions were explored using a questionnaire delivered both before and after the telerehabilitation session as per prior research [12]. This contained 14 items that examined perceptions regarding (1) level of comfort with telerehabilitation (3 questions), (2) audio and video quality (2 questions), and (3) general considerations regarding telerehabilitation consultation (9 questions) (detailed in Table 1). The questions in the pre- and postquestionnaire were matched to explore patient perceptions before and after the telerehabilitation session (e.g., before: "I *will have* no difficulty seeing the online speech pathologist"; after: "I *had* no difficulty seeing the online speech pathologist"). Responses were rated using a five-point scale (1: strongly disagree, 2: disagree, 3: unsure, 4: agree, 5: strongly agree).

Perceptions of the clinicians were explored through (a) a satisfaction questionnaire completed at the end of every session and (b) a single semistructured interview completed once at the end of testing the 100 patients. The satisfaction questionnaire has been published previously [2] and addressed (1) satisfactions with the system (4 questions), (2) the perceived level of patient-clinician rapport (1 question), (3) satisfaction with the level of service provided to the patient (1 question), and (4) suitability of a telerehabilitation assessment for the individual patient (2 questions) (detailed in Table 2). Satisfaction was rated on a five-point scale (1: strongly disagree, 3: unsure, 5: strongly agree). The semistructured clinician interview took approximately 15 minutes and involved reflecting on elements which helped make the clinic successful/unsuccessful.

2.5. Data Analysis. Levels of exact agreement between the O-SP and FTF-SP decisions for the three patient outcomes were calculated using percentages. A level of ≥80% exact agreement (for nominal/categorical data) was used to represent clinically acceptable levels of agreement, as per prior research [1–5, 13]. Session statistics were analysed descriptively. Patient perceptions before and after the session were collapsed into 3 groups (disagree/strongly disagree, unsure, and agree/strongly agree) and are reported descriptively. Comparison between proportion change over time was analysed using Chi-square or Fisher's exact test. Significance was set at $P < 0.05$. Results of the postsession clinician satisfaction questionnaires were compiled descriptively. The content of

the semistructured clinician interview was interpreted live by the interviewer who made notes during the interview. At the end of the interview, the interviewer summarized the key points and checked the accuracy of these with the interviewee.

3. Results

Analysis of patient outcomes revealed that 100% of sessions reached a clinical decision regarding patient intake status. Level of PEA between the O-SP and FTF-SP was 99% for the decision to place the patient oral or nonoral. For the 1 patient where the oral/nonoral decision was in disagreement, the FTF clinician had placed the patient completely on nonoral intake, while the teleclinician had essentially made the same decision, though they had allowed the person small sips of thickened fluids under speech pathology supervision in addition to nonoral supplementation. Level of agreement for safe fluid and food consistencies was 98% and 92%, respectively. For the 2 disagreements for fluid ratings and the 8 for food consistency ratings, these differed by no more than one fluid/diet level and no decision could be considered unsafe. Regarding the need for review/ongoing management, there was 88% exact agreement. Overall the O-SP recommended that 66 patients should be reviewed again within 1 week (to check safety on recommended diet or for ongoing reassessment), 27 in >1 week but <1 month, 1 in 3 months, and 6 were discharged. All incidences of disagreement were examined to explore any potential bias for either the O-SP or FTF-SP ratings. There was no clear pattern observed to support more conservative decision making or a particular pattern of error/disagreement occurring in either environment.

Session statistics revealed an average duration of 45 minutes (SD: 13, mode: 46, range 22–80). The first quartile of the cohort (i.e., the shortest times) ranged from 22 to 37 minutes and contained 80% normal or mildly dysphagic patients. The top 25% (i.e., longest session durations) ranged between 48 and 80 minutes and contained 68% moderate or severe patients. Disconnections were rare, occurring in only 10% of the sessions with the maximum number of disconnections in any session being 2. However, clinicians reported difficulties at times during sessions with periods of reduced audio (long delays) and/or visual quality (heavy pixilation) in 22% of the sessions. These audio and visual quality issues were identified as difficulties by clinicians; however, they did not prevent successful completion of the assessment. Only 6 assessments were cancelled outright and rescheduled due to equipment issues (camera frozen and not enabling zoom capabilities; system audio not functional), though trouble shooting and/or replacement equipment enabled subsequent patient assessments within the scheduled clinic to be completed.

Although all 100 patients were successfully assessed in the clinic, eighteen participants were cognitively unable to complete the patient questionnaires before or after the session. Examination of the questionnaire data from the other 82 revealed that greater than two-thirds agreed/strongly agreed with most questions before the session (Table 1). However,

TABLE 1: Pre- and postassessment patient questionnaire ($n = 82$).

Item	Preassessment			Postassessment			X^2 or fisher	P
	Strongly disagree/disagree n (%)	Unsure n (%)	Strongly agree/agree n (%)	Strongly disagree/disagree n (%)	Unsure n (%)	Strongly agree/agree n (%)		
(1) I will be (am#) comfortable to use telehealth if it is available in the hospital or healthcare facility nearest to my place of residence.	1 (1)	8 (10)	73 (89)	0 (0)	2 (2)	80 (98)	3.78	0.209
(2) I am (was) comfortable to undergo an assessment for my swallowing disorder via the internet.	3 (4)	3 (4)	76 (93)	0 (0)	1 (1)	81 (99)	0.08	1.000
(3) I will be (was) comfortable being online and would consider using the internet for the rehabilitation of my swallowing.	1 (1)	12 (15)	69 (84)	0 (0)	3 (4)	79 (96)	6.75	0.090
(4) I will have (I had) no difficulty in seeing the online speech pathologist.	26 (32)	26 (32)	30 (37)	15 (18)	1 (1)	66 (80)	11.38	**0.008**
(5) I will have (I had) no difficulty hearing the online speech pathologist.	23 (28)	27 (33)	32 (39)	19 (23)	3 (4)	60 (73)	3.00	0.601
(6) I would rate the online assessment as being equal to an assessment conducted traditionally in the face-to-face method.	4 (5)	31 (38)	47 (57)	3 (4)	11 (13)	68 (83)	11.66	0.030
(7) The instructions during the online assessment will be (were) clear and easy to follow.	1 (1)	26 (32)	55 (67)	2 (2)	3 (4)	77 (94)	7.13	0.075
(8) I will have (had) sufficient time to execute the instructions given during the assessment.	2 (2)	25 (30)	55 (67)	0 (0)	1 (1)	81 (99)	2.31	0.329
(9) I will have (had) opportunities to clarify any doubts during the online assessment.	0 (0)[a]	14 (17)	67 (88)	0 (0)	0 (0)	82 (100)	n/a[b]	n/a[b]
(10) Telehealth can replace a face-to-face assessment.	10 (12)	25 (30)	47 (57)	7 (9)	18 (22)	57 (70)	36.06	**<0.005**
(11) Telehealth will allow easy access to healthcare.	0 (0)	11 (13)	71 (87)	0 (0)	7 (9)	75 (91)	5.71	**0.047**
(12) Telehealth will save me travelling time and money.	2 (2)[a]	5 (6)	74 (91)	0 (0)	3 (4)	79 (96)	12.42	0.082
(13) Telehealth may benefit all patients alike.	1 (1)[a]	19 (23)	61 (75)	2 (2)	8 (10)	72 (88)	15.04	**0.003**
(14) I would prefer to have a traditional consultation with the speech pathologist despite possible costs and inconveniences.	19 (23)[a]	30 (37)	32 (40)	33 (40)	19 (23)	30 (37)	29.29	**<0.005**

Note: #: italics and brackets indicate pre-/postwording changes between the pre- and postassessment conditions. [a] $n = 81$; [b] not enough variation in the data to complete statistical analysis. Bold indicates significance at $P < 0.05$.

TABLE 2: Clinician perceptions of the telehealth session ($n = 100$).

	Strongly disagree (%)	Disagree (%)	Unsure (%)	Agree (%)	Strongly agree (%)
I was satisfied with the level of service the computer system allowed me to provide my clients	0	7	1	57	35
I am happy with the level of client-clinician rapport generated during this session	0	4	4	42	50
I found the computer and computer system easy to use during the session	0	4	1	41	54
The audio quality of the system was appropriate for the session	1	14	3	44	38
The visual quality of the system was appropriate for the assessments performed	0	12	5	65	18
I feel that I was able to satisfactorily and competently assess the client to the best of my abilities using the system	1	9	3	46	41
I feel that the telerehabilitation system would be a more efficient means of service delivery for this patient	0	12	12	23	53
I feel the telerehabilitation system would be a useful service delivery tool for patients with swallowing disorders	0	0	2	21	77

there were some patients who were unsure or disagreed with the questions relating to being able to see and hear the online clinician, if they believed instructions would be clear, if they would have sufficient time to execute tasks, or if the online assessment would be equal to or able to replace face to face sessions. There were also over 77% of patients who indicated that they were either unsure or agreed that they would prefer a traditional assessment in their presession questionnaire.

Patient perceptions immediately following the telerehabilitation session, however, revealed many of these negative positions had changed significantly (Table 1). A significant shift from 37 to 80% of patients agreed they had no difficulty seeing the online clinician. A significant change from 57% to 83% felt the online assessment was equal to a FTF assessment after the session. Significantly more patients felt that telerehabilitation could replace a FTF session, allowing easy access to healthcare, and could benefit all patients. There was also a change regarding preference for a traditional assessment with significantly more patients disagreeing they would prefer a traditional assessment. However, 37% continued to agree that they would prefer a traditional assessment (Table 1). Although responses to other questions were not significantly different from the presession perceptions, patterns of nonsignificant shifts towards agreeing with all statements were noted.

The postsession questionnaires completed by the clinicians revealed that over 90% who agreed/strongly agreed were happy with the service they could provide via the system, their level of rapport with patients, the ease of use of the system, their ability to assess the patient, and the usefulness of telerehabilitation as a service delivery option (Table 2). In 18% of sessions the clinicians did not agree that the audio quality was appropriate and in 17% of sessions they felt the video image was not adequate. For 24% of sessions, clinicians either were unsure (12%) or disagreed (12%) that telerehabilitation

would be a more efficient means of service delivery for that patient. Where they disagreed, these were sessions with patients with severely reduced vocal volume (making detecting clinical signs of aspiration difficult) and those with an inability to follow commands and instructions, excess body movements, significant hearing or vision impairment, fatigue, distress/agitation, and/or overall severe medical state.

The clinician interview allowed reflection on issues that had been problematic and factors which facilitated optimal functioning of the clinic. These fell into the 3 categories: patient considerations, general organisational issues, and staff roles. "Patient considerations" included multifactorial issues relating to the patients health and suitability for the clinic. Referrals need to be screened for suitability (i.e. to exclude patients with very low levels of alertness, or those with highly unstable medical states) prior to the clinic. Clinicians also noted the importance of ensuring that there are clear patient details and case history information provided to allow the online clinician and assistant to prepare for the session and to plan how to manage any patient factors (hearing impairment, cognitive deficits) which could raise challenges during the online assessment.

"General organisation" issues raised the importance of allowing 1 hour for each patient appointment to accommodate longer/more complex assessments and potential technology/connection issues. Preclinic setup (testing equipment, etc.) was seen as essential to the clinic running smoothly, as were advance bookings for porterage to transport inpatients to and from the telehealth room on time. Good communication between the booking site (patient end) and the hub site (O-SP end) to confirm appointments and any changes was critical. Clear protocols for referrals, appointments and session reporting at both the patient end and online clinician site needed to be established. Attendance at the clinic was also maximised by ensuring the appointment and patient status/suitability was re-confirmed the morning prior to the assessment clinic.

Clinicians noted that staff skills assisted the functioning of the clinic. The importance of having an assistant with good patient skills and manual handling skills was necessary for establishing rapport with the patient and repositioning during the session. They also commented that as they became more experienced, their ability to conduct the online session more efficiently improved. Convenient access to technical staff for equipment issues and ensuring that the staff involved in the clinic are trained in equipment operation and basic trouble shooting were also seen as important.

4. Discussion

The mixed methodology employed by the current study enabled examination of both the feasibility and consumer acceptance of a dysphagia telerehabilitation clinical service. Overall the data revealed a viable clinical service model which had good patient outcomes and minimal technical issues. Patient perceptions and clinician perceptions were also positive. For those clinicians who provide dysphagia services across multiple locations, or outreach services to rural locations, the current data supports the potential feasibility of using a telerehabilitation clinic model to enhance patient access to services.

Equipment and technical problems were minimal. The clinic adhered to published technical recommendations for telerehabilitation [11] and staff stressed that developing good technical trouble shooting skills and having access to technical staff were integral to the clinic's success. Only 6 individual assessment sessions needed to be cancelled and rescheduled due to equipment malfunction/technical issues. However, these technical issues were quickly rectified allowing continuation of the clinic and subsequent assessment sessions. Despite some reduced audio and/or visual quality at times during 22% of sessions, all assessments which were commenced were completed and a clinical decision regarding patient safety for oral intake was determined. It was not unexpected that some visual and auditory quality issues were experienced during sessions, as testing took place at intentionally controlled low bandwidths used to ensure the clinic's feasibility at the absolute minimum bandwidth available within the health network. Future service functionality has capacity to occur at much higher bandwidths. Hence, this will reduce the instances of audio delays and image pixillation experienced at low bandwidths.

Despite the presence of some slight reductions in visual or auditory quality, overall the quality of the clinical decisions between the O-SP and FTF-SP was found to be highly comparable, falling well above the 80% agreement criteria set in this study. This result is consistent with previous research [1–3] and supports the validity of clinical decisions made within the online environment. Where discrepancies occurred between the O-SP and FTF-SP, there was also no clear pattern observed to suggest that the online clinician made more conservative judgments or any particular pattern of errors in decision making. As such, the differences observed between the two raters appear to be best explained by simply the natural variability which exists between clinical decisions made by two professionals.

Session durations, however, were slightly longer than a traditional FTF assessment. On average, the assessment took three quarters of an hour, though this was shorter for less complex patients (who completed tasks more quickly and required fewer food/fluid trials). Considering the time needed to change/adjust the equipment during the session, the need for interaction between the online clinician and assistant, occasional technical difficulties, and the need to orientate patients to the online session, this slightly increased session duration is to be expected. It is also not excessively beyond the 20–30 minutes typically taken, in our clinical experience, to complete a thorough FTF CSE session. The 4-hour clinic model was also easily incorporated within the departments' speech pathology service. Following the format of other specialist speech pathology clinics (e.g., an instrumental dysphagia assessment clinic), having a routine, weekly clinic, helped with the organization of staff, equipment, rooms, and referrals.

Patient perceptions of the clinical service were positive and 98% felt comfortable receiving services via telerehabilitation to assess their swallowing disorder. Although prior to the session there was a proportion of patients who were unsure about some aspects of the service (e.g., visual or auditory quality), significantly less were concerned about these issues after the session. Indeed, as has been observed in other clinical groups [12, 14, 15], across all questions there was a shift toward even greater acceptance of the telerehabilitation modality after just one session. However, it was noted that whilst 99% felt comfortable with their assessment, 37% indicated they would prefer a traditional consultation. A number of studies have found similar results, with a small proportion of patients having a preference for traditional clinical models [16–18]. Although reasons for this decision were not examined, there is growing interest in exploring the demographics of users of various types of teleservices [19], and this is an area of future research.

Clinicians were positive about the clinic and felt satisfied with the levels of service and patient rapport established in over 90% of sessions. Whilst certain patient characteristics were noted which enhanced the complexity of assessing a patient in the online environment, clinical decisions were achieved for all patients and the quality of decision making remained comparable to the FTF clinician. This finding is consistent with previous studies which have noted that assessing patients of greater severity may be more complex, but is not impossible to achieve via telerehabilitation [3, 13]. Key factors that clinicians felt contributed to the success of the sessions and the clinic overall included the importance of appropriate referrals, sufficient clinical notes about each patient to enable adequate preparation (particularly for more complex patients), having a team of trained staff, and clear procedures.

5. Conclusion

The current trial provided valuable insight into the service issues associated with implementing a dysphagia assessment clinic via telerehabilitation. Overall the clinic was found to run with acceptable efficiency, with minimal technical difficulty, and with comparable primary patient outcomes to FTF assessment. Patient satisfaction was high and clinicians were satisfied with the service in over 90% of the assessments conducted. It is acknowledged, however, that this was a short-term trial clinic and used a simulated service model. Future studies of actual remote clinical implementation will enable exploration of additional factors such as changes to waiting time for services, impact on clinician and/or patient travel time, and evaluation of the economic cost-benefits of service models within various different clinical contexts (e.g., outpatient services, residential aged care services) [20].

Acknowledgments

The authors acknowledge the National Health and Medical Research Council (NHMRC) grant funding (APP1002472) which supported this research. They also thank the staff of the Speech Pathology Department of the Royal Brisbane and Women's Hospital for their role in the recruitment of participants for this study and the participants of this study for their time, patience, and cooperation. Additional thanks are due to Dr. Monique Waite and Laurelie Wall who assisted in paper preparation. This research was conducted at the Speech Pathology Department of The Royal Brisbane and Women's Hospital, Brisbane, Australia, and The University of Queensland, Brisbane, Australia.

References

[1] S. Sharma, E. C. Ward, C. Burns, D. Theodoros, and T. Russell, "Assessing swallowing disorders online: a pilot telerehabilitation study," *Telemedicine Journal and e-Health*, vol. 17, no. 9, pp. 688–695, 2011.

[2] E. C. Ward, S. Sharma, C. Burns, D. Theodoros, and T. Russell, "Validity of conducting clinical dysphagia assessments with patients with normal to mild cognitive impairments via Telerehabilitation," *Dysphagia*, vol. 27, pp. 460–472, 2012.

[3] E. C. Ward, C. L. Burns, D. G. Theodoros, and T. Russell, "Impact of dysphagia severity on clinical decision making via telerehabilitation," *Telemedicine Journal and e-Health*. In press.

[4] E. C. Ward, J. Crombie, M. Trickey, A. Hill, D. Theodoros, and T. Russell, "Assessment of communication and swallowing post-laryngectomy: a telerehabilitation trial," *Journal of Telemedicine and Telecare*, vol. 15, no. 5, pp. 232–237, 2009.

[5] L. Ward, J. White, T. Russell et al., "Assessment of communication and swallowing function post laryngectomy: a telerehabilitation trial," *Journal of Telemedicine and Telecare*, vol. 13, no. 3, supplement 3, pp. 88–91, 2007.

[6] A. L. Perlman and W. Witthawaskul, "Real-time remote telefluoroscopic assessment of patients with dysphagia," *Dysphagia*, vol. 17, no. 2, pp. 162–167, 2002.

[7] G. A. Malandraki, G. McCullough, X. He, E. McWeeny, and A. L. Perlman, "Teledynamic evaluation of oropharyngeal swallowing," *Journal of Speech, Language, and Hearing Research*, vol. 54, no. 6, pp. 1497–1505, 2011.

[8] G. A. Malandraki, V. Markaki, V. C. Georgopoulous, J. L. Bauer, I. Kalogeropoulos, and S. Nanas, "An international pilot study of asynchronous teleconsultation for oropharyngeal dysphagia," *Journal of Telemedicine and Telecare*, vol. 19, pp. 75–79, 2013.

[9] E. C. Ward, S. Sharma, C. Burns, D. G. Theodoros, and T. Russell, "Managing patient factors in the assessment of swallowing via telerehabilitation," *Internation Journal of Telemedicine and Applications*, vol. 2012, Article ID 132719, 6 pages, 2012.

[10] K. H. O'Neil, M. Purdy, J. Falk, and L. Gallo, "The dysphagia outcome and severity scale," *Dysphagia*, vol. 14, no. 3, pp. 139–145, 1999.

[11] D. M. Brennan, L. Tindall, D. Theodoros et al., "A blueprint for telerehabilitation guidelines—October 2010," *Telemedicine Journal and e-Health*, vol. 17, no. 8, pp. 662–665, 2011.

[12] S. Sharma, E. C. Ward, C. Burns, D. G. Theodoros, and T. Russell, "Assessing dysphagia via telerehabilitation: patient perceptions and satisfaction," *International Journal of Speech Language Pathology*, vol. 15, pp. 176–183, 2013.

[13] A. J. Hill, D. G. Theodoros, T. G. Russell, E. C. Ward, and R. Wootton, "The effects of aphasia severity on the ability to assess language disorders via telerehabilitation," *Aphasiology*, vol. 23, no. 5, pp. 627–642, 2009.

[14] K. Cranen, R. H. I. Veld, M. Ijzerman, and M. Vollenbroek-Hutten, "Change of patients' perceptions of telemedicine after brief use," *Telemedicine Journal and E-Health*, vol. 17, no. 7, pp. 530–535, 2011.

[15] S. M. Finkelstein, S. M. Speedie, G. Demiris, M. Veen, J. M. Lundgren, and S. Potthoff, "Telehomecare: quality, perception, satisfaction," *Telemedicine and e-Health*, vol. 10, no. 2, pp. 122–128, 2004.

[16] A. Allen and J. Hayes, "Patient satisfaction with teleoncology: a pilot study," *Telemedicine Journal*, vol. 1, no. 1, pp. 41–46, 1995.

[17] J. L. Huston and D. C. Burton, "Patient satisfaction with multi-specialty interactive teleconsultations," *Journal of Telemedicine and Telecare*, vol. 3, no. 4, pp. 205–208, 1997.

[18] M. H. Lowitt, I. Z. Kessler, C. L. Kauffman, F. J. Hooper, E. Siegel, and J. W. Burnett, "Teledermatology and in-person examinations: a comparison of patient and physician perceptions and diagnostic agreement," *Archives of Dermatology*, vol. 134, no. 4, pp. 471–476, 1998.

[19] A. Mehrotra, S. Paone, G. D. Martich, S. M. Albert, and G. J. Shevchik, "Characteristics of patients who seek care via eVisits instead of office visits," *Telemedicine Journal and e-Health*, vol. 19, no. 7, pp. 1–5, 2013.

[20] C. L. Burns, E. C. Ward, A. J. Hill et al., "A pilot trial of a speech pathology telehealth service for head and neck cancer patients," *Journal of Telemedicine and Telecare*, vol. 18, pp. 443–446, 2012.

8

Usability Study of a Wireless Monitoring System among Alzheimer's Disease Elderly Population

Stefano Abbate,[1] Marco Avvenuti,[2] and Janet Light[3]

[1] Institute of Informatics and Telematics, National Research Council, Via G. Moruzzi 1, 56124 Pisa, Italy
[2] Department of Information Engineering, University of Pisa, L. Lazzarino 1, 56122 Pisa, Italy
[3] Department of Computer Science & Applied Statistics, University of New Brunswick, Saint John, NB, Canada E2L 4L5

Correspondence should be addressed to Stefano Abbate; stefano.abbate@iit.cnr.it

Academic Editor: Fei Hu

Healthcare technologies are slowly entering into our daily lives, replacing old devices and techniques with newer intelligent ones. Although they are meant to help people, the reaction and willingness to use such new devices by the people can be unexpected, especially among the elderly. We conducted a usability study of a fall monitoring system in a long-term nursing home. The subjects were the elderly with advanced Alzheimer's disease. The study presented here highlights some of the challenges faced in the use of wearable devices and the lessons learned. The results gave us useful insights, leading to ergonomics and aesthetics modifications to our wearable systems that significantly improved their usability and acceptance. New evaluating metrics were designed for the performance evaluation of usability and acceptability.

1. Introduction

Healthcare technology using wireless sensors has reached a high level of maturity and reliability and hence these devices are now being deployed in homes/nursing homes for use in managing people's health. To take full advantage of the penetration of these pervasive systems in people's well-being and reap their full benefits, the technologies must be minimally invasive and must be accepted by users willingly.

A necessary condition for acceptance is the awareness of benefits to the user population in using the system. Since young adults are well acquainted with modern sensor devices, they willingly accept the introduction of new technologies in their care process. In contrast, among the elderly, who are the main beneficiary population of these monitoring devices, there is still reluctance on their part to use them. Even though an increasing number of the elderly are aware of the advantages of a pervasive health monitoring system, they rarely understand how it works.

With the increase in Alzheimer's disease (AD) among the elderly population, there is a crucial need for technological support in their care process. Since there is no cure yet to reverse the cognitive decline among these individuals, technology could contribute to safely perform their normal living activities.

Unfortunately, people affected by AD have difficulties in understanding their health conditions, and the use of a device or systems that could help in their day-to-day activities. Some of them have a different perception of objects and are prone to forget using them or be adamant in not using them. In our initial study we found that even the simplest interactive devices such as wristband buttons or call buttons to alert a caregiver in an emergency situation are unlikely to be used by them.

Despite the technological maturity of healthcare devices and networking, little effort has been done to assess their usability and acceptability before deployments in homes and nursing homes. Health monitoring platforms developed so far have mainly focused on the functionalities using specific sets of sensors, vendor specific software, and protocols, for which usability issues have not been sufficiently addressed.

We addressed this gap by undertaking this exploratory study on how to increase the usability and acceptability of our wearable monitoring system to a small group of elderly affected by AD. In the study, we used the wireless accelerometer and electroencephalograph (EEG) logger integrated in our minimally invasive monitoring sensor (MIMS) system [1], with the aim of detecting possible falls and their preconditions. The wireless monitoring system used did not require any interaction with the subjects. However, the living environment should include a network infrastructure with wired alert systems to connect to central nurse care stations and/or wireless networks to hand-held devices carried by the nurses.

We defined ad hoc usability and acceptability parameters and evaluated them during a month long field test with long-term nursing home residents. The results gave us some important insights, leading to ergonomics and aesthetics modifications to our system that significantly improved its usability and acceptance.

2. Related Work

A number of systems engaged in health monitoring are surveyed here to compare our approach to those of others. Though every system studied here has been in deployment for a long period of time, it was disappointing to observe that none of them reported about user's acceptability of the system. Only technology descriptions were made public about these systems.

For example, Cao et al. survey of enabling technologies for wireless body area networks [2] discussed the network characteristics, such as the type of wireless connection (Bluetooth, ultrawideband, ZigBee) and path loss of the signal sent by body sensors according to their placement on the body and to the radio frequency used. Performance evaluation and their usability study results are missing.

A wearable monitoring system called SATIRE [3] collects the motion and location information of a subject. SATIRE requires sensors inserted in the garment worn by the user without the need of user's interaction. The sensors collect and store data locally. Periodically, the data is uploaded to a base station for further analysis and archive. The paper presents the design which includes a layered architecture (for both the base station and the sensors). Real-world testing and adaptability study of this system are not known.

The MIThril LiveNet system [4] is another distributed mobile system for real-time monitoring and analysis of the health status of an individual. The MIThril architecture offers many features to perform distributed sensing, classification in real-time, and context aware applications. It makes use of a PDA which should be worn by the patient at all times: body worn sensors send data through a network infrastructure for exchange of information and a machine learning infrastructure is used for classification of gathered data. Again, the usability and adaptability results are not reported.

Finally, the experience gained by the authors in developing fall monitoring systems presented in [5, 6] definitely proved that a usability study is important to provide the required metrics to evaluate the performance of a health monitoring system in real-world applications, especially with the elderly population.

3. Materials and Methods

The equipment we used for the usability study was based on the MIMS system described in [1]. We developed MIMS with the aim of providing a flexible and scalable platform for building a comprehensive and customizable health monitoring system, which guarantees interoperability among different sensor systems. MIMS can be easily integrated with any wireless communication system already in place and with any existing networked alert system. Figure 1 shows the complete monitoring system, consisting of four sensing systems.

System 1 is a fall detector. It consists of a wireless sensor node (based, in our case, on the Shimmer 2R platform [7]) able to sense human movements using an embedded accelerometer. The microcontroller (MSP430 family) can perform on-chip analysis and communicate with a base station using a Bluetooth module or IEEE 802.15.4 radio, as shown in Figure 2. Being battery powered, small, and lightweight, the device can be conveniently worn near the waist. The device runs a simple yet very reliable algorithm for fall detection described in [6]. In a nutshell, every time the acceleration reaches a given threshold, samples belonging to a fixed time window around the event are sent to the base station, which in turn analyzes the pattern of accelerations and decides whether the event was due to an activity of daily living (i.e., a false alarm) or to a real fall. In the case of a real fall, the system informs the caregiver through the alert system.

System 2 consists of a wireless electrophysiology sensor (based, in our case, on the Enobio platform [8]) which is able to capture the brain activity of a person in real time. Four digital electrodes are attached to the Enobio communication module and placed in the Enobio headband. Data from such electrodes/channels are wirelessly transferred to a base station using the IEEE 802.15.4 low power radio standard. The base station is represented by the Enobio USB receiver connected to a PC. Two wired ear clip electrodes (potential ground and potential ground feedback) act as references for sensed signals. Enobio (see Figure 3) is worn like a hat and can record not only brain activity but also heart activity through an electrocardiogram (ECG) and eye movements through an electrooculogram (EOG). The Enobio software is a Java application that allows (i) wireless communication between the Enobio and PC; (ii) data recording; (iii) data display; (iv) forwarding of data to other clients. Data is coded as simple ASCII file of tab delimited columns and can also be exported to the very common scientific format EDF (European Data Format). We used System 2 to analyze EEG potentials during the different stages of sleep, with the aim of studying brain signal patterns preceding a fall.

System 3 is composed of ambient sensors such as pressure pads, which are placed in the care environment to monitor lying on a bed or sitting on a chair, and volumetric motion detectors, which cover an area of 10.7 × 9.1 meters and are used to detect motion and activities such as entering/leaving a room. Door sensors are placed on the top of doors, windows, and drawers to detect when they are opened or closed; the toilet mat sensor detects both presence on or near the toilet to monitor bathroom activity and potential safety issues such as falls near to the toilet; emergency buttons can be placed

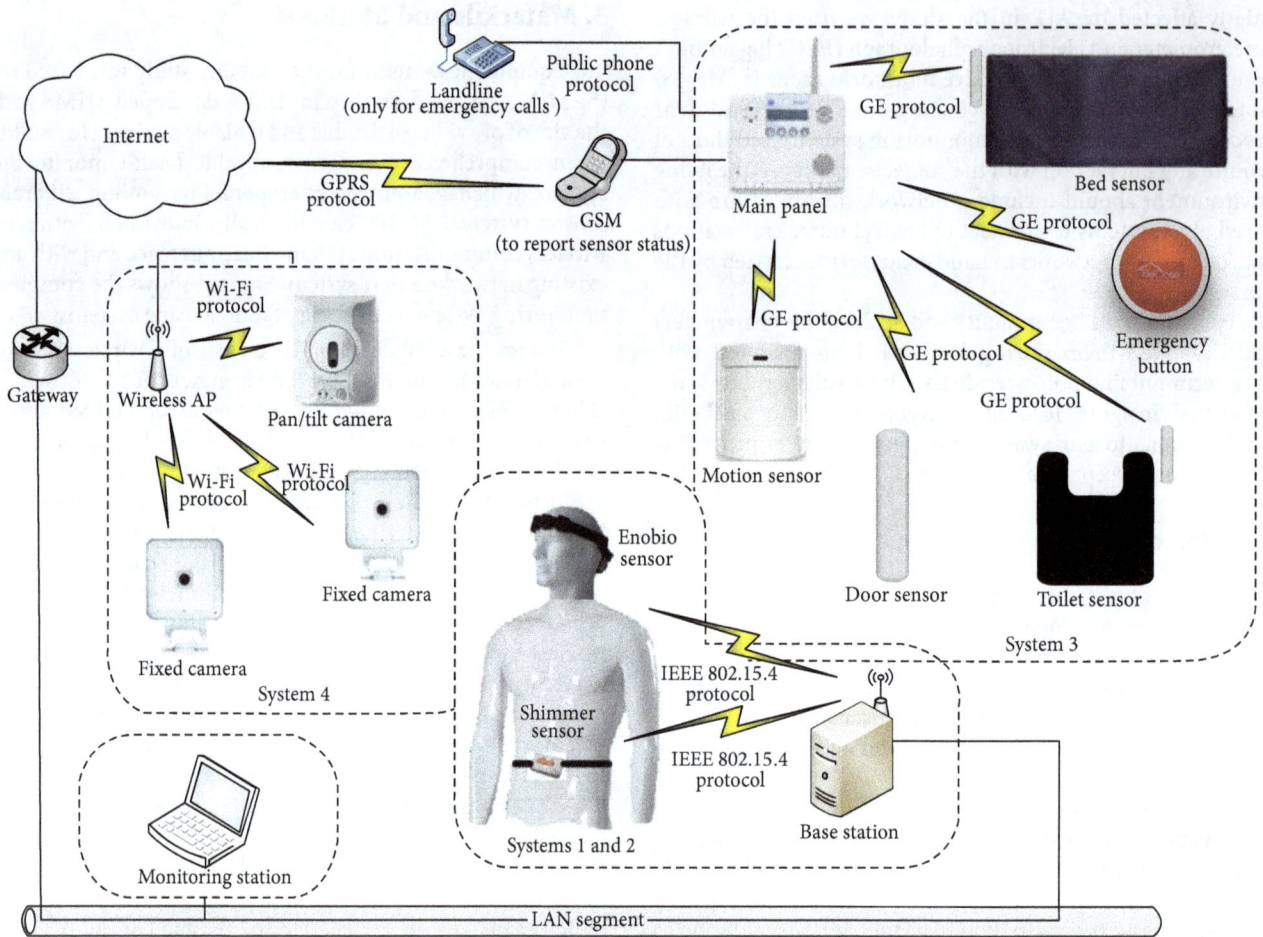

FIGURE 1: System overview.

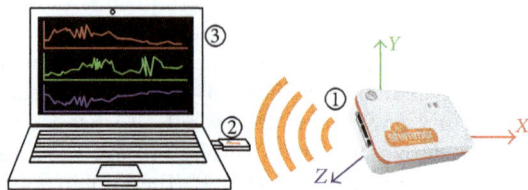

FIGURE 2: System 1—fall detector. (1) Shimmer 2R with accelerometer. (2) 802.15.4 receiver. (3) Base station.

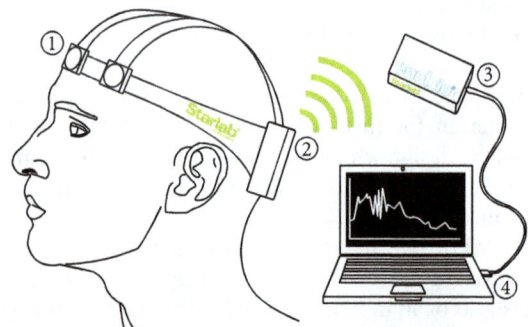

FIGURE 3: System 2—EEG analyzer. (1) Electrodes. (2) Battery pack/transmitter. (3) 802.15.4 receiver. (4) Base station.

where accidents are likely to happen; they are 7.6 centimeters in diameter; when pressed, they send an alert to the caregiver or to an emergency response service. The main panel acts as a base station and collects data from sensors exploiting the radio channel and a proprietary protocol (General Electric); the base station has battery backup and is equipped by a GSM transceiver and an interface to the landline.

System 4 is a camera-based monitoring system using the internet to continuously stream the video recording human activity (visual motion detection) over a selective region and over a specified observation period (e.g., at nighttime). Two types of cameras have been used: a fixed wireless camera (ADCV510) and a pan/tilt camera (ADC-V610PT). They both

have the live resolution options 640 × 480, 320 × 240, and 176 × 144, whereas the recording resolution options are 640 × 480 and 320 × 240; the recording compression is based on MPEG-4. The video motion detection can be configured with three different windows having adjustable sensitivity and thresholds. The streaming of video to the internet relies on a wireless Wi-Fi router and standard encryption (WEP, WPA, or WPA2); cameras can also be connected using a standard Ethernet connection. They are designed to work with the *Alarm.com* hosted video service which provides a surveillance solution. High-quality live and recorded videos are available to customers through web browsers or via mobile apps. Users can set and recall "preset" views or manually pan and tilt the camera remotely.

In the case of resource constraints for sensing, processing, storing, and communicating, some computational operations are delegated to the Virtual Hub, which is a base station running on a smart phone environment. The Virtual Hub receives data from the subsystems and is connected to the local healthcare information system through a friendly graphical user interface. A thorough description of the MIMS platform can be found in [1].

System 1 and System 2 are examples of active monitoring sensor system (AMSS). As they are based on wearable devices, they offer advantages in terms of continuous monitoring, cost, and efficiency. However, their acceptability strongly depends on the level of usability. System 3 and System 4, instead, were not considered in this study as they are environmental systems, whose major concerns are intrusion and privacy rather than usability.

3.1. Measuring Usability and Acceptability. According to the human engineering principles [9], the design of a system must follow the users' needs, fear, mental models, self-learning ability, social behavior, lifestyle, and fashion tastes. In fact, an accurate knowledge of end users can be achieved only by observing them closely.

In the case of monitoring people with AD/dementia living in a home or a nursing home, providing suitable care to them requires 24 × 7 continuous monitoring of their everyday activities [10]. Some of their regular daily activities are walking in a corridor, watching television, and, with the help of caregivers, having breakfast, lunch, dinner, and medication; some subjects have a small nap in the afternoon. They are prone to disorientation and wandering at any time of the day or night, and statistics show that they are more prone to falls compared to general elderly population [11]. To compensate psychomotor deficiencies, variant medical equipment is used such as canes, crutches, and wheelchairs. However, not all the subjects are able to understand (or remember) that they need to use them during their walking activity to prevent fall.

In this context, we define usability as the level at which a device can assist a user without interfering with his/her normal activities of daily living. Acceptability is defined as the constraints which guide the designer to realize factors that satisfy one's need and therefore people's willingness to use. The following are the evaluation criteria we developed to measure usability and acceptability:

(1) willingness to use (WTU),

(2) easiness to learn (ETL),

(3) time to accept (TTA),

(4) willingness to keep (WTK),

(5) number of errors (NOE) due to incorrect interactions,

TABLE 1: Usability and acceptability parameters.

Metrics	Levels		
WTU	Low	Medium	High
ETL	Low	Medium	High
TTA	Short	Average	Long
WTK	Low	Medium	High
NOE	None	Few	Many
LOS	Low	Indifferent	High
IWA	None	Low	High

(6) level of satisfaction (LOS),

(7) interference with activities of daily living (IWA).

The ranking of evaluation criteria is shown in Table 1.

Results of a Nielsen's research [12] have shown that a usability study can be suitably performed with up to 5 subjects, because the behavior of users does not change significantly as their number increases. This matches the obvious fact that performing small tests does not require huge investments for devices, and it makes the test feasible when, as in our case, it is done on a very critical population such as the elderly affected by AD. Of course, this does not hold for statistical studies, but here we are interested in only qualitative results, as the goal is to gain insights for improving the design of wearable devices based on feedback received by users to increase the usability and adaptability.

Based on these observations, we tried to get the maximum benefit-cost ratio by delivering the usability and acceptability test to four subjects affected by AD with advanced age. The four subjects involved in the test were from 75 to 92 years old. All of them were at staggering stages of dementia progression and associated abnormal behaviors, thus limiting the usability study. In particular, AD subjects were at levels 5/6 of Reisberg stage and they resulted below a score of 12 out of 30 (severe cognitive impairment) of the MMSE (Folstein test). All the patients were in long-term care.

It should be mentioned here that, for 24 × 7 monitoring of AD individuals, a number of trials had to be conducted before a full data collection is accomplished, with the result that some of these tests could not be completed in consecutive days. Some contributing factors to the difficulty in monitoring were age, disease, and associated behavior. Nevertheless, the observations were invaluable.

4. Results and Discussion

Table 2 summarizes the results of the study using Systems 1 and 2 of the MIMS platform. Experiences and reactions of the subjects in adapting to the wearable devices and to the monitoring sessions are reported in terms of the usability and acceptability criteria described above, together with observed reactions from the subjects.

In the overall, the study showed that with a few modifications to the way devices are placed, colored, or integrated with clothing, and after some convincing story about the importance of wearing the devices, AD individuals eventually wore and benefited from the monitoring technologies. Since

TABLE 2: Behavior of the subjects towards new monitoring systems.

System 1	Subject 1	Subject 2	Subject 3	Subject 4
Day 1	WTU: low ETL: high TTA: n/a WTK: low NOE: low LOS: low IWA: none Did not want to wear it. After 30 minutes the subject forgot about it and was happy to remove it at the end of day.	WTU: n/a ETL: low TTA: short WTK: high NOE: many LOS: high IWA: none No resistance. Then the patient removed it and played with it. At the end, he did not want to give it back.	WTU: n/a ETL: high TTA: short WTK: medium NOE: none LOS: indifferent IWA: none No resistance.	WTU: high ETL: high TTA: short WTK: high NOE: none LOS: indifferent IWA: none No resistance. The patient was already using a pouch around the waist.
Day 2	WTU: medium WTK: medium NOE: low LOS: indifferent Light resistance to wear it initially.	WTU: high NOE: few Happy to wear it.	LOS: none Totally indifferent.	WTK: medium Indifferent.
Day 3	WTU: high TTA: long WTK: high NOE: none Happy to wear it. The family members convinced the subject to wear it saying it was meant for stomach pain relief.	NOE: none LOS: indifferent Indifferent.		

System 2	Subject 1	Subject 2	Subject 3
Night 1	WTU: high ETL: low TTA: n/a WTK: low NOE: few LOS: low IWA: high No resistance at the beginning (the patient loves hats). The patient removed it after some time.	WTU: medium ETL: low TTA: n/a WTK: low NOE: high LOS: low IWA: none The patient kept for some minutes then removed it. After three times the patient did not want to wear it anymore.	WTU: low ETL: high TTA: short WTK: medium NOE: none LOS: low IWA: low No resistance but the patient did not like it.
Night 2	NOE: many IWA: low The subject wore it but moved it many times.	WTU: low WTK: low NOE: high Removed it many times during night.	WTU: medium WTK: medium LOS: medium No resistance.
Night 3	ETL: medium TTA: average WTK: medium NOE: none LOS: indifferent The subject was willing to wear it and did not move at all during night.	TTA: average WTK: medium NOE: none LOS: indifferent The subject was monitored from bedside all night to make sure she wore it.	

the Shimmer sensor has to be placed on the waist, System 1 achieved higher usability and acceptance than System 2. From the study, we found that integrating the sensor with clothing, so that it could be considered as an everyday accessory, made it better accepted. In doing so, the device must be prevented from choking the individual, and the difference in dress code between women and men must be considered. Since the device is sensitive to movements, careful wearing practices must be observed while placing/removing the device, and touching, meddling, or breaking the device should be prevented during specific activities such as lying on a bed (during the afternoon nap) or sitting on a chair.

Therefore, we adopted the following two solutions.

(1) The device was integrated onto a belt buckle (see Figure 4(a)). A leather style gave the buckle a retro aesthetic that made it suitable for both men and women.

(2) The device was attached to a Velcro stripe belt. Two small stripes were crossed to hold the device firm and properly placed on the waist (Figure 4(b)). For women, the device was hidden under the shirt/vest.

A significant effort was necessary to improve the usability of System 2, as the Enobio sensor must be worn like a hat during night sleep. The main problem arose from the presence of a bulky battery pack and transmitter on the user's nape, and this initially made it almost impossible to carry out sleep tests. During the study, we repeatedly modified the device in order to improve its acceptability (measured by WTU) and to make it as least intrusive as possible in order to avoid the user feeling embarrassed while wearing it (measured by WTK).

To improve the ergonomics of the Enobio sensor, we moved the battery/transmitter from the back of head/neck to the top of the head on a belt. For acceptability, we observed that the elderly enjoy wearing caps in the night to keep them warm; so we worked on the aesthetic side by embedding the sensor in a bonnet style cap with a light texture to prevent sweating (see Figure 5). However, it happened that some users took the hat off before getting into a deep sleep. This problem was partially solved by asking them to wear the hat without the sensing device during daytime. In this way, they got acquainted with wearing the hat and no longer noticed the sensing device was embedded in the hat during the sleep time.

An important factor to be considered here is the color of the device's enclosure. Colors have different impacts and meanings in one's space or environment. Bright colors or color combinations can help visually impaired people in understanding the surroundings. Warm colors such as orange red, pink, yellow, brown, and their shades are favorable for identifying objects. Cool colors such as blue, green, purple, and their shades are useful to give an impression of coolness, discretion, and serenity. The study gave us evidence that when a device comes in one's favorite colors, it is easier to make it acceptable, as it happened with subject 1 to whom we provided the Enobio with a pink cap.

5. Conclusions

Technologies applied to healthcare are meant to improve the wellness among people. However, not everyone easily accepts such technologies as designed by engineers. The usability study showed that the design and development of a monitoring device must consider its target users' preferences before it can be broadly deployed. Nontechnical factors depending on both the users and the environment must be considered for quick adaptability and reap the benefit to improved care.

The wireless sensor devices developed within our fall monitoring project were tested to assess their usability among AD elderly in a long-term care home. This rare opportunity gave us many insights leading to positive changes in our system in terms of ergonomics and aesthetics, as well as some modifications to our system architecture. Though the sample size was small due to the complexity in conducting the tests and the difficulty to manage AD subjects for test during day and night, we were able to achieve a qualitative usability assessment.

Patient's unawareness of the system's benefits is a major concern. For example, the Enobio EEG wearable sensor was formerly tested with healthy subjects informed of the sleep study. Even though they reported a slight discomfort, they were always conscious of wearing the hat and often restricted their movements while being in the bed. During the study, our patients showed different reactions. They did not understand about the sleep tests performed. Some of them thought that the hat was to keep them warm. While someone did not move at all in the bed, assuming a supine position for the entire night, others kept removing the hat. As a result, their sleep was interrupted by the testing, as the hat had to be put back to the correct position several times.

The study suggests that ergonomic and aesthetic modifications are necessary to improve the level of usability and acceptability, especially in an elderly user population. Analysis of the users' dress code was fundamental to figure out a comfortable and easily wearable solution. Typically, the elderly are attached to a specific aesthetic dress code, characteristic of their likes/dislikes. They prefer simple, loose, and comfortable dress and therefore the focus should be on a retro style. Unfortunately, such loose dresses make it difficult to put wearable devices close to the body in order to monitor accurately. At the same time, care must be taken such that these devices should not cause itching, rashes, or skin diseases if worn too tight.

From a manufacturing point of view, the devices worn by a patient must be robust and waterproof to avoid accidental damages (e.g., the sensor can fall to a sink full of water, or it can be thrown away or tampered). The device should also provide a switch or a special combination of buttons in order to be activated and deactivated by the nurse before placing it. A battery indicator is another element that would help nurses to identify if the device needs to be charged. The caregivers interface is fundamental to understand how to assign each sensing node to a person, to check the history and general status. In particular, the sensing devices should periodically send a message to signal that they are working correctly and,

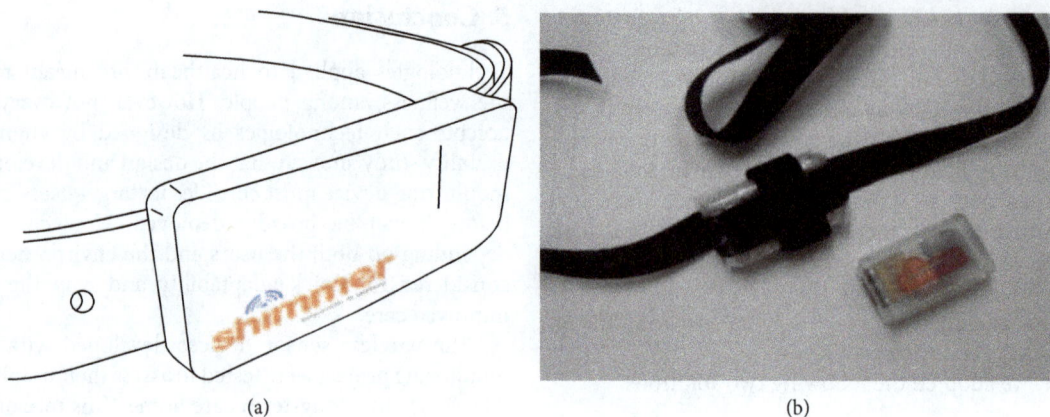

(a)   (b)

FIGURE 4: Shimmer integrated into a belt buckle (a). Shimmer attached to a Velcro stripe (b).

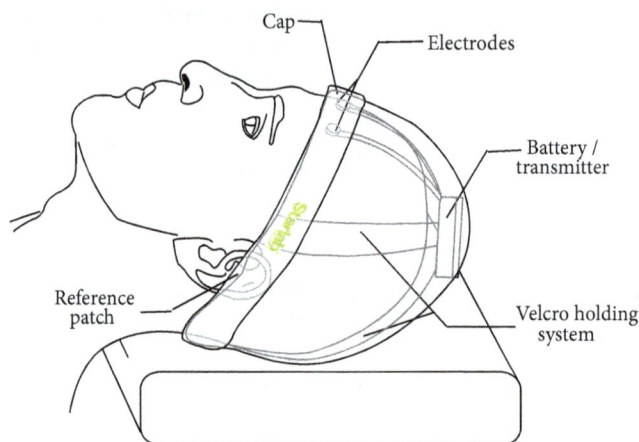

FIGURE 5: The modified cap was more comfortable during sleeping/going to bed.

in this case, they will also provide an update to a localization system.

From the technical point of view, it was found that the deployment of a monitoring system should consider existing communication network infrastructure and the range of sensors in a pretesting phase. Feedback from such testing would enable modifications to system's functions in order to improve its performance and adaptability. For example, in designing the Shimmer-based prototype we initially set the sensors to work within a 100-meter range from the base station, without considering that our subjects were used to walk back and forth along the corridors even far from their bedrooms. After the study, we realized the need of extending the coverage of the sensors for continuous monitoring. A possible solution would have been to adopt a multihop routing protocol, with each node running a message forwarding program besides the monitoring one. However, this would have drastically reduced the nodes' battery lifetime and, in the end, the system's usability. We identified the right solution by distinguishing nodes into two types: *sensing nodes*, worn by the individuals, and *forwarding nodes*, connected to power outlets at fixed locations in the nursing home. Sensing nodes send data to the base station through the forwarding nodes,

by selecting the closest node at one-hop distance. Forwarding nodes run a routing algorithm that guarantees no packet loss, which is a critical requirement because the system cannot tolerate undelivered alarms.

As final remarks, even though a cost analysis is beyond the scope of this paper, we would like to stress on the fact that, as argued by analysts addressing the problem of why technology innovation tends to increase the cost of healthcare rather than making things simpler and cheaper [13], the best way technology can save costs is if it is used to better organize the healthcare system. In this sense, systems like the MIMS platform offer an automatic and seamless monitoring system, enabling continuous data collection otherwise very difficult or even impossible to obtain. The bare technological cost of the MIMS equipment used for our experiments, which glues together known and mature technologies, is in the order of 200 USD and 2,000 USD for Systems 1 and 2, respectively. However, we must be aware that the market cost of such systems is driven by healthcare stakeholders other than the research laboratories, whose role is only to propose proof-of-concept, innovative healthcare systems. In commercial use, the entire set of the ambient monitoring systems shown in Figure 1 are being deployed by healthcare companies in homes and nursing homes of some North American provinces, for an approximate cost of 100 USD for a month. So, when deployed in large numbers, there are considerable savings in healthcare cost with manageable equipment cost.

Acknowledgments

The authors wish to express their appreciation for the administrators, nurses, and families of the residents from the Kings Way Care, New Brunswick, Canada, who participated in the study. The environment monitoring equipment support provided to the researchers by industries Care Link Advantage and BeClose was valuable for the study. This work was partially funded by the Fondazione Cassa di Risparmio di Lucca, Italy, under the project "Fall Detection Alarm System for Elderly People" (FiDo). Special thanks are due to Arnoud Simonin and Anais Zeifer, the intern students from the U of Limoges, for their help during testing and in the ergonomic development of the hat solution.

References

[1] S. Abbate, M. Avvenuti, and J. Light, "MIMS: a minimally invasive monitoring sensor platform," *IEEE Sensors Journal*, vol. 12, no. 3, pp. 677–684, 2012.

[2] H. Cao, V. Leung, C. Chow, and H. Chan, "Enabling technologies for wireless body area networks: a survey and outlook," *IEEE Communications Magazine*, vol. 47, no. 12, pp. 84–93, 2009.

[3] R. K. Ganti, T. F. Abdelzaher, P. Jayachandran, and J. A. Stankovic, "SATIRE: a software architecture for smart AtTIRE," in *Proceedings of the 4th International Conference on Mobile Systems, Applications and Services (MobiSys '06)*, pp. 110–123, ACM, June 2006.

[4] M. Sung and A. S. Pentland, "Livenet: health and lifestyle networking through distributed mobile devices," in *Proceedings of the Workshop on Applications of Mobile Embedded Systems (WAMES '04)*, Boston, Mass, USA, 2004.

[5] S. Abbate, M. Avvenuti, F. Bonatesta, G. Cola, P. Corsini, and A. Vecchio, "A smartphone-based fall detection system," *Pervasive and Mobile Computing*, vol. 8, no. 6, pp. 883–899, 2012.

[6] S. Abbate, M. Avvenuti, G. Cola, P. Corsini, J. Light, and A. Vecchio, "Recognition of false alarms in fall detection systems," in *Proceedings of the IEEE Consumer Communications and Networking Conference (CCNC '11)*, pp. 23–28, January 2011.

[7] Shimmer Research, 2010, http://www.shimmer-research.com.

[8] Enobio by Starlabs, 2010, http://starlab.es.

[9] S. J. Guastello, *Human Factors Engineering and Ergonomics: A System Approach*, Lawrence Erlbaum Associates, New York, NY, USA, 2006.

[10] M. Avvenuti, C. Baker, J. Light, D. Tulpan, and A. Vecchio, "Non-intrusive patient monitoring of Alzheimer's disease subjects using wireless sensor networks," in *Proceedings of the World Congress on Privacy, Security, Trust and the Management of e-Business (CONGRESS '09)*, pp. 161–165, IEEE, August 2009.

[11] R. V. Pedroso, F. G. D. M. Coelho, R. F. Santos-Galduróz, J. L. R. Costa, S. Gobbi, and F. Stella, "Balance, executive functions and falls in elderly with Alzheimer's disease (AD): a longitudinal study," *Archives of Gerontology and Geriatrics*, vol. 54, no. 2, pp. 348–351, 2012.

[12] J. Nielsen, "How Many Test Users in a Usability Study?" Jakob Nielsen's Alertbox, 2012, http://www.useit.com/alertbox/number-of-test-users.html.

[13] J. S. Skinner, "The Costly Paradox of Health-Care Technology," MIT Technology, 2013, http://www.technologyreview.com/news/518876/the-costly-paradox-of-health-care-technology/.

9

Medical Image Watermarking Technique for Accurate Tamper Detection in ROI and Exact Recovery of ROI

R. Eswaraiah and E. Sreenivasa Reddy

Department of Computer Science and Engineering, Acharya Nagarjuna University, Guntur 522510, Andhra Pradesh, India

Correspondence should be addressed to R. Eswaraiah; eswar_507@yahoo.co.in

Academic Editor: Fei Hu

In telemedicine while transferring medical images tampers may be introduced. Before making any diagnostic decisions, the integrity of region of interest (ROI) of the received medical image must be verified to avoid misdiagnosis. In this paper, we propose a novel fragile block based medical image watermarking technique to avoid embedding distortion inside ROI, verify integrity of ROI, detect accurately the tampered blocks inside ROI, and recover the original ROI with zero loss. In this proposed method, the medical image is segmented into three sets of pixels: ROI pixels, region of noninterest (RONI) pixels, and border pixels. Then, authentication data and information of ROI are embedded in border pixels. Recovery data of ROI is embedded into RONI. Results of experiments conducted on a number of medical images reveal that the proposed method produces high quality watermarked medical images, identifies the presence of tampers inside ROI with 100% accuracy, and recovers the original ROI without any loss.

1. Introduction

Telemedicine eliminates distance hurdle and provides access to medical services available at far-away locations. It allows transmission of medical data from one location to another and enables handy and faithful interactions between patients and medical staff. This exchange of medical images imposes an important prerequisite that the medical images were not modified by unauthorized users. This prerequisite is called maintaining integrity of medical images. Conversely transmission of medical image and patient data independently through commercial networks leads to more cost and transmission time [1]. Watermarking is used to deal with the above two concerns.

Based on the medium used for hiding data inside an image, watermarking techniques are classified into two categories, namely, spatial domain and frequency domain. In spatial domain watermarking techniques [2–5], data is embedded directly into host image. In frequency domain techniques [6–8], data is embedded into transformed host image.

Another classification of watermarking techniques is reversible techniques and irreversible techniques.

The original image can be obtained without loss from watermarked image with reversible watermarking techniques [7–10], while lossless recovery of original image is not possible with irreversible watermarking techniques [6]. Reversible watermarking is more suitable for medical images [11].

Based on application, watermarking techniques are categorized as robust, fragile, and hybrid. Robust watermarking techniques [6–8, 12] are used in applications where protection of copyright information of images is required, as robust watermarks sustain intentional or unintentional attacks on images. Fragile watermarking techniques [2–5, 13] are used in applications which require detection of tampers caused by unauthorized persons during transmission of images and also authorization of source of image. Hybrid watermarking techniques [14–16] are used in applications that require both privacy control and integrity control of images. These are the amalgamation of fragile and robust watermarking techniques. Here, robust watermarks are used for privacy control and fragile watermarks are used for the integrity control of image.

Most of the medical images contain two parts called ROI and RONI. From diagnosis point of view ROI part is more important. Care should be taken while hiding data into ROI part so that visual quality will not be degraded. At the same time any tampering with ROI must be identified and the original ROI must be recovered in order to avoid misdiagnosis and retransmission of medical image. The recovery data of ROI is generally embedded into RONI [3–5, 8, 16–18]. When any tamper is detected inside ROI of received watermarked medical image the tampered area of ROI is replaced with the recovery data embedded inside RONI.

In this paper, we propose a novel block based fragile medical image watermarking technique to achieve the following objectives.

(1) Identifying tampered blocks inside ROI accurately using both average and variance values of blocks.

(2) Recovering original ROI with zero loss, when it is tampered.

(3) Detecting tampers inside ROI and recovering original ROI with simple mathematical calculations.

(4) Avoiding the process of checking ROI of watermarked medical image for the presence of tampers when the ROI is not tampered.

(5) Avoiding distortion in ROI of watermarked medical image by not embedding any data inside ROI.

The rest of the paper is organized into four sections. Section 2 covers review literature, the proposed method is explained in Section 3, results are illustrated in Section 4, and finally conclusion is in Section 5.

2. Literature Review

So far many block based watermarking techniques were developed for identifying tampered areas inside ROI of medical images and recovering original ROI when any tamper is detected inside it. Zain and Fauzi [2] proposed a scheme, where the medical image is segmented into 8×8 blocks and then a mapping is established between the blocks for embedding the recovery information of each block into its corresponding mapped block. Later, each block is further divided into four subblocks of size 4×4 and then a 9-bit watermark is generated for each subblock. The generated 9-bit watermark of each subblock is embedded into LSBs of the first 9 pixels of the subblock in the corresponding mapped block. At receiver's end, the watermarked medical image is divided into blocks of 8×8 size and then the mapping between the blocks is calculated as done in embedding procedure. Later, each block is further divided into four subblocks of 4×4 size and then a 2-level detection scheme is applied for detecting tampered blocks. This 2-level detection scheme identifies tampered blocks, where level-1 detection is applied to subblocks of blocks and level-2 detection is applied to blocks. When a tampered block is detected, the corresponding mapped block is identified and then recovery data embedded in mapped block is extracted. This recovery data is used to replace the pixels in tampered block. Major drawbacks of this method are as follows. (1) If both block A and its mapped block B are tampered then it will not be

possible to recover original image. (2) This method does not use any authentication data for the entire medical image to check directly whether the image is tampered. So, all blocks in the image have to be checked one after another to detect the presence of tampers. This checking process leads to wastage of time when the image is not tampered. (3) A tampered block cannot be recovered with original pixels of the block as this method uses average of pixels inside the block for recovering the pixels in the tampered block.

Wu et al. [6] developed two block based methods. In the second method, JPEG bit-string of the selected ROI is generated and then divided into fixed length segments. Later, the medical image is divided into blocks and then hash bits are calculated for each block excluding the block with ROI. These hash bits are used as authentication data of the blocks. In each block of image, hash bits of the block and one segment of JPEG bit-string of ROI are both embedded using robust additive watermarking technique. Then all blocks are combined to get watermarked medical image. At receiver's end, the watermarked medical image is divided into blocks as done in embedding procedure. From each block, hash bits of the block and a segment of JPEG bit-string are both extracted. For each block, hash bits are calculated and then compared with the extracted hash bits to check whether the block is tampered or not. If the block with ROI is identified as tampered then the JPEG bit-string segments extracted from all blocks are used to recover the ROI. Disadvantages of this method are as follows: (1) it is not possible to get original ROI as JPEG bit-string of ROI is used to recover ROI when it is tampered and (2) this method requires more calculations to generate recovery data of ROI and embed it into all blocks of medical image.

Chiang et al. [7] proposed two block based methods based on symmetric key cryptosystem and modified difference expansion (DE) technique. The first method has the ability to recover the whole medical image, whereas the second method has the ability to recover only ROI of medical image. In the first method, the medical image is divided into 4×4 size blocks and then average of each block is calculated. Later, the average values of all blocks are concatenated and then encrypted using two symmetric keys $k1$ and $k2$ in order to increase the degree of security. Then, Haar wavelet transform is applied to all blocks to identify smooth blocks. The encrypted average values of all the blocks are embedded in the identified smooth blocks. At the receiver's end, the embedded data is extracted from watermarked image and then decrypted using the keys $k1$ and $k2$ to get the average values of all blocks. Later, average values are calculated for all blocks and then compared with extracted average values to detect tampered blocks. When a tampered block is detected the pixels in tampered block are replaced with the extracted average of that block. The second method is the same as the first method except that the bits of pixels in blocks of ROI are embedded instead of average values of all blocks in the entire image. Pitfalls of these schemes are as follows: (1) the two methods require more time for embedding data into medical image as all blocks of the medical image have to be transformed into frequency domain and then smooth blocks have to be identified for embedding data and (2) the two methods are not using any authentication data for the entire ROI or the entire image to check directly whether the ROI or the entire image is tampered. So, all blocks in the ROI or in the entire image have to be checked one after another to detect the presence of tampers. This checking process leads to wastage of time when the image is not tampered.

Liew et al. [3, 4] developed two reversible block based methods. In the first method, the medical image is segmented into two regions: ROI and RONI. Later, ROI and RONI are divided into nonoverlapping blocks of sizes 8×8 and 6×6, respectively. Then, a mapping is formed between blocks of ROI to embed recovery information of each block into its mapped block. Each block in ROI is mapped to a block in RONI. This mapping is used to embed LSBs of pixels in a ROI block into its mapped RONI block. Then, the method implemented by Zain and Fauzi [2] is applied only to ROI part of the medical image for detecting tampers inside ROI and recovering original ROI. The LSBs of pixels inside ROI are replaced with its original bits that were stored inside RONI to make the scheme reversible. The second method is the same as the first method except that the removed LSBs of pixels in blocks of ROI are compressed using Run Length Encoding technique before embedding into RONI blocks. Drawbacks of the two methods are as follows. (1) If both block A and its mapped block B inside ROI are tampered then it will not be possible to recover original ROI. (2) The two methods do not use any authentication data for the entire ROI to check directly whether the ROI is tampered. So, all blocks in the ROI have to be checked one after another to detect the presence of tampers. This checking process leads to wastage of time when the ROI is not tampered. (3) A tampered block cannot be recovered with original pixels of the block as these methods are using average of pixels inside the block for recovering the pixels in the tampered block.

Memon et al. [15] implemented a hybrid watermarking method. In this method, the medical image is segmented into ROI and RONI. Then, a fragile watermark is embedded into LSBs of ROI. RONI is divided into blocks of size $N \times N$ and then a location map indicating embeddable blocks is generated. A robust watermark is embedded into embeddable blocks of RONI using integer wavelet transform (IWT). Later, the location map is embedded into LL_3 of each block using LSB substitution method. Finally, ROI and RONI are combined to get watermarked image. At receiver's end, the watermarked medical image is segmented into ROI and RONI. Then, the robust watermark is extracted from RONI and is used for checking authentication of image. Fragile watermark is extracted from ROI and checked visually to know the presence of tampers inside ROI. Two disadvantages of this method are as follows: (1) there is no specification of how the original ROI is recovered when the ROI is tampered and (2) the time complexity of this method is more as it has to generate location map before embedding data.

Tjokorda Agung and Permana [5] developed a reversible method for medical images whose ROI size is more compared to size of RONI. In this method, the original LSBs of all pixels in medical image are collected and then LSB in each pixel is set to zero. Later, the medical image is segmented into ROI and RONI regions. Then, ROI and RONI are

divided into blocks of sizes 6×6 and 6×1, respectively. A mapping is formed between blocks of ROI for storing recovery information of each ROI block into its mapped ROI block. The removed original LSBs are compressed using RLE technique and then embedded into 2 LSBs of 6×1 blocks in RONI. At receiver's end, the watermarked medical image is segmented into ROI and RONI as done in embedding procedure. Then, the method proposed by Zain and Fauzi [2] is applied only to ROI part to detect tampers inside ROI and recover original ROI. The original LSBs that were embedded in RONI are extracted and then restored to their positions to get the original medical image. This method has the same drawbacks as the methods proposed by Liew et al. [3, 4].

Al-Qershi and Khoo [8] developed a reversible ROI-based watermarking scheme. At sender's end, the medical image is segmented into ROI and RONI. Later, data of patient and hash value of ROI are both embedded into ROI using the technique developed by Gou et al. Compressed form of ROI, average values of blocks inside ROI, embedding map of ROI, embedding map of RONI, and LSBs of pixels in a secret area of RONI are embedded into RONI using the technique of Tian. Finally, information of ROI is embedded into LSBs of pixels in a secret area. At receiver's end, ROI information is extracted from a secret area and is used to identify ROI and RONI regions. From the identified RONI region compressed form of ROI, average values of blocks inside ROI, embedding map of ROI, embedding map of RONI, and LSB of pixels in secret area are extracted. Using the extracted location map of ROI, patient's data and hash value of ROI are extracted from ROI. Then, hash value of ROI is calculated and compared with extracted hash value. If there is a mismatch between the two hash values then the ROI is divided into 16×16 blocks. For each block, the average value is calculated and compared with the corresponding average value in the extracted average values. If they are not equal then the block is marked as tampered and replaced by the corresponding block of the compressed form of ROI. Two disadvantages of this method are (1) extracting the embedded data from RONI without knowing the embedding map of RONI and (2) use of compressed form of ROI as recovery data for the ROI.

Al-Qershi and Khoo [17] proposed a scheme based on two-dimensional difference expansion (2D-DE). At sender's end, the medical image is divided into three regions: ROI pixels, RONI pixels, and border pixels. Later, the concatenation of patient's data, hash value of ROI, bits of pixels inside ROI, and LSBs of border pixels are compressed using Huffman coding and then embedded into RONI using 2D-DE technique. This embedding generates a location map which will be concatenated with information of ROI and then embedded into LSBs of border pixels. At receiver's end, from border pixels in the watermarked medical image both information of ROI and location map are extracted. Using this ROI information, ROI and RONI are identified. The extracted location map is used to extract patient's data, hash value of ROI, bits of pixels inside ROI, and LSBs of border pixels from RONI. The process for detecting tampered blocks is the same as the one used in [8]. Each tampered block is replaced by the corresponding block of pixels in the extracted ROI. The LSBs of border pixels are replaced using the extracted LSBs from RONI. A major drawback of this scheme is that it is applicable to only medical images whose ROI size is very less (up to 12% of size of the entire image).

Al-Qershi and Khoo [16] developed a hybrid ROI-based method. At sender's end, the medical image is divided into three regions: ROI, RONI, and border pixels. Later, patient's data and hash value of ROI are embedded inside ROI using modified DE technique. The ROI location map along with compressed form of ROI and average intensities of blocks inside ROI is then embedded into RONI using DWT technique. Then, size of watermark that is inserted into RONI and ROI information is embedded inside border pixels using the same DWT technique. At receiver's end, ROI information is extracted from border pixels and is used to identify ROI and RONI regions. Compressed form of ROI, average intensities of blocks in ROI, and location map of ROI are extracted from the identified RONI region. Using the extracted location map of ROI, patient's data and hash value of ROI are extracted from ROI. The procedure for detecting tampered blocks and recovering ROI is the same as in [8]. Two disadvantages of this method are (1) use of compressed form of ROI as recovery information for the ROI and (2) applicability to only images whose size is at least 512×512.

Deng et al. [9] developed a region-based tampering detection and recovering method based on reversible watermarking and quadtree decomposition. In this method, original image is divided into blocks with high homogeneity using quadtree decomposition and then a recovery feature is calculated for each block using linear interpolation of pixels. The recovery features of all blocks are embedded as the first watermark using invertible integer transformation. Quadtree information as the second layer watermark is embedded using LSB replacement. In the authentication phase, the embedded watermark is extracted and the original image is recovered. The similar linear interpolation technique is utilized to get each block's feature. The tampering detection and localization can be achieved through comparing the extracted feature with the recomputed one. The extracted feature can be used to recover those tampered regions with high similarity to their original state. One drawback of this scheme is that original image cannot be recovered when it is tampered.

Kim et al. [19] developed a region-based tampering detection and restoring scheme for authentication and integrity verification of images based on image homogeneity analysis. This method divides the image into variable-sized blocks using quadtree decomposition and then chooses the average value of each block as the recovery feature. Some of the drawbacks identified with this method are as follows: (1) the original image cannot be recovered exactly when the region with recovery information is tampered and (2) computational complexity of the algorithm is high.

Tan et al. [20] proposed a dual layer reversible watermarking technique with tamper detection capability for medical images. This method embeds source information and encrypted location signal as layer 1 watermark into the medical image. CRC values of blocks in the medical image are used for detecting tampers and are embedded as the

TABLE 1: A 4×4 block in a medical image.

66	70	84	71
71	83	72	65
79	68	74	69
80	73	80	75

TABLE 2: Modified 4×4 block of the medical image.

80	64	73	68
80	69	79	73
66	82	71	70
77	83	82	63

second layer watermark. This method is not specifying how the tampered blocks are recovered to get original image.

Most of the reviewed schemes are detecting the tampered blocks in the watermarked medical image based on average intensity of the blocks. These schemes fail in identifying the changes or tampers in any block if the values of pixels in that block are modified without changing the average value of the block. For example, if the values of pixels of a block in a watermarked medical image are as shown in Table 1 then the average intensity of the block will be 72. There is a possibility to achieve the same average intensity for the block as shown in Table 2 by changing the values of pixels. By comparing only the average values of original and modified blocks it is not possible to detect modifications done in the block accurately. So there is a need to develop a system that can detect the tampers accurately even when only the pixel values of the block are changed by keeping the average value the same.

3. Proposed Method

To achieve the above-mentioned objectives, we propose a novel medical image watermarking method. A medical image may contain several disjoint ROI areas in different shapes. Each ROI area is marked by a physician or by a clinician interactively and is represented by an enclosing polygon. The enclosing polygon is characterized by the number of vertices and their coordinates. In the present work, we consider medical images containing a single ROI, though the proposed method can be used with medical images containing multiple ROI areas. The outer three lines of pixels in the image are used as border of image.

In the proposed method, the medical image is segmented into three sets of pixels, ROI pixels, RONI pixels, and border pixels as shown in Figure 1. Later, hash code of ROI is calculated using SHA-1 technique and is used to authenticate ROI. Even a change in single bit of ROI is identified using this hash code, as SHA-1 generates a unique code of size 160 bits for any input. ROI and RONI of medical image are divided into nonoverlapping blocks of sizes 4×4 and 8×8, respectively. Then, each block in ROI is mapped to a block in RONI using (1). This mapping is based on the assumption that the number of blocks in ROI is less than the number of blocks in RONI and is used to embed recovery information

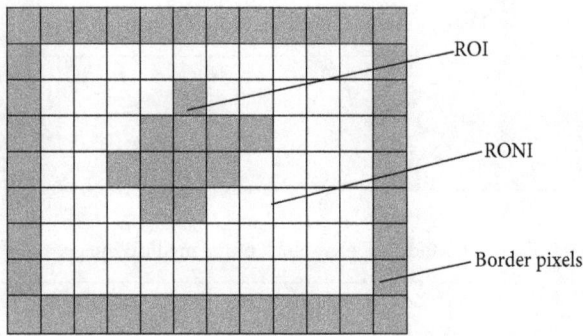

FIGURE 1: Division of medical image into three regions.

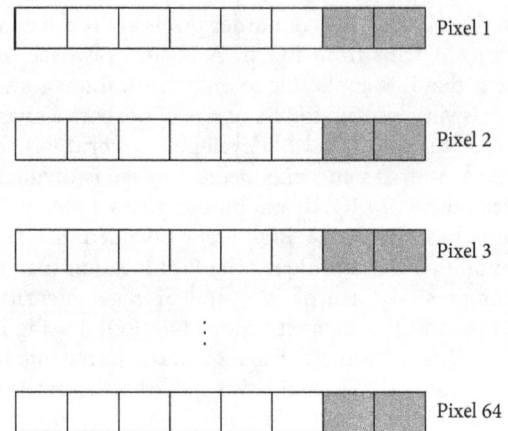

FIGURE 2: Embedding the recovery data of a ROI block into 2 LSBs of pixels in mapped RONI block.

of each ROI block into its corresponding mapped RONI block. For each ROI block, recovery data is generated by collecting the bits of pixels inside the block. The recovery data of each ROI block is embedded into LSBs of pixels inside the corresponding mapped RONI block. Consider

$$B_{\text{RONI}} = [(k \times B_{\text{ROI}}) \bmod N_b] + 1, \qquad (1)$$

where B_{RONI} is block number in RONI, k is a secret key and is a prime number between 1 and N_b, B_{ROI} is block number in ROI, and N_b is the number of blocks in ROI.

For each 4×4 block of ROI in 8-bit medical images, the size of recovery data is 128 bits (collection of bits of pixels inside the ROI block). Two LSBs of each pixel in mapped RONI block are used to embed this recovery data as shown in Figure 2. Similarly, in 12-bit and 16-bit medical images the sizes of recovery data are 192 and 256 bits, respectively. Three and four LSBs of pixels in mapped RONI block are used to embed recovery data of each ROI block in 12-bit and 16-bit medical images. Finally, the information of ROI and the hash value of ROI are embedded into LSBs of border pixels, where information is defined as the number of vertices and coordinates of vertices of an enclosing polygon and border is defined as the outer three lines of pixels in the image. The detailed embedding algorithm is explained as follows.

3.1. Embedding Algorithm

(1) Segment the medical image into three sets of pixels called ROI pixels, RONI pixels, and border pixels.

(2) Calculate hash value of ROI (h1) using SHA-1 technique.

(3) Divide ROI into nonoverlapping blocks of size 4×4 pixels.

(4) Divide RONI into nonoverlapping blocks of size 8×8 pixels.

(5) Map each ROI block to a block in RONI using (1), assuming that the number of blocks in ROI is less than the number of blocks in RONI.

(6) Collect bits of 16 pixels inside each ROI block as recovery data.

(7) Embed recovery data of each ROI block into 2 or 3 or 4 LSBs of pixels in mapped RONI block, depending on bit depth.

(8) Encrypt the collection of bits indicating hash value (h1) and information of ROI by a secret key k1.

(9) Embed the encrypted bits into the LSBs of border pixels.

The watermarked medical image is now ready to send through network to other medical practitioners at remote locations.

At receiver's end, both information and hash value of ROI are extracted from LSBs of border pixels of the received watermarked medical image. With the extracted ROI information, pixels of ROI and RONI are identified in the watermarked medical image. Then, hash value of ROI is calculated and compared with extracted hash value in order to detect the presence of tampers inside ROI of received medical image. If there is a match between the two hash values then the received medical image is authentic and is directly used for making diagnosis decisions. Mismatch between the two hash values indicates the presence of tampers inside ROI of received watermarked image. To detect tampered areas inside ROI and recover the original ROI, ROI and RONI of received watermarked image are divided into nonoverlapping blocks of sizes 4×4 pixels and 8×8 pixels, respectively, as done in embedding procedure. For each ROI block, the mapped RONI block is identified using (1). Then, bits of pixels of each ROI block are extracted from LSBs of corresponding mapped RONI block. Both average and variance of each ROI block are calculated and compared with average and variance of pixels extracted from corresponding RONI block. When a block in ROI is detected as tampered block, the extracted bits of pixels are used to recover the original ROI block. The detailed extraction algorithm is explained as follows.

3.2. Extraction Algorithm

(1) Extract the encrypted bits from the LSBs of border pixels.

TABLE 3: Results of embedding data in three medical images of different modalities.

Modality	Size of image	Bit depth	Size of ROI	Number of blocks in ROI	PSNR	WPSNR	MSSIM	TPE
CT	336×406	12 bits	144×168	1512	53.36	54.15	0.9575	0.0549
MRI	480×512	16 bits	208×216	2808	51.52	53.44	0.9327	0.0828
US	309×255	8 bits	132×106	874	56.82	58.13	0.9854	0.0346

TABLE 4: Average performance of the proposed method.

Modality of image	Average PSNR	Average WPSNR	Average MSSIM	Average TPE
CT scan	50.26	52.81	0.9325	0.0490
MRI scan	52.13	54.65	0.9246	0.0682
Ultrasound	55.47	56.42	0.9612	0.0301

(2) Decrypt the extracted bits to obtain information of ROI and hash value of ROI (h1).

(3) Identify ROI pixels and RONI pixels in the received medical image by using information of ROI.

(4) Calculate hash value of ROI (h2) using SHA-1 technique.

(5) Compare h1 with h2.

(6) Stop the extraction procedure, if h1 = h2, otherwise.

(7) Divide ROI and RONI into blocks of sizes 4×4 and 8×8, respectively.

(8) Repeat steps 8 to 11 for each block (B) inside ROI in order to identify tampered ROI blocks.

(9) Calculate average (a1) and variance (v1) values of block B.

(10) Extract bits of pixels of ROI block B from 2 or 3 or 4 LSBs of pixels in mapped RONI block, depending on bit depth.

(11) Calculate average (a2) and variance (v2) of extracted pixels values.

(12) Mark the ROI block B as tampered if a1 $\neq$ a2 or v1 $\neq$ v2.

(13) Replace each tampered ROI block B with the bits of pixels, extracted from corresponding mapped RONI block, to get the original ROI block.

Now the medical image is ready for making diagnosis decisions.

4. Experimental Results

Experiments are conducted on around hundred medical images of 8-bit, 12-bit, and 16-bit depth and of different modalities like CT scan, MRI scan, ultrasound, and so on. Out of the hundred images, 40 medical images are CT scan, 30 medical images are MRI scan, and the remaining 30 images are ultrasound. We used the metrics called peak signal-to-noise ratio (PSNR) and weighted peak signal-to-noise ratio (WPSNR) [21] for measuring the quality of generated watermarked medical images. The formula for PSNR is as follows:

$$PSNR\,(dB) = 10 * \log \left(\frac{255^2}{MSE} \right)$$

$$MSE = \sum_{i=1}^{x} \sum_{j=1}^{y} \frac{\left(\left| A_{ij} - B_{ij} \right| \right)}{x * y}, \tag{2}$$

where x and y are the width and height of the image. A_{ij} is original medical image and B_{ij} is watermarked medical image.

Higher value of PSNR and WPSNR indicates less distortion in the watermarked images. A metric called mean structural similarity index (MSSIM) [22] is used to measure the similarity between the original and the watermarked medical images. The value of MSSIM is between −1 and 1. Value 1 of MSSIM designates that the original and watermarked images are similar. To know the level of degradation in the watermarked medical image, total perceptual error (TPE) [23] metric is used. Lower value of TPE designates less degradation in the watermarked image.

Figure 3 shows some of the medical images used in our experiments. These images are CT scan of brain, MRI scan of shoulder, and ultrasound image of abdomen. For simulating the proposed technique, a rectangular shaped ROI is considered in each medical image. Figure 3 also shows the watermarked medical images and the reconstructed medical images. There is no considerable visual difference between original, watermarked, and reconstructed images. Table 3 depicts the results of experiments conducted on the three medical images that are shown in Figure 3. The average results obtained by conducting experiments on the hundred medical images are shown in Table 4.

In the proposed technique, the values of PSNR and WPSNR of watermarked and reconstructed medical images are greater than 40 dB. If the PSNR and WPSNR values of the watermarked and reconstructed medical image are above 40 dB then the medical image watermarking technique is said to be effective [24]. The apparent change in the structural information of the watermarked medical images is immaterial as the MSSIM values of all medical images are

Original image   Watermarked image   Reconstructed image

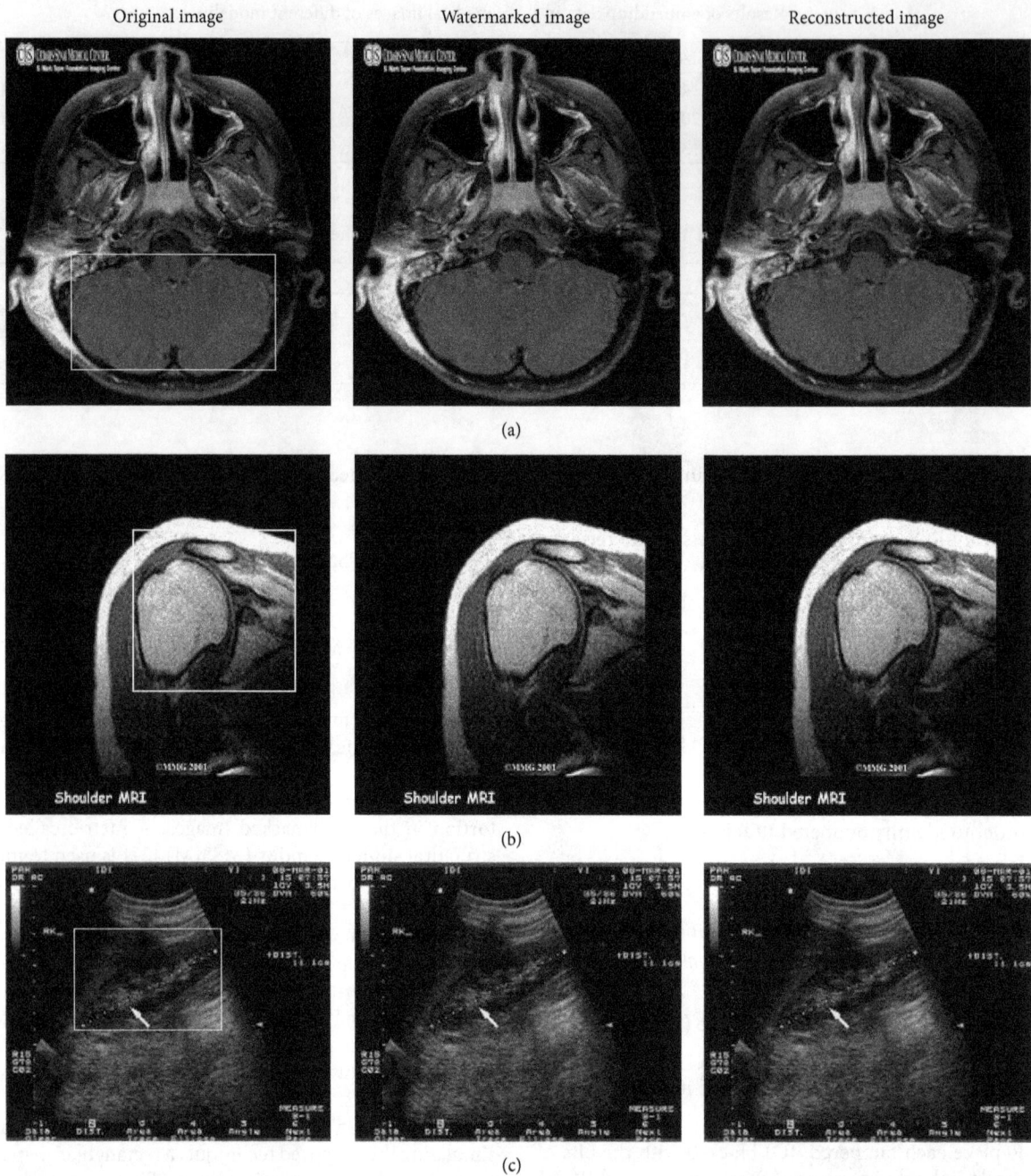

(a)

(b)

(c)

FIGURE 3: Original, watermarked, and reconstructed medical images. From top to bottom: CT scan, MRI scan, and ultrasound images.

very near to 1. Similarly, the low TPE values indicate less degradation in the watermarked medical images.

The intruders are prevented from obtaining hash value and information of ROI by encrypting it with a secret key before embedding inside border. Some of the state-of-the-art techniques [2–5] are not using any authentication data like hash value of ROI to check directly whether the ROI is tampered or not. So, all blocks inside ROI have to be checked one after the other to detect the presence of tampers. This checking process leads to wastage of time when the watermarked medical image is not tampered. Such wastage of

time is not incurred in the proposed method as it is using hash value of ROI to directly check whether the ROI is tampered.

As shown in Figure 4, we induced some tampers into ROI of the watermarked medical images for testing the performance of the proposed scheme in terms of detecting tampered or modified areas inside ROI and recovering original ROI. The proposed method identified all the tampered locations inside ROI with 100% accuracy and recovered the original ROI with no loss as shown in Figure 5. In medical images, the LSBs of pixels inside RONI and border are zero. So, the LSBs of pixels in RONI and border are set to 0

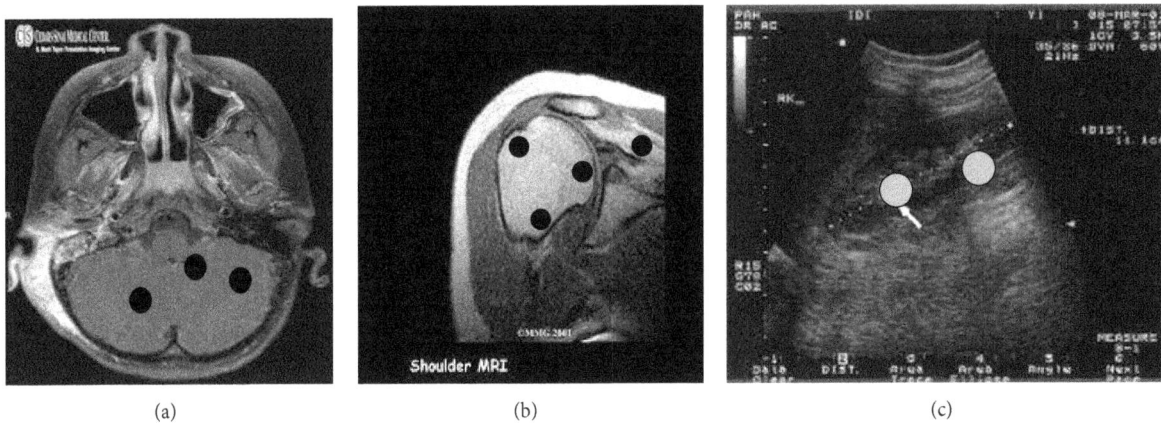

FIGURE 4: Watermarked medical images (from left to right: CT scan, MRI scan, and ultrasound) with tampers inside ROI.

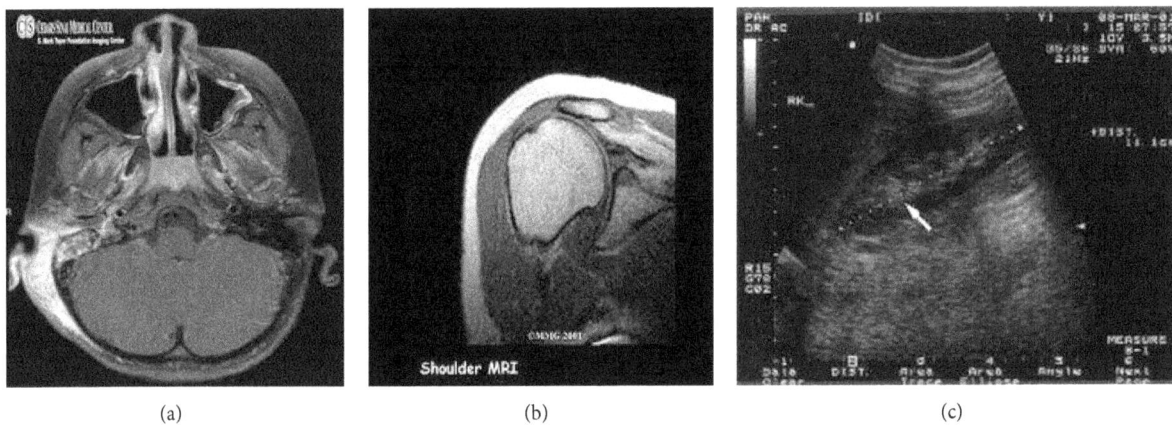

FIGURE 5: Recovered medical images (from left to right: CT scan, MRI scan, and ultrasound).

after extracting the embedded data from them. Table 5 shows comparison between the proposed scheme and the reviewed schemes.

The proposed method is developed on the assumption that the intruders generally try to modify only the significant part, ROI, in the medical images during their transmission. So, identifying changes inside ROI and recovering original ROI must be done before using the medical image for making diagnosis decisions. The proposed method can be used with medical images whose pixels are represented using 8 or 12 or 16 bits and with medical images of different modalities like CT scan, MRI scan, ultrasound, and so on. The RONI and border parts are not recovered exactly as LSBs of all pixels in RONI and border are set to bit 0 after extracting embedded data from them. This limitation does not affect the efficiency of the method as RONI and border parts of medical images are insignificant in the process of diagnosis decision making. It can only be used with medical images whose ROI size is small (up to 25% of the entire medical image). It is not robust against common attacks and image manipulation operations. This method can recover original ROI only when the RONI and border of the watermarked medical image are not attacked or modified by intruders. As intruders generally try to modify the ROI of the medical images during their transmission, this method emerges as a significant alternative in the field of medical image transmission.

5. Conclusion

In this paper, we proposed a block based fragile medical image watermarking technique for tamper detection and recovery. It is evident from the values of PSNR, WPSNR, MSSIM, and TPE that the proposed method produces high quality watermarked medical images. Embedding distortion inside ROI of watermarked medical images is zero as no data is embedded into ROI. The proposed method accurately identifies and localizes tampered blocks inside ROI using average and variance values of blocks. Original ROI with zero loss is recovered as the pixels in tampered blocks are replaced with original pixel values. The proposed method uses simple mathematical calculations for generating authentication and recovery data, identifying tampered blocks inside ROI, and recovering original ROI. This scheme does not check the presence of tampers inside ROI when the extracted hash value of ROI matches recalculated hash value of ROI. But some of the reviewed schemes are checking the presence of tampers without ascertaining whether or not the ROI or the entire medical image is tampered.

TABLE 5: Comparison between the proposed scheme and reviewed schemes.

Scheme	ROI-based	Embedding distortion inside ROI	Spotting tampers inside ROI	Accurate identification of tampered blocks	Recovery of tampered blocks inside ROI or image
Zain and Fauzi [2]	No	—	No	No	With average intensity of blocks
Wu et al. [6]	Yes	No	No	No	With JPEG compressed form of ROI
Chiang et al. [7]	Yes	No	No	No	With average intensity of blocks
Liew and Zain [3], Liew et al. [4]	Yes	Yes	No	No	With average intensity of blocks
Memon et al. [15]	Yes	Yes	No	No	No
Tjokorda Agung and Permana [5]	Yes	Yes	No	No	With average intensity of blocks
Al-Qershi and Khoo [8]	Yes	Yes	Yes	No	With compressed form of ROI
Al-Qershi and Khoo [17]	Yes	No	Yes	No	With original pixels of blocks
Al-Qershi and Khoo [16]	Yes	Yes	Yes	No	With compressed form of ROI
Deng et al. [9]	No	—	No	No	With linear interpolation of pixels of blocks
Kim et al. [19]	No	—	No	No	With average intensity of blocks
Proposed method	Yes	No	Yes	Yes	With original pixels of blocks

For future enhancement, we try to extend the method for medical images with large size ROI and to sustain common attacks and image manipulations.

References

[1] G. Coatrieux, J. Montagner, H. Huang, and C. Roux, "Mixed reversible and RONI watermarking for medical image reliability protection," in *Proceedings of the 29th Annual International Conference of IEEE-EMBS, Engineering in Medicine and Biology Society (EMBC '07)*, pp. 5653–5656, Lyon, France, August 2007.

[2] J. M. Zain and A. R. M. Fauzi, "Medical image watermarking with tamper detection and recovery," in *Proceedings of the 28th Annual International Conference of the IEEE Engineering in Medicine and Biology Society (EMBS '06)*, pp. 3270–3273, September 2006.

[3] S.-C. Liew and J. M. Zain, "Reversible medical image watermarking for tamper detection and recovery," in *Proceedings of the 3rd IEEE International Conference on Computer Science and Information Technology (ICCSIT '10)*, pp. 417–420, July 2010.

[4] S.-C. Liew, S.-W. Liew, and J. M. Zain, "Reversible medical image watermarking for tamper detection and recovery with Run Length Encoding compression," *World Academy of Science, Engineering & Technology*, no. 50, pp. 799–803, 2011.

[5] B. W. Tjokorda Agung and F. P. Permana, "Medical image watermarking with tamper detection and recovery using reversible watermarking with LSB modification and Run Length Encoding (RLE) compression," in *Proceedings of the IEEE International Conference on Communication, Networks and Satellite (COMNETSAT '12)*, pp. 167–171, Bali, Indonesia, July 2012.

[6] J. H. K. Wu, R.-F. Chang, C.-J. Chen et al., "Tamper detection and recovery for medical images using near-lossless information hiding technique," *Journal of Digital Imaging*, vol. 21, no. 1, pp. 59–76, 2008.

[7] K.-H. Chiang, K.-C. Chang-Chien, R.-F. Chang, and H.-Y. Yen, "Tamper detection and restoring system for medical images using wavelet-based reversible data embedding," *Journal of Digital Imaging*, vol. 21, no. 1, pp. 77–90, 2008.

[8] O. M. Al-Qershi and B. E. Khoo, "Authentication and data hiding using a reversible ROI-based watermarking scheme for DICOM images," in *Proceedings of International Conference on Medical Systems Engineering (ICMSE '09)*, pp. 829–834, 2009.

[9] X. Deng, Z. Chen, F. Zeng, Y. Zhang, and Y. Mao, "Authentication and recovery of medical diagnostic image using dual reversible digital watermarking," *Journal of Nanoscience and Nanotechnology*, vol. 13, no. 3, pp. 2099–2107, 2013.

[10] B. Lei, E. L. Tan, S. Chen, D. Ni, T. Wang, and H. Lei, "Reversible watermarking scheme for medical image based on differential evolution," *Expert Systems with Applications*, vol. 41, no. 7, pp. 3178–3188, 2014.

[11] X. Luo, Q. Cheng, and J. Tan, "A lossless data embedding scheme for medical images in application of e-diagnosis," in *Proceedings of the 25th Annual International Conference of the IEEE Engineering in Medicine and Biology Society*, pp. 852–855, September 2003.

[12] J. J. Eggers, R. Bauml, R. Tzschoppe, and B. Girod, "Scalar Costa scheme for information embedding," *IEEE Transactions on Signal Processing*, vol. 51, no. 4, pp. 1003–1019, 2003.

[13] A. M. Nisar and S. A. M. Gilani, "NROI watermarking of medical images for content authentication," in *Proceedings of the 12th IEEE International Multitopic Conference (INMIC '08)*, pp. 106–110, Karachi, Pakistan, December 2008.

[14] A. Giakoumaki, S. Pavlopoulos, and D. Koutsouris, "Multiple image watermarking applied to health information management," *IEEE Transactions on Information Technology in Biomedicine*, vol. 10, no. 4, pp. 722–732, 2006.

[15] N. A. Memon, A. Chaudhry, M. Ahmad, and Z. A. Keerio, "Hybrid watermarking of medical images for ROI authentication and recovery," *International Journal of Computer Mathe-*

matics, vol. 88, no. 10, pp. 2057–2071, 2011.

[16] O. M. Al-Qershi and B. E. Khoo, "Authentication and data hiding using a hybrid ROI-based watermarking scheme for DICOM images," *Journal of Digital Imaging*, vol. 24, no. 1, pp. 114–125, 2011.

[17] O. M. Al-Qershi and B. E. Khoo, "ROI-based tamper detection and recovery for medical images using reversible watermarking technique," in *Proceedings of the IEEE International Conference on Information Theory and Information Security (ICITIS '10)*, pp. 151–155, Beijing, China, December 2010.

[18] H. Nyeem, W. Boles, and C. Boyd, "Utilizing least significant bit-planes of RONI pixels for medical image watermarking," in *Proceedings of the International Conference on Digital Image Computing: Techniques and Applications (DICTA '13)*, IEEE, November 2013.

[19] K.-S. Kim, M.-J. Lee, J.-W. Lee, T.-W. Oh, and H.-Y. Lee, "Region-based tampering detection and recovery using homogeneity analysis in quality-sensitive imaging," *Computer Vision and Image Understanding*, vol. 115, no. 9, pp. 1308–1323, 2011.

[20] C. K. Tan, J. C. Ng, X. Xu, C. L. Poh, Y. L. Guan, and K. Sheah, "Security protection of DICOM medical images using dual-layer reversible watermarking with tamper detection capability," *Journal of Digital Imaging*, vol. 24, no. 3, pp. 528–540, 2011.

[21] N. Ponomarenko, S. Krivenko, K. Egiazarian, J. Astola, and V. Lukin, "Weighted MSE based metrics for characterization of visual quality of image denoising methods," in *Proceedings of the 8th International Workshop on Video Processing and Quality Metrics for Consumer Electronics (VPQM '14)*, Scottsdale, Ariz, USA, 2014.

[22] Z. Wang, A. C. Bovik, H. R. Sheikh, and E. P. Simoncelli, "Image quality assessment: from error visibility to structural similarity," *IEEE Transactions on Image Processing*, vol. 13, no. 4, pp. 600–612, 2004.

[23] A. B. Watson, "DCT quantization matrices visually optimized for individual images," in *Human Vision, Visual Processing, and Digital Display IV*, vol. 1913 of *Proceedings of SPIE*, pp. 202–216, San Jose, Calif, USA, 1993.

[24] K. Chen and T. V. Ramabadran, "Near-lossless compression of medical images through entropy-coded DPCM," *IEEE Transactions on Medical Imaging*, vol. 13, no. 3, pp. 538–548, 1994.

mHealth in Sub-Saharan Africa

Thomas J. Betjeman,[1] **Samara E. Soghoian,**[2] **and Mark P. Foran**[2]

[1] Ben Gurion University of the Negev, Medical School for International Health, New York, NY 10032, USA
[2] NYU School of Medicine, Bellevue Hospital Center, New York, NY 10016, USA

Correspondence should be addressed to Mark P. Foran; mark.foran@gmail.com

Academic Editor: Jocelyne Fayn

Mobile phone penetration rates have reached 63% in sub-Saharan Africa (SSA) and are projected to pass 70% by 2013. In SSA, millions of people who never used traditional landlines now use mobile phones on a regular basis. Mobile health, or mHealth, is the utilization of short messaging service (SMS), wireless data transmission, voice calling, and smartphone applications to transmit health-related information or direct care. This systematic review analyzes and summarizes key articles from the current body of peer-reviewed literature on PubMed on the topic of mHealth in SSA. Studies included in the review demonstrate that mHealth can improve and reduce the cost of patient monitoring, medication adherence, and healthcare worker communication, especially in rural areas. mHealth has also shown initial promise in emergency and disaster response, helping standardize, store, analyze, and share patient information. Challenges for mHealth implementation in SSA include operating costs, knowledge, infrastructure, and policy among many others. Further studies of the effectiveness of mHealth interventions are being hindered by similar factors as well as a lack of standardization in study design. Overall, the current evidence is not strong enough to warrant large-scale implementation of existing mHealth interventions in SSA, but rapid progress of both infrastructure and mHealth-related research in the region could justify scale-up of the most promising programs in the near future.

1. Introduction

Mobile phones are increasingly accessible worldwide. There are an estimated 6.8 billion mobile phones being used in the world in 2013, compared to 1 billion in 2002, corresponding to penetration rates of approximately 96% globally: 128% in developed countries and 89% in developing countries [1]. In sub-Saharan Africa (SSA), the penetration of cell phones is estimated to be 63% in 2013 and projected to pass 70% by 2015 [2]. Hundreds of millions of people in SSA who never gained access to traditional landlines for telecommunication now use mobile phones on a regular basis [3]. In many developing countries, wireless technology is less expensive and more readily available than wired technology [4]. This technology has unique potential to reach large numbers of people living in resource-limited or remote locations.

Mobile health (mHealth) is the use of mobile phone technology for health-related purposes. This relatively new, dynamic, and rapidly evolving field includes the development and study of mobile phone applications such as short messaging service (SMS), voice calling, and wireless data transmission to collect or disseminate health-related information or to direct care. Recently, there has been an explosion in mHealth activities globally [5]. Early evidence from grey literature and peer-reviewed publications suggests that mobile phone-based platforms can be effectively and efficiently used for a variety of health-related purposes. However, the vast majority of published reports are program or project process evaluations. Scholarly articles describing health outcomes or analysing the cost-effectiveness of mHealth interventions remain few in number [6]. Further, there is a lack of standardization with regard to mobile device application design, which renders comparative studies looking at specific variables difficult [7]. Most mHealth research to date has been conducted in high-income countries with advanced mobile and information infrastructure. However, an increasing number of mHealth interventions are being developed and applied to disease prevention and control in more resource-limited contexts. Applications of mHealth within the field of global health include medication adherence, health worker communication, health education, and emergency and disaster response. Given its relatively large rural populations, varied landscape, limited transportation infrastructure, and rapidly expanding wireless network coverage, sub-Saharan Africa (SSA) is well positioned to benefit from the promise of remote medical service delivery. This review aims to provide a summary of key articles, published on or before March 16, 2013, from the peer-reviewed scientific literature describing current progress on mHealth initiatives in SSA and to explore potential future applications of mHealth in the region.

2. Methods

An initial search of original research and review articles was conducted via PubMed on March 16, 2013 using "mHealth" in the title or abstract. Since Professor Robert Istepanian first coined the term "mHealth" in 2004 [8], it has become a widely recognized and utilized term. The search was limited to this term to narrow the focus of the review. The initial search resulted in 109 articles. The articles were handsearched for reference to Sub-Saharan Africa, developing countries, or disaster response. This selection process yielded 21 articles. Articles not directly pertaining to health were removed, as were articles greater than ten-year old. This screening yielded 18 articles. Additional web searches provided background information relevant to the review. Articles were sorted by topic and findings summarized below.

3. Medication Adherence

Although many mHealth initiatives in SSA are still in the development and pilot phases, a growing number of applications have been implemented. To date, the majority of studies on mHealth interventions in the region have been small-scale pilot or feasibility studies evaluating SMS based messaging systems for improved disease management. Preliminary results are promising, especially in the area of medication adherence among patients being treated for HIV and/or tuberculosis (TB).

SIMpill is a pill dispensing system that embeds a SIM card in a small pill bottle, which registers and sends an SMS text to a central server each time the bottle is opened [9]. Each text message is time-stamped and contains a unique identification code linked to the patient's mobile phone number. If the central server does not receive text messages before a preset time, a reminder text is automatically sent to the patient's mobile phone. If there is no response, an alert is then sent to the patient's healthcare provider who can followup directly with the patient. A pilot study of 155 patients in Cape Town, South Africa, demonstrated treatment success rates of 94% with that system, up from 22–60%. SIMmed is a less expensive system that simply asks patients to dial into a central server each time they take their medications [9]. Again, if no communication is received from the patient by a designated time each day, the system sends a reminder text message to the patient, and alerts a healthcare provider if the patient again fails to respond. A SIMmed pilot showed compliance rates of 90%, but health outcomes such as treatment success rates have not yet been studied [9]. Nevertheless, such demonstrated improvements in treatment success rates with SIMpill and

compliance rates with SIMmed are promising and could warrant further investigation and consideration on behalf of policy makers.

A similar product, Wisepill, was tested for technical feasibility and functionality in rural southwest Uganda [10]. Wisepill devices are also designed to promote medication adherence by transmitting data to a central server each time a patient's pill bottle is opened. The study compared use of a standard cellular network-based general packet radio service (GPRS) with one that added SMS service for real-time communication. The primary outcome tested was the number of network failures per person-month: (Network failures were defined as transmission interruptions of >48 hours due to lack of network connectivity). Among the 157 participants, there were 1.5 and 0.3 network failures per person-month for GPRS and GPRS + SMS, respectively. The additional cost for having SMS was approximately 1 USD per participant per month if one SMS was sent daily and GPRS was about 1.25 USD for the SIM card and 0.80 USD for 3 months of airtime to transmit data. The study concluded that the addition of SMS to cell networks serving remote areas significantly enhances the functionality of real-time mHealth applications in those areas [10]. Effects on patient adherence and treatment outcomes were not studied.

A mobile directly observed therapy (MDOT) model for tuberculosis studied in Kenya uses a combination of video and text messaging to encourage medication adherence [11]. The goal of this system is to improve treatment of TB among patients residing in rural locations and to decrease the burden of directly observed therapy (DOT) on patients and the healthcare system, without sacrificing effectiveness. The MDOT model has patient's relatives or friends capture video images of the patient taking his or her medication. Each day the new video is sent via mobile messaging service (MMS) to a central database where it is time and date stamped and logged. Medical nurses review the videos and can follow up if they were inadequate or not received. Video and SMS text messages containing health promotion messages and reminders are also sent out to patients regularly. A feasibility study in 13 patients found high degrees of interest and receptivity among both patients and nurses. However, about 50% of messages were not received, mostly as a result of technical issues and lost phones, and one patient was lost to follow-up [11]. In addition to these technical challenges, the high costs associated with MMS messaging and mobile phones capable of video communication may be a major limitation for the widespread adoption of this sort of system. However, current projections estimate that multimedia-messaging costs will decline and infrastructure will improve rapidly in the coming years. Further study with larger sample sizes and measurement of adherence and health outcomes may be warranted.

The WelTel Kenya1 study was designed to promote antiretroviral (ARV) medication adherence using a simpler and much less resource intensive system of weekly SMS text messages inquiring about patients' general wellbeing [12]. Patients are expected to respond within 48 hours. If a patient reports symptoms of poor health or does not respond, then healthcare providers follow up by phone. A randomised control trial of 538 participants, SMS intervention ($n = 273$) and standard care ($n = 265$), found significantly higher rates of self-reported medication adherence (relative risk for non-adherence 0.81; $P < 0.006$) and better rates of viral suppression (relative risk of viral load suppression failure 0.85; $P < 0.04$) in an intention to treat analysis [12]. The system costs under $8 USD per patient per year. Considering the cost of adding second-line therapy for patients who fail treatment, this application holds promise as a cost-effective strategy. Importantly, the WelTel Kenya1 trial did not incorporate specific daily or timed medication reminders and feedback, suggesting that improved communication and linking with healthcare providers alone may encourage patients to stick with long-term therapies.

Pop-Eleches et al. showed that automated text message reminders could be useful in improving HIV medication adherence in Kenya [13]. The study involved 431 adult patients who had initiated ARV treatment within 3 months. Participants in the intervention groups received SMS reminders that were either short or long and sent at a daily or weekly frequency. Adherence was measured using the medication event monitoring system on the pill bottle of one of the drugs prescribed and it was extrapolated that adherence with one drug most likely indicated adherence with all drugs. In intention-to-treat analysis, 53% of participants receiving weekly SMS reminders achieved adherence of at least 90% during the 48 weeks of the study, compared with 40% of participants in the control group ($P < 0.03$). Participants in groups receiving weekly reminders were also significantly less likely to experience treatment interruptions exceeding 48 hours during the 48-week follow-up period than participants in the control group (81 versus 90%, $P < 0.03$). Overall weekly short reminders seemed to be the most effective based on adherence rates in that subgroup. The results indicate that a simple and cheap intervention such as automated reminders for HIV patients on ARV therapy can significantly increase adherence. Further, this study suggests that short reminders are more effective than long reminders, which could inform future program design and effectiveness trails.

Based on the evidence from these short-term trails, SMS reminders could be a cost-effective way to improve medication adherence in SSA. This would especially be the case in areas that have preexisting wireless network coverage with SMS capabilities. Although much of the current research evaluating the impact of mHealth interventions on medication compliance in SSA has been promising, more work is needed to assess long-term impact. Longitudinal and follow-up studies will be an important addition to the current literature in this area.

4. Health Worker Communication

In addition to direct communication and support for patients, a number of mHealth applications have been designed as tools to increase community health worker (CHW) access to health information, decision making, and/or logistical support. For example, SMS-based communication and professional networking to support CHWs were studied in rural

areas of Malawi [14]. The authors used a mixed methods approach to determine the frequency of SMS use, the most common reasons for use, and CHW feedback on the extent to which SMS capabilities facilitated and improved the quality of medical care that they could provide. Communication costs and efficiency were compared between one geographic area with SMS capabilities and two areas of similar demographics that did not have SMS or other cell phone service. In this study, CHWs most often used SMS to report medical supply shortages, followed by texts to obtain or communicate general information, and then by texts about patients with emergencies. The average cost per communication was about five times less expensive using SMS than in areas without SMS service. Communication via SMS took an average of nine minutes, whereas health workers in areas without SMS generally had to report any issues in person and this took an average of 24 hrs. Further, the CHWs using SMS claimed that they received more respect and confidence from the communities that they served and had to make fewer referrals to district hospitals since they could handle more problems on their own. It remains yet to be studied whether SMS actually reduced the incidence of supply stockouts or patient transfers [14].

An earlier retrospective study, also conducted in rural Malawi, used a free open source program called Frontline SMS to assist in the activities of 75 CHWs whose primary tasks were to manage HIV and TB patients [15]. The program uses automated responses based on key words in received text messages. Common uses were patient referral, drug dosing information, emergency support, and reporting patient mortality. Over the course of six months, it was found that the fuel savings alone (combined with those of the TB coordinator) heavily outweighed the operational costs of the FrontlineSMS network (a $2,750 net savings over six months). Similarly, the free time gained by hospital staff (2,048 hours) enabled higher resolution in data reporting (16.67 reports/week versus 25 reports/month prepilot) and expanded healthcare delivery capacity (100 additional TB patients put on treatment).

Ngabo et al. published a study on a mobile phone-based system designed and implemented in Rwanda using RapidSMS, a free and open-sourced software development framework, with the aim of monitoring pregnancy and reducing bottlenecks in communication associated with maternal and infant deaths [16]. The RapidSMS system was customized to allow interactive communication between the CHW following mother-infant pairs in their community, a national centralized database, the local health facility, and, in the case of an emergency alert, the ambulance driver. Over a 12-month period a total of 432 CHWs were trained and equipped with mobile phones by the Ministry of Health. During this time there was a registered 27% increase in facility-based delivery from 72% twelve months before to 92% at the end of the twelve-month pilot phase. The system was also found to promote prenatal visits since only registered pregnancies could be entered into the database. Further, the program facilitated the monitoring of CHW activities by remote supervisors. At the time the paper was published the project had rolled out to 18 out of the 30 districts nationwide with a total of 15,000 phones distributed to more than 7000

CHWs who were subsequently trained. Key elements that enabled the project to function were a strong commitment from the national government which provided the phones as well as covering programming fees, collaboration between the public and private sectors whereby the cost of sending text messages decreased 10-fold for all messages used in the program, and a previously well-established CHW program with good distribution of workers. Major challenges were telephone maintenance and replacement, especially in areas without electricity that were far from the nearest health centre.

A formative mixed methods study conducted by Chang et al. looks at some quantitative as well as qualitative (assessed on a Likert scale) aspects of mHealth using smartphones at a community-based HIV care organization in Uganda [17]. Interviews were conducted with 20 participants (6 CHW, 4 clinic staff, and 10 patients) and 6 focus groups. The study revealed that almost all of the participants had cell phones (not specifically smart phones) (93%), whereas almost none (4%) had access to the Internet at their homes. Most of the participants thought that using smartphones would improve the work of CHWs especially by allowing them to be monitored more effectively using GPS, photo, and video functions. Among CHWs, the main concern expressed was that the introduction of new technology might threaten their job security. Weaknesses of the study included a small sample size as well as not differentiating qualitative responses according to the role of the participant (i.e., CHW, clinic staff, and patient).

A cost analysis by Chang showed costs per patient per year in Uganda of $8.75 for a peer health worker (PHW) program versus $2.35 for an mHealth support program [18]. Both interventions were found to be reasonable for the budgetary requirements of many AIDS care programs. The effectiveness in averting virologic failure and loss to follow-up were shown for the PHW intervention with the addition of mHealth; however, a comparison of effectiveness of PHWs with and without mHealth was not performed.

Looking at the studies cited dealing with mHealth in health worker communication, it is evident that basic mobile phone use along with SMS capabilities can improve CHW efficiency while potentially reducing overall program costs. Utilization of smartphones may also be beneficial but necessitates more initial investment and has not yet shown clear advantages over basic cell phones + SMS.

5. eHealth

MHealth is one major component of eHealth, which refers to the utilization of information and communication technology for health more broadly, including data transmission and video telecommunication via the Internet. MHealth and Internet-based healthcare (eHealth) interventions are being used in many of the countries in SSA participating in the Millennium Villages Project. The Millennium Villages Project is using an open source eHealth platform, Global Network (MVG-Net), to track overall progress toward health-related outcomes and to help inform clinical decision making and management [19]. Key health indicators being measured include patient coverage relative to the overall population, immunizations, malnutrition screenings, and improvements in health-related outcomes. Focus is placed on the implementation of ChildCount+ (a point of care decision support SMS-based mobile phone system) and OpenMRS (a web-based, open source electronic medical record (EMR) platform). Results of the complete study are not released, but the pilot showed significant advances in the parameters described previously for those using the ChildCount+ system. Community health workers claimed to have more difficulty using the OpenMRS system indicating that more time and resources will need to be invested into training on this system before its efficacy can demonstrated. This preliminary study suggests that in SSA, the effectiveness and implementation of mHealth interventions will likely outpace eHealth. It is important to note the potential synergistic relationship between mHealth implementation and the adoption and utilization of EMR. mHealth programs being used in concert with an EMR system could potentially facilitate coordination of patient care, health worker efficiency, and data collection and analysis. However, the lack of existing infrastructure in many areas of SSA, as well as the lack of background familiarity with EMR platforms among health care workers, poses significant obstacles to the adoption of EMR systems in many areas where mHealth may be currently viable.

6. Health Education

A study conducted by Chib et al. in Uganda was critical of the current enthusiasm for mHealth with respect to disseminating health education materials [20]. The study focused on a Text to Change Project in the Aura district of Uganda that took place in 2009. An SMS quiz on HIV awareness was sent to 10,000 cell phone subscribers from a single provider. Questions dealt with knowledge of HIV transmission as well as questions promoting visits to the clinic for HIV testing and counselling. Of the 10,000 mobile numbers who were sent messages, 2,363 numbers responded, of which 1,954 answered the quiz questions (the rest responded to the gender and/or age questions only). Most of those who responded were men (of those who answered the gender question 421 were male versus 202 female). This was probably because men tended to be the ones with ownership of a cell phone and a higher literacy rate. This phenomenon presented a significant obstacle to the effectiveness of the program since the information was failing to reach those who are most vulnerable, that is, poor females. The study was critical of such technological interventions that fail to reach those most in need. Further, it was found that, of the question answers that were received, people tended only to answer questions that they knew the correct answer to and skip those they might not have. Thus, the amount of new information gained was likely to be limited.

7. eEmergency and Disaster Response

The search process used for this literature review did not reveal any formal studies of mHealth in disaster response in

SSA, but there were several studies conducted in developing countries elsewhere in the world. The lessons learned in those areas could prove valuable for future applications of mHealth technology in disasters in SSA. Furthermore, in most of these studies mHealth was utilized by international humanitarian response teams, which could consider implementing these applications in future disasters in SSA.

eEmergency, or internet-based provision of emergent medical and disaster care, is expanding rapidly. Examples of the use of mobile technology in disaster response include remote triage and monitoring, telemonitoring, medical image transmission (mainly X-ray and FAST), decision support applications, field hospital IT systems, and patient and health care worker tracking. Two notable recorded instances in which mobile technologies (specifically field hospital IT systems and teleradiology) were implemented in actual disasters were the US military in Pakistan in response to the 2005 earthquake and the Israeli Defence Forces in response to the 2010 earthquake in Haiti. Both cases showed that the electronic system in use helped with management of resources, identification and tracking of patients, and continuity of care and effective discharge [21].

Another implementation study was performed on a novel electronic patient medical record and tracking system used in postearthquake Haiti in 2010 [22]. The system used iPhones and the application iChart and was implemented at the Fond Parisien (FDP) Disaster Rescue Camp for all patients registered from January to March 2010. According to the majority of the approximately 150 medical care providers who used the program, handheld EMR and tracking systems could potentially reduce workload, but the iChart program was too "cumbersome" to fulfil that need [22]. That said, the program did facilitate continuity of care and patient hand-offs by providing a centralized database (the alternatives were handwritten files or nonnetworked computers) with standardized spellings of people's names and flags for those patients that required complicated postsurgical care. Further, iChart's online database was used to generate (albeit limited) aggregate census information for real-time analysis and reporting.

It was found that important features when considering a mobile health technology to be used in disaster situations are that it be readily available (many volunteers already have iPhones), not require much training to use (iPhone apps are generally very intuitive), and have adequate data management and security (in this case the app required a user ID and pass code to log in, although the option for tiered access and permissions was not available). Another important consideration is the ability to utilize mobile devices without continuous internet connectivity, and sync when connectivity is available, preferably to a cloud-based central system [22].

Interestingly, surveys looking at user satisfaction with mHealth in disaster simulations showed that those with administrative roles tended to favour the usage of mHealth whereas providers working in the field were not as satisfied and felt that mHealth was being used to monitor them as opposed to helping them perform their duties [22]. It was also learned that mHealth technologies for disaster response would be most effective if they are utilized for everyday purposes before a disaster. Overall, more data is required to demonstrate the effectiveness of mHealth in disaster medicine, especially in less developed countries [22].

8. Challenges

Despite great promise, there is currently limited evidence for improved health outcomes or the costeffectiveness of mHealth in SSA. In particular, more research needs to be conducted regarding the costeffectiveness of mHealth and eHealth programs compared to other health interventions in the region. This is especially the case for underrepresented areas such as francophone Africa. Establishing feasibility still remains a priority for the field. Given the varying infrastructure throughout SSA, it is important to test the feasibility of mHealth interventions over a broad geographic distribution. Lack of standardization of mHealth applications and studies is another serious obstacle to the provision of reliable studies and data to warrant industry scaleup. The WHO has recommended moving from computer-based research, focusing on usability, to a health outcomes-based approach facilitating randomized control studies and standardized replicable study designs [5]. Another challenge is that the majority of mHealth research is being conducted in high-income countries with advanced telecommunication infrastructure, which is not yet as widely available in SSA, especially broadband internet access. This poses many problems in feasibility especially with regard to more complex mHealth programs using smart phones as well as EMRs. Some of the technical and ethical challenges facing mHealth in SSA include transmission error detection and management, ensuring patient privacy during wireless transmission [23], phone security and sharing, inconsistent or limited network availability, and specific technical issues such as movement artefact in biomonitoring [4]. Information security is of particular concern and can only be adequately addressed once there is large enough industry buy-in to facilitate standardization and policy implementation. As of yet, most existing trials are small scale with varying degrees of security measures such as firewalls and tiered password access. A study of the prospects for scaleup of mHealth specifically in South Africa by Leon et al. showed that there are barriers in the following areas: strategic leadership, learning environment, capacity for implementation, culture of information use, technology usability, interoperability, privacy and security, sustainable funding, and cost effectiveness [24]. Most prominent among these are the weaknesses in organisational capacity, culture of using health information for management, and a relatively less developed ICT environment. According to a survey by the WHO all member states in Africa, barriers to investment, and scaleup of mHealth programs in the region are primarily due to operating costs, knowledge, infrastructure, and policy (in order of magnitude) [5]. Of note, globally the primary barriers that were identified were priorities, knowledge, policy, and cost effectiveness.

9. Conclusions

Mobile technology has significant potential for positive impact on healthcare in SSA. Mobile infrastructure has leapfrogged land-based telecommunication infrastructure in much of the region, and mobile penetration is now high, even in low-income and remote areas. In rural areas, where population densities are lowest and access to healthcare personnel often limited, mHealth offers potential solutions for maximizing healthcare worker impact and efficiency. Areas of mHealth where the most promise has been shown to date are in medication adherence and healthcare worker communication though the evidence is not yet sufficient to warrant large-scale investment and policy change. The use of mHealth in disseminating health education anonymously has been much less successful largely due to lack of adequate penetration to the most vulnerable groups of people. Such issues of access are not so apparent in other applications of mHealth such as medication adherence and CHW communication since participants are identified beforehand and provided with the appropriate technology if they do not already have it. Internet-based applications within the scope of eHealth remain largely unfeasible in much of SSA as of yet due to lack of infrastructure as well as issues with familiarity and usability. Isolated usage of mHealth in coordination with EMR systems during disaster scenarios has had mixed results but shows great potential for coordinating patient information and improving patient care, especially if such systems are made part of day-to-day healthcare provision and thus familiar to users. While operating, costs and infrastructure remain primary obstacles to the adoption and implementation of mHealth in SSA versus other areas of the globe, the rapid expansion of market-driven telecom infrastructure in the region could overcome these hurdles in the not too distant future. Likewise, challenges resulting from lack of cultural familiarity with wireless technology are disappearing with the introduction of cell phone access in even the most remote areas of SSA. Further, the rise of 3G access and smart phones could facilitate more complex mHealth and eHealth applications as well as synchronization with EMRs even in remote areas where traditional access to the Internet has been cost prohibitive. Further progress in the field of mHealth in SSA will rely on large-scale studies demonstrating feasibility and cost effectiveness over a broad geographic distribution. Policies that, incentivize telecom companies to provide their services for mHealth programs at reduced rates would be one way of facilitating larger studies. Standardization of mHealth studies is also essential if large-scale comparative analyses are to be performed and steps should be taken by international health organizations as well as academic and industry institutions to address this challenge.

References

[1] "The World in 2013: ICT Facts and Figures," 2013, http://www.itu.int/en/ITU-D/Statistics/Documents/facts/ICTFacts-Figures2013.pdf.

[2] Deloitte, "Sub-Saharan Africa Mobile Observatory 2012," 2012, http://www.gsma.com/publicpolicy/wp-content/uploads/2013/01/gsma_ssamo_full_web_11_12-1.pdf.

[3] "The world factbook 2009," 2009, https://www.cia.gov/library/publications/the-world-factbook/.

[4] G. D. Clifford and D. Clifton, "Wireless technology in disease management and medicine," *Annual Review of Medicine*, vol. 63, pp. 479–492, 2012.

[5] World Health Organization, "mHealth: new horizons for health through mobile technologies," in *WHO: Global Observatory for eHealth Series*, vol. 3, World Health Organization, 2011.

[6] D. West, "How mobile devices are transforming healthcare," in *Brookings: Issues in Technology Innovation*, Brookings, 2012.

[7] M. Tomlinson, M. J. Siedner, M. J. Rotheram-Borus, L. Swartz, and A. C. Tsai, "Scaling up mHealth: where is the evidence?" *PLoS Medicine*, vol. 10, no. 2, Article ID e1001382, 2013.

[8] R. S. H. Istepanian, E. Jovanov, and Y. T. Zhang, "Introduction to the special section on m-Health: beyond seamless mobility and global wireless health-care connectivity," *IEEE Transactions on Information Technology in Biomedicine*, vol. 8, no. 4, pp. 405–414, 2004.

[9] E. Barclay, "Text messages could hasten tuberculosis drug compliance," *The Lancet*, vol. 373, no. 9657, pp. 15–16, 2009.

[10] M. J. Siedner, A. Lankowski, D. Musinga et al., "Optimizing network connectivity for mobile health technologies in sub-Saharan Africa," *PLoS One*, vol. 7, no. 9, Article ID e45643, 2012.

[11] J. A. Hoffman, J. R. Cunningham, A. J. Suleh et al., "Mobile direct observation treatment for tuberculosis patients. A technical feasibility pilot using mobile phones in Nairobi, Kenya," *The American Journal of Preventive Medicine*, vol. 39, no. 1, pp. 78–80, 2010.

[12] R. T. Lester, P. Ritvo, E. J. Mills et al., "Effects of a mobile phone short message service on antiretroviral treatment adherence in Kenya (WelTel Kenya1): a randomised trial," *The Lancet*, vol. 376, no. 9755, pp. 1838–1845, 2010.

[13] C. Pop-Eleches, H. Thirumurthy, J. P. Habyarimana et al., "Mobile phone technologies improve adherence to antiretroviral treatment in a resource-limited setting: a randomized controlled trial of text message reminders," *AIDS*, vol. 25, no. 6, pp. 825–834, 2011.

[14] N. V. Lemay, T. Sullivan, B. Jumbe, and C. P. Perry, "Reaching remote health workers in Malawi: baseline assessment of a pilot mHealth intervention," *Journal of Health Communication*, vol. 17, supplement 1, pp. 105–117, 2012.

[15] N. Mahmud, J. Rodriguez, and J. Nesbit, "A text message—based intervention to bridge the healthcare communication gap in the rural developing world," *Technology and Health Care*, vol. 18, no. 2, pp. 137–144, 2010.

[16] F. Ngabo, J. Nguimfack, F. Nwaigwe et al., "Designing and Implementing an Innovative SMS-based alert system (RapidSMS-MCH) to monitor pregnancy and reduce maternal and child deaths in Rwanda," *The Pan African Medical Journal*, vol. 13, p. 31, 2012.

[17] L. W. Chang, V. Njie-Carr, S. Kalenge et al., "Perceptions and acceptability of mHealth interventions for improving patient care at a community-based HIV/AIDS clinic in Uganda: a mixed methods study," *AIDS Care*, vol. 25, no. 7, pp. 874–880, 2013.

[18] L. W. Chang, J. Kagaayi, G. Nakigozi et al., "Cost analyses of peer health worker and mHealth support interventions for improving AIDS care in Rakai, Uganda," *AIDS Care*, vol. 25, no. 5, pp. 652–656, 2012.

[19] P. Mechael, B. Nemser, R. Cosmaciuc et al., "Capitalizing on the characteristics of mHealth to evaluate its impact," *Journal of Health Communication*, vol. 17, supplement 1, pp. 62–66, 2012.

[20] A. Chib, H. Wilkin, L. X. Ling, B. Hoefman, and H. van Biejma, "You have an important message! Evaluating the effectiveness of a text message HIV/AIDS campaign in Northwest Uganda," *Journal of Health Communication*, vol. 17, supplement 1, pp. 146–157, 2012.

[21] T. Case, C. Morrison, and A. Vuylsteke, "The clinical application of mobile technology to disaster medicine," *Prehospital and Disaster Medicine*, vol. 27, no. 5, pp. 473–480, 2012.

[22] D. W. Callaway, C. R. Peabody, A. Hoffman et al., "Disaster mobile health technology: lessons from Haiti," *Prehospital and Disaster Medicine*, vol. 27, no. 2, pp. 148–152, 2012.

[23] H. S. Fraser and J. Blaya, "Implementing medical information systems in developing countries, what works and what doesn't," *AMIA Annual Symposium Proceedings*, vol. 2010, pp. 232–236, 2010.

[24] N. Leon, H. Schneider, and E. Daviaud, "Applying a framework for assessing the health system challenges to scaling up mHealth in South Africa," *BMC Medical Informatics and Decision Making*, vol. 12, article 123, 2012.

Teleultrasound: Historical Perspective and Clinical Application

Adilson Cunha Ferreira,[1,2,3] **Edward O'Mahony,**[1] **Antonio Hélio Oliani,**[2]
Edward Araujo Júnior,[4] **and Fabricio da Silva Costa**[1,3]

[1]Department of Obstetrics and Gynaecology and Department of Perinatal Medicine, Pregnancy Research Centre,
 Royal Women's Hospital, University of Melbourne, Melbourne, VIC 3207, Australia
[2]School of Medicine, University of São José do Rio Preto, São José do Rio Preto, SP, Brazil
[3]Monash Ultrasound for Women, Melbourne, VIC, Australia
[4]Department of Obstetrics, Paulista School of Medicine-Federal University of São Paulo (EPM-UNIFESP),
 05303-000 São Paulo, SP, Brazil

Correspondence should be addressed to Adilson Cunha Ferreira; adilsonteleultrassonografia@gmail.com

Academic Editor: Sotiris A. Pavlopoulos

The health care of patients in rural or isolated areas is challenged by the scarcity of local resources, limited patient access to doctors and hospitals, and the lack of specialized professionals. This has led to a new concept in telemedicine: teleultrasonography (or teleultrasound), which permits ultrasonographic diagnoses to be performed remotely. Telemedicine and teleultrasonography are effective in providing diagnostic imaging services to these populations and reduce health care costs by decreasing the number and duration of hospitalizations and reducing unnecessary surgical procedures. This is a narrative review to present the potential clinical applications of teleultrasonography in clinical practice. The results indicate that although barriers persist for implementing teleultrasonography in a more universal and routine way, advances in telecommunications, Internet bandwidth, and the high resolution currently available for portable ultrasonography suggest teleultrasonography applications will continue to expand. Teleultrasound appears to be a valuable addition to remote medical care for isolated populations with limited access to tertiary healthcare facilities and also a useful tool for education and training.

1. Introduction

Under the WHO definition of telemedicine, "the delivery of health care services, where distance is a critical factor," it is intended for the exchange of valid information for the diagnosis, prevention, and treatment of disease and for the continuing education of health service providers, as well as for research and evaluation purposes [1]. Ultrasonography is very useful diagnostic tool because it is a noninvasive, generally nonexpensive, and highly portable method that does not use ionizing radiation [2]. However, generating and interpreting ultrasound images are highly operator-dependent. As a result, performance and interpretation of these examinations have traditionally been limited to medical specialists [3, 4]. Although some remote areas have access to basic primary care services, including X-rays and ultrasound, they frequently lack specialized radiologists and ultrasonographers [5]. This lack of experienced doctors or qualified technicians has led to a new concept in telemedicine: teleultrasonography (or teleultrasound), which permits ultrasonographic examinations to be performed remotely in a synchronous (real-time) or asynchronous fashion. Over the past decade, research on teleultrasonography has evolved incrementally, especially with regard to technology, which is why most of the work has been published in technical engineering and medical informatics journals. However, few studies have been published on training doctors and technicians from remote or isolated areas.

This paper presents a narrative review of the potential clinical applications of teleultrasound in clinical practice.

2. Historical Perspectives

The committee formed by the collaboration between ACR, American College of Radiology, and NEMA, National Electrical Manufacturers Association in 1983, aimed to solve the problem of the Babel of files formats, images, and information generated by different manufacturers and equipment and to define the parameters for the transmission of distance medical images in an asynchronous way. From this point onwards, several studies were carried out in order to prove the diagnostic accuracy of this type of transmission, which is well established today [6–8].

Among the different areas of teleradiology, teleultrasonography is potentially the safest and least expensive area because it does not utilize ionizing radiation and is affordable [3, 4]. Investigators in the United States, the United Kingdom, Canada, and Australia were the pioneers in this research and in carrying out pilot studies [5–9]. The majority of these projects were based on the use of hardware and software packages which required high speed broadband connections and were associated with a high cost of implementation [5].

3. Transmission Modes

The asynchronous method is noninteractive. In this mode, data are collected, stored, and then forwarded to a sonologist for interpretation. This system can capture and store images as well as audio and text. This mode eliminates the need for the doctor and patient to be present at the same time in the same place and is widely used in countries where technicians instead of doctors perform ultrasound examinations [7, 10]. It is also widely used in university hospitals where trainees perform the examination and save the images, which are then evaluated together with the supervising physician [7, 11]. This type of service increases population access to services that are not locally available and is currently the most widespread mode of using teleultrasonography [11, 12]. In the synchronous mode, data transmission takes place in real time, that is, while the examination is being performed. This mode enables more experienced doctors to remotely supervise any person who is operating the ultrasound equipment, including technicians, medical residents, and personnel in training [12]. This system reduces the need for face-to-face consultations and allows for earlier detection of problems, which may further reduce the costs associated with the delocalization of specialized personnel. In the medical field, this modality involves a real-time interaction between the patient, the person operating the ultrasound equipment, and the interpreting specialist who will report the final diagnosis. This mode is not only possible but is well accepted by the physicians and patients involved. With the widespread use of the Internet across the world and increased communication via fixed or wireless broadband Internet access, the synchronous mode should become an important tool for clinical practices and educational purposes [13–15].

4. Research Categories and Themes

Research on teleultrasonography can be divided into studies that use synchronous (real-time) (Figure 1) and asynchronous

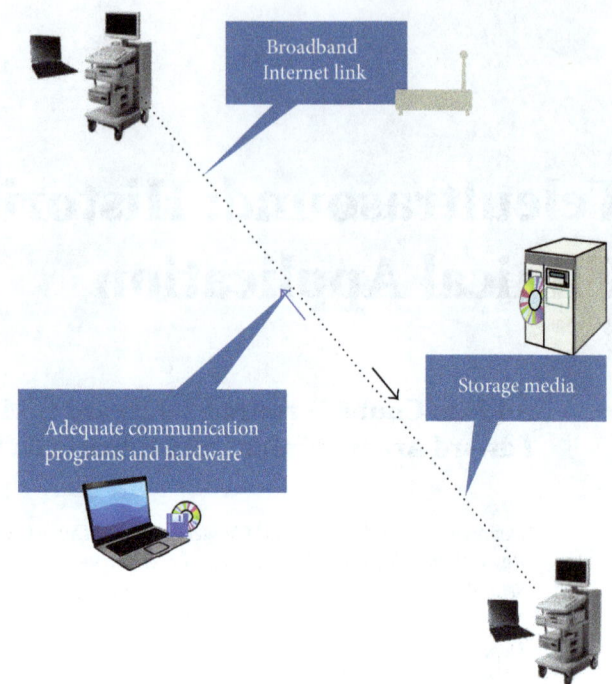

FIGURE 1: Illustrative description of the system utilized to real-time transmission of video clips and images between different centers.

(store-and-forward) transmission. Within these two categories of research, there are three recurring themes that are relevant to the successful implementation of a teleultrasonography system: (a) the quality of the transmitted images; (b) clinical applications; (c) the nontechnical and technical barriers to implementation [4].

Opinions in the literature are divided with regard to the transmission system involved in teleultrasonography. Some authors consider that good image quality can only be obtained with the use of asynchronous transmission, which, in addition to good diagnostic accuracy, allows for the training and professional supervision to produce a satisfactory level of clinical competence [6–8, 10, 12]. Other studies have sought to demonstrate the accuracy of the teleultrasonography performed in real time between a tertiary center and a remote area. The authors argue that the image quality was not very clear when teleultrasonography first started but that current telecommunication and image compression technologies have made high-quality synchronous and asynchronous transmissions feasible [5, 16]. Other authors argue in favour of real-time transmissions because the asynchronous mode only allows images and videos to be stored for future analysis and their interpretation may be incomplete or diagnostically inaccurate if some important information is missing and cannot be recovered [17]. However, the increasingly routine use of real-time transmission is still associated with high costs, and various studies have proposed alternatives to reduce these costs [5, 18–20].

5. Image Quality

Studies focused on the quality of transmitted images have attempted to determine the minimum bandwidth required,

Image A
Transventricular
plane

Image B
Transthalamic plane

Image C
Transcerebellar plane

Image D
Measurement of the
atrium of the lateral
ventricles

(a)

(b)

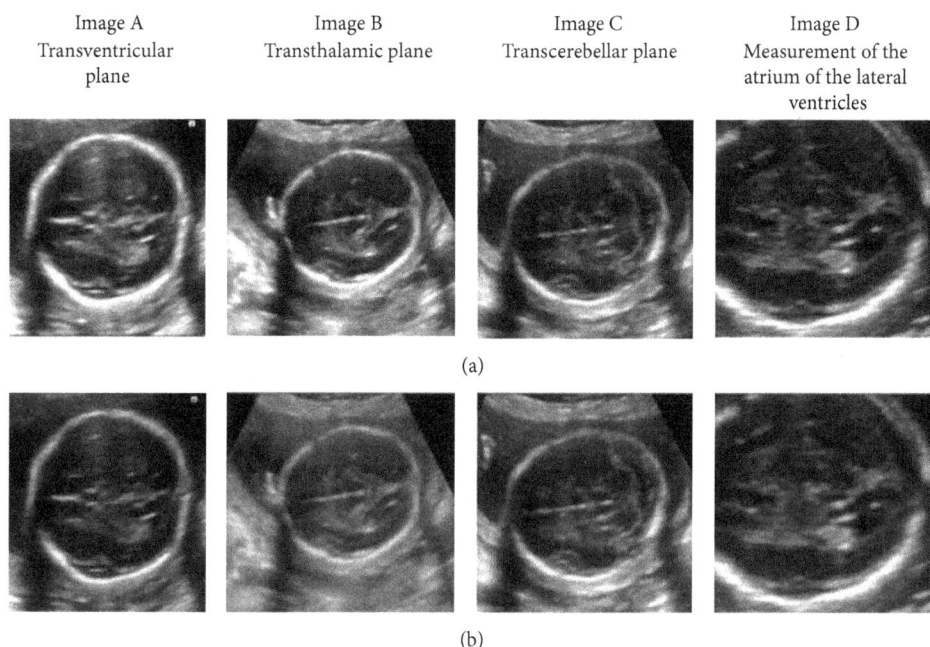

FIGURE 2: Transventricular, transthalamic, transcerebellar, and measurement of the atrium of the lateral ventricles; (a) original and (b) transmitted image planes of fetal central nervous system.

the most efficient processing signal, and the optimal compression system to generate an image with high diagnostic value [19]. The first studies on the quality of image in teleultrasound examined the transmission with the use of bandwidths such as 128 kbit/s, 256 kbit/s, and 384 kbit/s and suggested that the larger the bandwidth, the greater the amount of information received by the observer, which resulted in a more accurate diagnosis [21–25].

Whereas some researchers have evaluated the quality of transmitted images using analyses made by other radiologists, other researchers have measured image degradation using a careful analysis of the Fourier spectrum and contrast measurements [20]. Some studies have used a robotic arm for real-time transmissions. The results indicate that, although the duration of such tests is longer than that required for an in-person examination, the method could provide diagnostic information that is not available in remote or inaccessible areas [26, 27] (Figure 2).

6. Advances in Real-Time Transmission

More recently, a new type of image transmission has emerged under the name of Remote Task Scale, where the expert sees the images transmitted in real time with loss of quality but remotely receives the tests' recorded sequence of images with total quality. This modality can be implemented with the use of broadband technology of medium and high speed and with the use of streaming video [19, 20, 28].

With the advancement of open networks, image compression technology, and bandwidth levels in many countries, including developing countries, many locales have bandwidth that exceeds the minimum bandwidth recommended

for transmission in the initial studies published a decade ago on high-quality synchronous and asynchronous transmissions. Advances in telecommunications and signal processing and the relatively high resolution currently available for portable ultrasound equipment greatly increase the potential clinical applications of teleultrasonography. The remaining technical and logistical barriers include the availability of telecommunications in the desired areas and the training of medical professionals involved in the transmission, reception, and analysis of the images [4, 29].

7. Training and Education

According to the World Health Organization (WHO), diagnostic imaging is a necessary procedure for accurately treating at least 25% of patients worldwide. However, there is currently a lack of imaging services in vast areas of the world, especially in developing countries [1]. Where they do exist, these services are often of poor quality, resulting in misdiagnoses or nondiagnoses [20]. This is because the diagnostic quality of ultrasound images is extremely dependent on the physician and requires a certain level of expertise to obtain all the image planes necessary and interpret their meaning [11, 17]. Thus, even having the appropriate technology at their disposal, many patients in geographically or socially isolated areas may remain disadvantaged by the lack of a trained professional to operate them [17]. In reality, many small medical centers and isolated locations do not have well-trained sonographers to perform the initial assessments that provide an accurate diagnosis. However, although there have been advances in research in the field of teleultrasonography, studies addressing the training of medical or technical personnel are scarce. In our review, only 5% of the literature on teleultrasonography evaluated education and training of operators. Yet these studies did not systematically quantify the degree to which the professionals involved had improved.

A study in Italy reported that, in relation to the use of teleultrasonography, at least one month of didactic and hands-on training should be performed by operators to ensure that they have acquired sufficient technical competence [30]. Other authors recommended that training should be performed in the workplace of the local doctors by radiologists or sonologists who will evaluate and interpret the images [10, 13, 24]. A more recent study proposed that remote guidance by a specialist be given in real time to instruct inexperienced doctors in acquiring and visualizing the appropriate planes during examinations. The authors considered this educational tool superior to verbal instruction while training doctors at a distance because it enables new skills to be acquired in half the time required using traditional educational practices [15].

Currently, there are no standard training protocols for sonographers in remote locations. To ensure a greater degree of quality control, the images produced locally should be continuously examined via the Internet by competent radiologists and sonologists to ensure that they are following the proper scanning protocols and that the images contain sufficient diagnostic value [3, 4]. The teleultrasonography and other forms of telemedicine continue to grow; it is important that high quality standards be maintained, or its use may be detrimental to the population. The establishment of a framework to address and examine telemedical errors has been proposed to ensure high levels of quality and safety [31]. Regarding teleultrasonography, gaps in quality include inappropriate scanning protocols, improper scanning technique, inadequate image collection, incomplete examinations, false diagnoses, and nondiagnoses [3, 4, 15].

8. Clinical Utility

A significant portion of teleultrasonography research has focused on its use on an outpatient basis with emphasis on the areas of obstetrics and fetal medicine, especially to confirm pregnancy, monitor fetal growth, and evaluate pregnancy related complications such as placenta previa or placenta accreta.

An increasing number of new applications for teleultrasonography have included investigations of almost every organ and system in various medical fields, including the diagnosis of clinical or surgical conditions, examining severely ill patients and guided procedures [2, 15]. In recent years, many systems have been developed for the paramedic care of trauma patients, both at the scene of an accident and during transport to the hospital, allowing medical teams to adequately prepare to perform required emergency procedures before the patient's arrival [17]. Despite the persistence of barriers in implementing teleultrasonography more broadly and routinely in the initial care administered at the site of trauma, the advances in telecommunications, Internet signal processing, and the high resolution currently available

for portable ultrasound equipment increase the scope of applications for teleultrasonography [29]. The remaining technical and logistical barriers are being solved on a daily basis and include improving the availability of telecommunications in desired areas, the reception and analysis of the images, and the training of medical professionals involved in transmission [4].

Several studies on teleultrasonography in remote areas of Australia and Canada have demonstrated its usefulness in gestational and fetal heart examinations [2]. However, most of these studies demonstrated a good correlation between diagnoses made locally and those made remotely [7, 21, 22, 24, 32–34]. One example of this correlation was reported in studies conducted in Queensland, Australia. This state, which had a population of 3.3 million, 55% of whom lived in rural areas, only had two specialized fetal-maternal echography centers, which were located at universities in the capital, Brisbane. The implementation of a teleultrasonography service showed good diagnostic accuracy and identified all of the existing fetal abnormalities in the cases examined. Clinicians for these patients stated that, in the absence of teleultrasonography, they would have sent 1/3 of these patients to the closest specialized ultrasonography center, which was located 1500 km away [13, 14, 35].

A similar study was conducted to review the usefulness, accuracy, and benefits of teleultrasonography in primary care hospitals in South Dakota (USA) that care for neonates with suspected congenital heart disease. Two primary hospitals established a telemedicine link with a tertiary center. A pediatric cardiologist interpreted the neonatal teleultrasound images, and the results and recommendations of the specialist were immediately reported to the attending physicians. The study concluded that teleultrasonography could accurately distinguish between neonates who needed immediate cardiac care and those with less critical heart disease, thereby providing immediate diagnoses and appropriate care [36].

9. Future Directions

Although it is clear that ultrasonography is an easily adaptable imaging technology, especially for use in developing countries, the mere presence of the equipment does not indicate improvements in patient care [17]. With the continuous development and democratization of the Internet and other information technologies, teleultrasonography has the potential to assist in the provision of specialist services to remote locations. In addition to typical teleultrasonography applications in routine clinical practice, emergency interventional procedures guided by teleultrasonography, such as thoracocentesis, pericardiocentesis, and paracentesis, are already being used experimentally in intensive care units. The routine use of these and other innovations should result in overall improvements in patient care in remote and isolated regions [17].

The future for the application of teleultrasound is potentially enormous, both for the developed countries and for the developing ones. Several efforts have been made in order to increase the simplification of the ultrasound equipment,

TABLE 1: Main findings about the published articles about teleultrasound.

Reference number	Author	Title and journal	Year	Main findings
[1]	World Health Organization–WHO	Telemedicine: opportunities and developments in Member States. Reports on the Second Global Survey on eHealth 2009. HYPERLINK "http://www.who.int/goe/publications/goe_telemedicine_2010.pdf"	2009	(1) Teleradiology currently has a 33% rate of established service provision globally. (2) While developing countries are more likely to consider resource issues such as high costs, underdeveloped infrastructure, and lack of technical expertise to be barriers to telemedicine, developed countries are more likely to consider legal issues surrounding patient privacy and confidentiality, competing health system priorities, and a perceived lack of demand to be barriers to telemedicine implementation. (3) Following the analysis of the survey results, WHO recommends steps member states can take to capitalize on the potential of ICTs. One such step is creation of national agencies to coordinate telemedicine and eHealth initiatives, ensuring they are appropriate to local contexts, cost-effective, consistently evaluated, and adequately funded as part of integrated health service delivery. Ultimately telemedicine initiatives should strengthen rather than compete with other health services.
[2]	Law and Macbeth	Ultrasound: From Earth to Space. MJM 2011; 13(2): 59–65.	2011	Ultrasound is a well-proven diagnostic modality on Earth and is becoming increasingly useful in space. Ultrasound shows much promise in benefitting both astronauts and patients on Earth.
[3]	Sutherland et al.	A comparison of telesonography with standard ultrasound care in a rural Dominican clinic. J Telemed Telecare. 2009; 15(4): 191–5.	2009	The pilot study demonstrated that store-and-forward telesonography reduced time of diagnosis and increased the continuity of care compared to the usual ultrasound referral system in the region of the Dominican Republic which was studied.
[4]	Sutherland et al.	Telesonography: foundations and future directions. J Ultrasound Med. 2011; 30(4): 517–22.	2011	Future projects may use telesonography to supplement the training of health care providers in remote locations in an effort to establish permanent sonography services for their respective communities.
[5]	Popov et al.	The feasibility of realtime transmission of sonographic images from a remote location over lowbandwidth Internet links: a pilot study. AJR Am J Roentgenol. 2007; 188(3): 219–22.	2007	Real-time transmission of sonographic images over low bandwidth Internet links offers the potential for sonography to be performed at a remote underdeveloped region and interpreted in real time at a distant site by trained radiologists, thereby extending the presence of physicians in virtual space.
[6]	Hersh et al.	The evidence base of telemedicine. J Telemed Telecare. 2006; 12(Suppl 2): S1-2.	2006	
[7]	Ferrer-Roca et al.	Tele-virtual sonography. J Perinat Med. 2006; 34(2): 123–9.	2006	(1) 3D reconstruction could reduce multiple explorations due to image constrains such as suboptimal fetal positioning among others. (2) Virtual sonography was important to reach confidence on distant diagnosis. (3) It was also considered a tool for offline local review of nontrained sonographer acquisitions.
[8]	Kasmai	Realtime Telesonography: Vision or Reality? Ultrasound. 2006;14(3): 152–4.	2006	It is now possible to configure and set up a streaming telesonography service with minimum cost and effort.

TABLE 1: Continued.

Reference number	Author	Title and journal	Year	Main findings
[9]	Afset and Lunde	Tele-echocardiography. Education in echocardiography via video conferences. Tidsskr Nor Laegeforen. 1994; 114(10): 1175–8.	1994	Teleechocardiography is a method that is suitable for basic training in echocardiography and the diagnostic precision is sufficient for the method to be applied clinically.
[43]	Afset et al.	Accuracy of routine echocardiographic measurements made by an inexperienced examiner through tele-instruction. J Telemed Telecare. 1996; 2(3): 148–54.	1996	The reproducibility and accuracy of routine echocardiographic measurements made by an inexperienced doctor using teleinstruction were comparable to those observed in reproducibility studies made under normal examination conditions. There were no systematic measurement errors. Teleinstructed echocardiography is also an excellent educational tool, allowing an inexperienced examiner gradually to take responsibility for the local echocardiographic service.
[44]	Trippi et al.	Emergency echocardiography telemedicine: an efficient method to provide 24-hour consultative echocardiography. J Am Coll Cardiol. 1996; 27(7): 1748–52.	1996	
[45]	Mulholland et al.	Application of a low cost telemedicine link to the diagnosis of neonatal congenital heart defects by remote consultation. Heart. 1999; 82(2): 217–21.	1999	Transmitted images were of sufficient quality to allow confirmation or exclusion of major congenital heart disease. The telemedicine link facilitated early diagnosis and initiation of appropriate management in patients with complex congenital heart disease and avoided the need for transfer in those where significant congenital heart disease was excluded.
[21]	Wootton et al.	The effect of transmission bandwidth on diagnostic accuracy in remote fetal ultrasound scanning. J Telemed Telecare. 1997; 3(4): 209–14.	1997	A study which found that, although there were no perceived differences in technical quality between recordings transmitted at 384 or 1920 kbit/s, diagnostic accuracy was marginally worse at the lower bandwidth. This suggests that the higher bandwidth conveys more detail and information to the observer, which in turn enables more accurate diagnosis. However, further work is required before a definitive choice can be made about the optimum transmission bandwidth for remote fetal ultrasound studies.
[22]	Hussain et al.	Evaluation of a training and diagnostic ultrasound service for general practitioners using narrowband ISDN. J Telemed Telecare. 1999; 5(Suppl1): S95–9.	1999	A pilot study which demonstrated that store-and-forward images are far superior to hard-copy images for technical quality.
[23]	Brebner et al.	The diagnostic acceptability of low-bandwidth transmission for tele-ultrasound. J Telemed Telecare. 2000; 6(6): 335–8.	2000	The quality of dynamic ultrasound images transmitted at 384 kbit/s was diagnostically acceptable but was unsatisfactory at 128 kbit/s.
[10]	Hussain et al.	The feasibility of telemedicine for the training and supervision of general practitioners performing ultrasound examinations of patients with urinary tract symptoms. J Telemed Telecare. 2004; 10(3): 180–2.	2004	Forwarded images were superior to hard-copy images.
[11]	Adambounou et al.	System of telesonography with synchronous teleconsultations and nchronous telediagnoses. Med Sante Trop. 2012; 22(1): 54–60.	2012	A successful pilot trial of a low cost synchronous teleultrasound system in a developing country.
[12]	Meuwly	Telesonography-Modern Solutions for an old Question. Ultraschall in Med 2010; 31(4): 421–3.	2010	As volume US acquisition seems to be rather independent of the skill of the local operator, asynchronous remote interpretation of reconstructed images from volume data sets appears to be a well-appropriate technical solution for telesonography, provided that suitable workstations for postprocessing will be available.
[13]	Chan et al.	Randomized comparison of the quality of realtime fetal ultrasound images transmitted by ISDN and by IP video conference. J Telemed Telecare. 2002; 8(2): 91–6.	2002	We compared the quality of real-time fetal ultrasound images transmitted using ISDN and IP networks. There were no significant interobserver variations. The most significant variable affecting the mean score was the bandwidth used. IP transmission in a private (nonshared) network is an acceptable alternative to ISDN for fetal teleultrasound and one deserving further study.
[14]	Lewis	A tele-ultrasound needs analysis in Queensland. J Telemed Telecare. 2006; 11(Suppl 2): S61–4.	2006	A teleultrasound needs analysis in Queensland which found that approximately 10% of cases would have benefited from telesonography and that there was a strong preference for store and forward transmission.

TABLE 1: Continued.

Reference number	Author	Title and journal	Year	Main findings
[15]	Sheehan et al.	Expert visual guidance of ultrasound for Telemedicine. J Telemed Telecare. 2010; 16(2): 77–82.	2010	An inexperienced ultrasonographer can be significantly assisted by EVG compared to verbal instruction alone. This could be useful for telementoring in rural hospitals as well as for teaching, both in person and at a remote site.
[16]	Yoo et al.	Performance of a web-based, realtime, tele-ultrasound consultations system over highspeed commercial telecommunications lines. J Telemed Telecare.2004; 10: 175–9.	2004	A Web-based, real-time teleultrasound consultation system was designed and tested by radiologists. A bit rate of more than 0.6 Mbit/s, at 30 frames/s, is suggested as the threshold for the maintenance of diagnostic image quality.
[17]	Pian et al.	Potential Use of Remote Telesonography as a Transformational Technology in Underresourced and/or Remote Settings. Emergency Medicine International. 2013. Article ID 986160, 9 pages. HYPERLINK "http://dx.doi.org/10.1155/2013/986160"	2013	This paper summarizes the current literature surrounding the development of teleultrasound as a transformational technology and its application to underresourced settings.
[18]	Ferlin et al.	Tele-obstetric ultrasound: analysis of first-trimester ultrasound images transmitted in realtime. J Telemed Telecare. 2012; 18(1): 54–8.	2012	Teleobstetric ultrasound: analysis of first-trimester ultrasound images transmitted in real-time; the quality of images transmitted via the Internet through the use of low-cost software appeared suitable for screening for chromosomal abnormalities in the first trimester of pregnancy.
[19]	Paulus and Thompson	Inexpensive, realtime teleultrasound using a commercial, web-based video streaming device. J Telemed Telecare. 2012; 18: 185–8.	2012	System was feasible; response times increased with increasing distance.
[20]	Bassignani et al.	Review of technology: planning for the development of telesonography. J Digital Imaging. 2004; 17(1): 18–27.	2004	With less compression, the bit rate rises, and the only way the encoder can contain bit rate within the set bandwidth is by lowering frame rate or reducing image quality. Review the relevant technologies and industry standard components that will enable low-cost telesonography.
[24]	Chan et al.	Realtime fetal ultrasound by telemedicine in Queensland. A successful venture? J Telemed Telecare. 2001; 7(Suppl 2): 7–11.	2001	A real-time fetal teleultrasound consultation service in Queensland, which uses ISDN transmission at 384 kbit/s, 1500 km away. All significant anomalies and diagnoses have been confirmed. A crude cost-benefit calculation suggests that the teleultrasound service resulted in a net saving which enabled almost four times the number of consultations to be carried out.
[25]	O'Neill et al.	The design and implementation of an off-the-shelf, standards-based tele-ultrasound system. J Telemed Telecare. 2000; 6(Suppl 2): S52–3.	2000	A feasible DICOM system, synchronous.
[26]	Arbeille et al.	Use of a robotic arm to perform remote abdominal telesonography. AJR Am J Roentgenol. 2007; 188(4): 317–22.	2007	Robotic telesonography can be used for reliable diagnosis without moving the patient. No false diagnoses were made in this study. A bandwidth of 250 Kbps via integrated services digital network or satellite is required for reliable diagnosis.
[27]	Courreges et al.	Clinical trials and evaluation of a mobile, robotic tele-ultrasound system. J Telemed Telecare. 2005; 11 Suppl 1: 46–9.	2005	Feasibility of a robotic teleultrasound system.
[28]	Martini et al.	A Cross-Layer Approach for Wireless Medical Video Streaming in Robotic Teleultrasonography. IEEE Eng Med Bio Conference.2007 (EMBC 2007), Lyon, France, August 2007.	2007	Successful performance of video streaming in a robotic teleultrasonography system through a cross-layer approach based on tailor made controller structures is presented.
[29]	Fuentes	Remote interpretation of ultrasound images. Clin Obstet Gynecol. 2003; 46(4): 878–81.	2003	In the near future, the ability to transmit volume rendered images over standard phone lines will enhance the application of telesonography.
[30]	Cavina et al.	Telesonography: technical problems, solutions and results in the routine utilization from remote areas. Studies Health Technol Informatics. 2001; 81: 81–9.	2001	

TABLE 1: Continued.

Reference number	Author	Title and journal	Year	Main findings
[31]	Demiris et al.	To telemedically err is human. Joint Commission. J Quality Safe. 2004; 30(9): 521–7.	2004	To address patient safety and provide high-quality care, a framework for addressing and examining telemedical errors needs to be established.
[32]	Lagalla	Telecommunications, health and radiology: potential synergies for the new millennium. Radiol Med. 2001; 102(1-2): 14–9.	2001	Italian paper to highlight the potentialities and limitations in the use of teleradiology and to provide a set of recommendations/guidelines.
[33]	Soong et al.	The fetal tele-ultrasound project in Queensland. Aust Health Rev. 2002; 25(3): 57–73.	2002	We report on some of our practical experiences and difficulties in establishing such a service.
[34]	Arbeille et al.	Fetal-tele-ecography using a robotic arm and a satellite link. Ultrasound Obstet Gynecol. 2005; 26(3): 221–6.	2005	Teleechography using a robotic arm provides the main information needed to assess fetal growth and the intrauterine environment within a limited period of time.
[36]	Awadallah et al.	Tele-echocardiography in neonates: utility and benefits in South Dakota primary care hospitals. S D Med. 2006; 59(3): 97–100.	2006	A study of teleechocardiography to assess neonates with suspected congenital heart disease. Teleechocardiography accurately distinguished neonates who required tertiary cardiac care from those with less critical cardiac disease fostering prompt diagnosis and appropriate care while subjecting a minimal number of patients to costly emergency transport.
[37]	Crawford et al.	How to set up a low-cost teleultrasound capable videoconference system with wide applicability. Critical Ultrasound J. 2012; 4: 13.	2012	A functional remote telementored ultrasound (RTUS) system was constructed with a laptop computer wireless Internet and/or was tethered through a smartphone. The RTUS system allowed real-time mentored teleultrasound to be conducted from a variety of settings via VOIP transmissions. Numerous types of ultrasound examinations were conducted such as abdominal and thoracic examinations with a variety of users mentored who had previous skills ranging from none to expert. Internet connectivity was rarely a limiting factor, with competing logistical and scheduling demands of the participants predominating.
[38]	Su et al.	Application of Tele-Ultrasound in Emergency Medical Services. Telemed e-Health. 2008; 14(8): 816–24.	2008	This study describes the development of teleultrasound for prediagnosis in a medical emergency setting which will enhance prediagnosis options for on-duty emergency physicians; emergency medical technicians can also obtain instructions from on-duty physicians to enhance damage and disaster control ability in critical moments.
[39]	Wootton	Telemedicine in the National Health Service. J Roy Soc Med 1998; 91: 614–21.	1998	Having become technically and economically feasible, telemedicine deserves investigation by well-conducted research, which is adequately funded.
[40]	World Health Organization	Telemedicine: opportunities and developments in member states report. In Second Global Survey on eHealth Global Observatory for eHealth Series. 2011, vol 2. WHO Press, Switzerland.	2011	

increasing their portability. These advances open new areas of potential applications [37]. In the future, these technologies will be common place and will be first-use technologies, providing rapid and accurate diagnoses and improving the quality of patient care, especially in remote communities [11]. These technologies have led some scholars to consider the tool of teleultrasonography as the "stethoscope of the future" [38].

The routine use of portable ultrasound equipment allied to technological advances may be used for educational purposes in practically any place in the world, providing training of quality and permanent updating for ultrasonography professionals living in remote or needy regions. These innovations combined with educational strategies and the introduction of strict training protocols for health care workers, primarily but not exclusively in remote communities, will allow teleultrasonography to be definitively established as an effective tool in health care and an important tool in educating and training individuals working with ultrasonography. With increased use of ultrasonography, the need for education and training of users becomes clear.

Notably, teleultrasonography has been studied very little for its use in the continuing education of health care providers. Future studies should be conducted not only to quantify the results of patient care but also to measure the degree of training of the professionals involved because performing supervised ultrasound examinations can be used as a tool for a second opinion, encouraging continuous and gradual improvement.

10. Barriers to the Implementation of Clinical Teleultrasound

In the 90s, Wooton summarized the critical questions that needed to be approached in order to develop a plan for the implementation of telemedicine: to evaluate the necessary structural changes to incorporate technology, develop an education and training process and formulate guidelines, quality control, and continuous audit [39]. These questions also apply to teleultrasound and are up-to-date even nowadays.

Teleultrasound is a specific type of telemedicine that uses the technological advances for the remote interpretation of ultrasound images. Nevertheless, software, hardware, and/or video-conferences platforms that are necessary for the transmission of images are still highly costly which is one of the main barriers for its implementation in the developing countries [37, 40].

Secondly, although the technological barriers for the development of teleultrasound are continuously disappearing, the nontechnological ones still persist. These barriers include deficits in training and operational protocols, complexity in the use of equipment, and concerns regarding the security and, by extension, the confidentiality of electronically transmitted information [3, 4, 41, 42].

Table 1 summarizes the main findings of published articles about teleultrasound.

11. Conclusions

Teleultrasound is a valuable addition to remote medical care for isolated populations with limited access to tertiary healthcare facilities. As some studies point out, the portability and the low cost of the equipment frequently make ultrasonography the only modality of image test available in remote places. The implementation of teleechography in remote or needy places allows for more timely detection of problems, facilitates the obtaining of a second opinion, and reduces the costs of moving. Educational strategies for health agents in remote or needy locations must be continuously researched and developed with the purpose of standardizing training protocols and providing quality assistance to these populations.

References

[1] World Health Organization, "Telemedicine: opportunities and developments in Member States. Reports on the Second Global Survey on eHealth," 2009, http://www.who.int/goe/publications/goe_telemedicine_2010.pdf.

[2] J. Law and P. B. Macbeth, "Ultrasound: from earth to space," McGill Journal of Medicine, vol. 13, no. 2, pp. 59–65, 2011.

[3] J. E. Sutherland, H. D. Sutphin, F. Rawlins, K. Redican, and J. Burton, "A comparison of telesonography with standard ultrasound care in a rural Dominican clinic," Journal of Telemedicine and Telecare, vol. 15, no. 4, pp. 191–195, 2009.

[4] J. E. Sutherland, D. Sutphin, K. Redican, and F. Rawlins, "Telesonography: foundations and future directions," Journal of Ultrasound in Medicine, vol. 30, no. 4, pp. 517–522, 2011.

[5] V. Popov, D. Popov, I. Kacar, and R. D. Harris, "The feasibility of real-time transmission of sonographic images from a remote location over low-bandwidth Internet links: a pilot study," The American Journal of Roentgenology, vol. 188, no. 3, pp. W219–W222, 2007.

[6] W. R. Hersh, D. H. Hickam, and M. Erlichman, "The evidence base of telemedicine: overview of the supplement.," Journal of Telemedicine and Telecare, vol. 12, pp. S1–S2, 2006.

[7] O. Ferrer-Roca, A. Kurjak, J. M. Troyano-Luque, J. B. Arenas, A. L. Mercé, and A. Diaz-Cardama, "Tele-virtual sonography," Journal of Perinatal Medicine, vol. 34, no. 2, pp. 123–129, 2006.

[8] B. Kasmai, "Realtime telesonography: vision or reality?" Ultrasound, vol. 14, no. 3, pp. 152–154, 2006.

[9] J. E. Afset and P. Lunde, "Tele-echocardiography. Education in echocardiography via video conferences," Tidsskrift for den Norske Laegeforening, vol. 114, no. 10, pp. 1175–1178, 1994.

[10] P. Hussain, A. Deshpande, P. Shridhar, G. Saini, and D. Kay, "The feasibility of telemedicine for the training and supervision of general practitioners performing ultrasound examinations of patients with urinary tract symptoms," Journal of Telemedicine and Telecare, vol. 10, no. 3, pp. 180–182, 2004.

[11] K. Adambounou, F. Farin, A. Boucher et al., "System of tel-esonography with synchronous teleconsultations and asynchronous telediagnoses," *Medecine et Sante Tropicales*, vol. 22, no. 1, pp. 54–60, 2012.

[12] J.-Y. Meuwly, "Telesonography—modern solutions for an old question," *Ultraschall in der Medizin*, vol. 31, no. 4, pp. 421–423, 2010.

[13] F. Y. Chan, A. Taylor, B. Soong et al., "Randomized comparison of the quality of realtime fetal ultrasound images transmitted by ISDN and by IP video conference," *Journal of Telemedicine and Telecare*, vol. 8, no. 2, pp. 91–96, 2002.

[14] C. Lewis, "A tele-ultrasound needs analysis in Queensland," *Journal of Telemedicine and Telecare*, vol. 11, pp. S61–S64, 2006.

[15] F. H. Sheehan, M. A. Ricci, C. Murtagh, H. Clark, and E. L. Bolson, "Expert visual guidance of ultrasound for telemedicine," *Journal of Telemedicine and Telecare*, vol. 16, no. 2, pp. 77–82, 2010.

[16] S. K. Yoo, D. K. Kim, S. M. Jung, E.-K. Kim, J. S. Lim, and J. H. Kim, "Performance of a Web-based, realtime, tele-ultrasound consultation system over high-speed commercial telecommunication lines," *Journal of Telemedicine and Telecare*, vol. 10, no. 3, pp. 175–179, 2004.

[17] L. Pian, L. M. Gillman, P. B. McBeth et al., "Potential use of remote telesonography as a transformational technology in underresourced and/or remote settings," *Emergency Medicine International*, vol. 2013, Article ID 986160, 9 pages, 2013.

[18] R. M. Ferlin, D. M. Vaz-Oliani, A. C. Ferreira, E. G. Tristão, and A. H. Oliani, "Tele-obstetric ultrasound: analysis of first-trimester ultrasound images transmitted in realtime," *Journal of Telemedicine and Telecare*, vol. 18, no. 1, pp. 54–58, 2012.

[19] Y. M. Paulus and N. P. Thompson, "Inexpensive, realtime tele-ultrasound using a commercial, web-based video streaming device," *Journal of Telemedicine and Telecare*, vol. 18, no. 4, pp. 185–188, 2012.

[20] M. J. Bassignani, S. J. Dwyer III, J. M. Ciambotti et al., "Review of technology: planning for the development of telesonography," *Journal of Digital Imaging*, vol. 17, no. 1, pp. 18–27, 2004.

[21] R. Wootton, J. Dornan, N. M. Fisk et al., "The effect of transmission bandwidth on diagnostic accuracy in remote fetal ultrasound scanning," *Journal of Telemedicine and Telecare*, vol. 3, no. 4, pp. 209–214, 1997.

[22] P. Hussain, D. Melville, R. Mannings, D. Curry, D. Kay, and P. Ford, "Evaluation of a training and diagnostic ultrasound service for general practitioners using narrowband ISDN," *Journal of Telemedicine and Telecare*, vol. 5, pp. S95–S99, 1999.

[23] J. A. Brebner, H. Ruddick-Bracken, E. M. Brebner et al., "The diagnostic acceptability of low-bandwidth transmission for tele-ultrasound," *Journal of Telemedicine and Telecare*, vol. 6, no. 6, pp. 335–338, 2000.

[24] F. Y. Chan, B. Soong, D. Watson, and J. Whitehall, "Realtime fetal ultrasound by telemedicine in Queensland. A successful venture?" *Journal of Telemedicine and Telecare*, vol. 7, no. 2, pp. S7–S11, 2001.

[25] S. K. O'Neill, D. Allen, and P. D. Brockway, "The design and implementation of an off-the-shelf, standards-based tele-ultrasound system.," *Journal of Telemedicine and Telecare*, vol. 6, pp. S52–S53, 2000.

[26] P. Arbeille, A. Capri, J. Ayoub, V. Kieffer, M. Georgescu, and G. Poisson, "Use of a robotic arm to perform remote abdominal telesonography," *The American Journal of Roentgenology*, vol. 188, no. 4, pp. 317–322, 2007.

[27] F. Courreges, P. Vieyres, R. S. H. Istepanian, P. Arbeille, and C. Bru, "Clinical trials and evaluation of a mobile, robotic tele-ultrasound system," *Journal of Telemedicine and Telecare*, vol. 11, no. 1, pp. S46–S49, 2005.

[28] M. G. Martini, R. S. Istepanian, M. Mazzotti, and N. Philip, "A cross-layer approach for wireless medical video streaming in robotic teleultrasonography," in *Proceedings of the 29th Annual International Conference of the IEEE Engineering in Medicine and Biology Society (EMBS '07)*, pp. 3082–3085, Lyon, France, August 2007.

[29] A. Fuentes, "Remote interpretation of ultrasound images," *Clinical Obstetrics & Gynecology*, vol. 46, no. 4, pp. 878–881, 2003.

[30] E. Cavina, O. Goletti, P. V. Lippolis, and G. Zocco, *Telesonography: Technical Problems, Solutions and Results in the Routine Utilization From Remote Areas*, vol. 81 of *Studies in Health Technology and Informatics*, 2001.

[31] G. Demiris, T. B. Patrick, J. A. Mitchell, and S. E. Waldren, "To telemedically err is human," *Joint Commission Journal on Quality and Safety*, vol. 30, no. 9, pp. 521–527, 2004.

[32] R. Lagalla, "Telecommunications, health and radiology: potential synergies for the new millennium," *Radiologia Medica*, vol. 102, no. 1-2, pp. 14–19, 2001.

[33] B. Soong, F. Y. Chan, S. Bloomfield, M. Smith, and D. Watson, "The fetal tele-ultrasound project in Queensland," *Australian Health Review*, vol. 25, no. 3, pp. 67–73, 2002.

[34] P. Arbeille, J. Ruiz, P. Herve, M. Chevillot, G. Poisson, and F. Perrotin, "Fetal tele-echography using a robotic arm and a satellite link," *Ultrasound in Obstetrics and Gynecology*, vol. 26, no. 3, pp. 221–226, 2005.

[35] F. Y. Chan, B. Soong, D. Watson, and J. Whitehall, "Realtime fetal ultrasound by telemedicine in Queensland. A successful venture?" *Journal of Telemedicine and Telecare*, vol. 7, no. 2, pp. 7–11, 2001.

[36] S. Awadallah, I. Halaweish, and F. Kutayli, "Tele-echocardiography in neonates: utility and benefits in South Dakota primary care hospitals," *South Dakota Medicine*, vol. 59, no. 3, pp. 97–100, 2006.

[37] I. Crawford, P. B. McBeth, M. Mitchelson, J. Ferguson, C. Tiruta, and A. W. Kirkpatrick, "How to set up a low cost tele-ultrasound capable videoconferencing system with wide applicability," *Critical Ultrasound Journal*, vol. 4, no. 1, p. 13, 2012.

[38] M.-J. Su, H.-M. Ma, C.-I. Ko et al., "Application of tele-ultrasound in emergency medical services," *Telemedicine and e-Health*, vol. 14, no. 8, pp. 816–824, 2008.

[39] R. Wootton, "Telemedicine in the National Health Service," *Journal of the Royal Society of Medicine*, vol. 91, no. 12, pp. 614–621, 1998.

[40] World Health Organization, *Telemedicine: Opportunities and Developments in Member States Report*, vol. 2 of *Second Global Survey on eHealth Global Observatory for eHealth Series*, WHO Press, Geneva, Switzerland, 2011, http://www.who.int/goe/publications/goe_telemedicine_2010.pdf.

[41] J. G. Anderson, "Social, ethical and legal barriers to E-health," *International Journal of Medical Informatics*, vol. 76, no. 5-6, pp. 480–483, 2007.

[42] K. S. Rheuban, "The role of telemedicine in fostering health-care innovations to address problems of access, specialty shortages and changing patient care needs," *Journal of Telemedicine and Telecare*, vol. 12, no. 2, pp. S45–S150, 2006.

12

Application of Teledermoscopy in the Diagnosis of Pigmented Lesions

C. B. Barcaui[1] and P. M. O. Lima ⓘ[2]

[1]Adjunct Professor of Dermatology, Faculty of Medical Sciences, State University of Rio de Janeiro,
  PhD in Medicine (Dermatology), by University of São Paulo, Dermatology Department, Pedro Ernesto University Hospital,
  Rio de Janeiro State University, Rio de janeiro, Brazil
[2]Physician Residing in Dermatology, Department of Dermatology, Pedro Ernesto University Hospital, State University of Rio de Janeiro,
  Rio de Janeiro, Brazil

Correspondence should be addressed to P. M. O. Lima; priscillameloolima@gmail.com

Academic Editor: Aura Ganz

Background. Dermatology, due to the peculiar characteristic of visual diagnosis, is suitable for the application of modern telemedicine techniques, such as mobile teledermoscopy. *Objectives*. To evaluate the feasibility and reliability of the technique for the diagnosis of pigmented lesions. *Methods*. Through the storage and routing method, 41 pigmented lesions were analyzed. After the selection of the lesions during the outpatient visit, the clinical and dermatoscopic images were obtained by the resident physician through the cellphone camera and sent to the assistant dermatologist by means of an application for exchange of messages between mobile platforms. Firstly, the assistant dermatologist described the visualized dermatoscopic structures and defined its diagnosis and conduct, based solely on the evaluation of the clinical and dermatoscopic images, without having the knowledge of the anamnesis data. Afterwards, the same assistant dermatologist evaluated the patient face to face, defining the dermatoscopic structures, diagnosis, and conduct. The data obtained through teledermoscopy and face-to-face assessments were compared and accuracy was defined as the concordance between the diagnoses. *Results*. A match rate of 90% between teledermoscopic and face-to-face diagnosis was demonstrated (McNemar's statistical analysis, whose p value was 0.1366, showed no evidence to support the inferiority of the teledermoscopic method).

1. Introduction

The reduction of the morbidity and mortality of nonmelanoma skin cancer and melanoma is the greatest current challenge for dermatology and, within this context, this includes the early diagnosis of melanoma, dermatoscopy, teledermatology, and teledermoscopy.

Early diagnosis results in a better prognosis for the patient (thin, <1mm, nonulcerated melanomas have a 95% survival rate within 5 years, whereas Breslow ulcerated melanomas> 4mm and lymph node metastasis have only 24% survival at 5 years), and dermoscopy is essential, since it consists of a more accurate method for the diagnosis of melanoma than the naked eye one, increasing the detection of early-stage melanoma by up to 49% [1].

Dermatology, due to the peculiar characteristic of visual diagnosis, is ideal for the application of modern telemedicine techniques, with several recent studies proving the viability and reliability of teledermatology and, in particular, teledermoscopy, with high levels of concordance in diagnosis and management plan in relation to face-to-face consultation [2].

The World Health Organization defines telemedicine as the use of health communication technologies for the exchange of medical information for diagnosis, treatment, prevention, research, evaluation, and education. One of the existent ways of telemedicine is teledermatology, which is already well established, whose publications began in 1995 and these ones have been growing exponentially. Within teledermatology, teledermoscopy appears as a promising area for the diagnosis and management of pigmented skin lesions, early detection of skin cancer, and screening [2].

Teledermatology has two distinct operation models, the synchronous, through videoconference and satellite communication, which occurs in real time and the asynchronous, through a storage and routing system, including the use of e-mail, web, and mobile teledermatology, and which provides high levels of diagnostic accuracy, with lower cost, greater convenience, and practicality [3].

Storage and routing teledermatology are constantly growing around the world with improvements in communication and imaging technologies, allowing expert judgment in situations in which access to a dermatologist might be difficult due to geographic distance or excessive demand.

Mobile teledermoscopy consists of a new application of teledermatology, in which clinical and dermatoscopic images are captured and transmitted by mobile devices (e.g., smartphones, tablets) [4]. The image quality of these devices has been improved and no longer represents a barrier in teledermatology [5].

In this mobile teledermoscopy study, the first one developed in Brazil, we aimed to study the feasibility and reliability of the technique for the dermatological diagnosis of pigmented lesions.

2. Methods

Patients were prospectively selected from the outpatient clinic of the Department of Dermatology from April to June 2017. The inclusion criteria consisted of men or women, of any age, with pigmented lesions, whether melanocytic or not. After the selection of the lesions during the outpatient visit, the clinical and dermatoscopic images were obtained by the resident physician and sent to the assistant dermatologist before face-to-face assessment.

The clinical images were obtained using the cell phone camera (Iphone 6 model A1549, with an integrated camera of 8 megapixels, resolution 3264x2448 pixel, digital stabilization, autofocus and without flash, with a good natural lighting) in two panoramic and macromodes (at an established distance of 20 cm from the lesion to be further studied). The dermatoscope which has been used was DermLite DL4 from 3Gen®, San Juan Capistrano, CA 92675, USA; and, for the acquisition of the dermatoscopic images, the camera lens was applied to the DermoLite® MagnetiConnect TM device of the 3Gen® Connection Kit for iPhone6 P / N: DLCKi6-MC, San Juan Capistrano, CA 92675, USA, with the dermatoscope at position 0, in polarized mode, without making use of flash or zoom camera assets. To the large lesions, we performed more than one dermatoscopic image.

At first, the images were sent via WhatsApp Messenger, a free messaging application available for the iPhone and other platforms, to the assistant dermatologist with extensive experience in dermatoscopy, which described the dermatoscopic structures visualized, as well as the analysis of patterns, when these ones were applicable; and the diagnosis and procedures were defined, based only on the evaluation of the clinical and dermatoscopic images, without the knowledge of the anamnesis data.

At the second moment, the same assistant dermatologist evaluated the patient face-to-face, using the same dermatoscope and having access to anamnesis data (sex, age, location and time of the injury evolution, local symptoms, personal or family history of melanoma, comorbidities, and relevant aspects of the anamnesis), defining the dermatoscopic structures and / or pattern analysis, diagnosis, and procedures.

The data obtained through teledermoscopy and face-to-face examinations were compared, the differences between them being analyzed and what was essential being defined, in face-to-face examination, for decision-making. The face-to-face examination was defined as the gold standard for the final procedure. The diagnostic accuracy was defined as the agreement between the teledermoscopic diagnosis and the gold standard. Clinical and dermatoscopic face-to-face diagnoses were considered suitable in patients with clinically and teledermoscopically benign and nonsuspected lesions and no biopsy procedure was performed. The lesions considered malignant or suspicious were studied histopathologically and were correlated with clinical-dermatoscopic diagnosis.

The diagnostic agreement between teledermatology/teledermoscopy and face-to-face assessment was calculated using the McNemar test, hypothesis test for paired data. This test works with two hypotheses: the null hypothesis, in which there is no difference between the representativeness between the diagnoses by the two methods and the alternative hypothesis, in which there is statistical difference. At the significance level of 5% (0.05), the null hypothesis is accepted when the p value is greater than 0.05.

3. Results

Forty-one lesions were studied in 31 patients, 22 females, and 9 males. The mean age was 56.5 years (11 to 78 years). The lesions were present for an average duration of 80.4 months (from 1 day to 40 years), excluding those not specifically determined, only reported as present ones since childhood or as time of unknown onset. The specific locations included back (11 lesions), hand (7 including palmar lesion), malar (4), upper eyelid (2), cervical (2), thorax (2), breast (2), thigh, plantar (2), infraorbital (1), temporal (1), nose (1), retroauricular (1), armpit (1), abdomen (1), and leg (1 lesion). Eight patients reported local symptoms in the lesions, which consisted of growth (4), bleeding (1), color change (2), and pruritus (1). No patient had previous history of melanoma, one of whom had a personal history of basal cell carcinoma and one that had a family history of melanoma (first degree relative). Nineteen patients reported comorbidities: psoriasis (3), systemic arterial hypertension (8), diabetes (3), bullous lupus (1), cystic fibrosis (1), renal transplantation (1), and Sjogren's syndrome (1). We highlight other relevant aspects in the anamnesis in 10 cases, which consisted of the use of immunosuppressants (2), immunobiological (1), smoking (1), outdoor work profession (1), contact with exogenous pigment (1), inflammatory pigmentation of the underlying disease (1), application of acid to the lesion (1), and nonapplication of acid to the lesion (1).

From the clinical images obtained, two were reported by the teledermatologist as not perfectly made ones in focus and

TABLE 1: Teledermoscopic and face-to-face diagnostics.

	Teledermoscopy	Face to face
Lesion 1	Pigmented basal cell carcinoma	Pigmented basal cell carcinoma
Lesion 2	Intradermal melanocytic nevus	Intradermal melanocytic nevus
Lesion 3	Intradermal melanocytic nevus	Intradermal melanocytic nevus
Lesion 4	Intradermal melanocytic nevus	Intradermal melanocytic nevus
Lesion 5	Intradermal melanocytic nevus	Intradermal melanocytic nevus
Lesion 6	Solar lentigo / seborrheic keratosis	Solar lentigo / seborrheic keratosis
Lesion 7	Benign melanocytic lesion	Benign melanocytic lesion
Lesion 8	Blue nevus	Blue nevus
Lesion 9	Intracorneal hematoma	Exogenous pigmentation
Lesion 10	Atypical melanocytic nevus	Atypical melanocytic nevus
Lesion 11	Intradermal nevus	Intradermal nevus
Lesion 12	Blue nevus	Blue nevus
Lesion 13	Seborrheic keratosis	Seborrheic keratosis
Lesion 14	Benign melanocytic lesion	Benign melanocytic lesion
Lesion 15	Benign melanocytic lesion	Benign melanocytic lesion
Lesion 16	Suspected melanocytic lesion	Benign melanocytic lesion
Lesion 17	Benign melanocytic lesion	Benign melanocytic lesion
Lesion 18	Pigmented basal cell carcinoma	Pigmented basal cell carcinoma
Lesion 19	Dermatofibroma	Dermatofibroma
Lesion 20	Intradermal nevus	Intradermal nevus
Lesion 21	Melanoma or atypical melanocytic nevus	Melanoma or atypical melanocytic nevus
Lesion 22	Seborrheic keratosis	Seborrheic keratosis
Lesion 23	Solar lentigo associated with blue nevus or melanocytic lesion with homogeneous eccentric pigmentation	Solar lentigo associated with blue nevus
Lesion 24	Benign melanocytic lesion	Benign melanocytic lesion
Lesion 25	Melanoma	Pigmented basal cell carcinoma
Lesion 26	Solar lentigo / seborrheic keratosis	Solar lentigo / seborrheic keratosis
Lesion 27	Congenital nevus	Congenital nevus
Lesion 28	Solar lentigo	Solar lentigo
Lesion 29	Melanoma	Melanoma
Lesion 30	Benign melanocytic lesion	Benign melanocytic lesion
Lesion 31	Benign melanocytic lesion	Benign melanocytic lesion
Lesion 32	Melanoma	Melanoma
Lesion 33	Solar lentigo	Solar lentigo
Lesion 34	Benign melanocytic lesion	Benign melanocytic lesion
Lesion 35	Pigmented basal cell carcinoma	Pigmented basal cell carcinoma
Lesion 36	Benign melanocytic lesion	Benign melanocytic lesion
Lesion 37	Benign melanocytic lesion	Benign melanocytic lesion
Lesion 38	Benign melanocytic lesion	Benign melanocytic lesion
Lesion 39	Suspected melanocytic lesion	Benign melanocytic lesion
Lesion 40	Lentigo maligna	Lentigo maligna
Lesion 41	Benign melanocytic nevus	Benign melanocytic nevus

in one of the other cases there was an equivocal perception of the lesion size. All the dermatoscopic images were considered excellent.

There was no injury to the teleanalysis of the lesions in any of the cases. Teledermoscopic diagnoses and those established after face-to-face analysis are shown in Table 1 (lesions 1 to 41).

The teledermoscopic diagnoses were pigmented basal cell carcinoma (3), intradermal nevus (6), seborrheic keratosis (4), benign melanocytic lesion (12), blue nevus (3), intracorneal hematoma (1), atypical nevus melanocytic suspicion (2), dermatofibroma (1), congenital nevus (1), solar lentigo (2), and melanoma (4).

On the other hand, the face-to-face diagnoses consisted of pigmented basal cell carcinoma (4), intradermal nevus (6), seborrheic keratosis (4), benign melanocytic lesion (14), blue nevus (3), exogenous pigmentation atypical nevus (2), dermatofibroma (1), congenital nevus (1), solar lentigo (2), and melanoma (3).

The anatomopathological study was performed on 8 lesions and 4 pigmented basal cell carcinomas (lesions 1, 18, 25, and 35), 1 junctional melanocytic nevus (lesion 21), and 3 melanomas (lesions 29, 32, and 40) were found.

The agreement between the evaluations was 90%, and this reduction of 10 percentage points was not considered statistically significant, once there was no difference between the representativeness of the cases, since the p value was 0.1366. In other words, even though there is a reduction in concordance for teledermoscopy, there is insufficient statistical evidence to prove that this method is inferior, which can be considered equivalent to the traditional method (face-to-face assessment).

Discordant results included exogenous pigmentation, a pigmented basal cell carcinoma, and two benign melanocytic nevi.

The exogenous pigment lesion (lesion 9) was present 1 day ago in the right second finger of a 57-year-old female patient with a family history of melanoma and consisted of a discontinuous brownish macula, with poorly defined limits and linear medial aspect of the proximal interphalangeal joint to the dorsal distal interphalangeal joint. Dermoscopy revealed spots and globules, some brownish and other blackish ones, in the center and periphery, irregularly distributed along the lesion, with areas without dermatoscopic structures. The teledermoscopic diagnosis was of intracorneal hematoma. In the anamnesis, the contact with synthetic paint was revealed and the diagnosis was of exogenous pigmentation. In this case, the determining factor for the decision making was the data obtained during the anamnesis, from contact with the exogenous pigment. The conduct was expectant.

One case of benign melanocytic nevus was a 66-year-old man with a diagnosis of bullous lupus, with a dark brown macula on the back, for an unknown time, with no local symptoms, and with no melanoma history (lesion 16). In the dermoscopy analysis, reticulum-globular pattern, irregular net, and globules were identified with the colors light brown, dark brown, and gray. The diagnosis was of suspected malignant melanocytic lesion and the decision-making to be taken would be the excisional biopsy. In face-to-face assessment, the knowledge of the underlying disease and its pathophysiology (damage to basal epidermal cells), as well as the presence of suggestive lesions of disease activity, has modified diagnosis and decision-making for benign melanocytic lesion with inflammatory pigmentation of the disease and clinical follow-up.

The third discordant case (lesion 25) was referred to the male patient, 62 years old, renal transplant, using immunosuppressants, with lumbar lesion for unknown time, whose telediagnostic conclusion was melanoma or recurrent nevi

(multicomponent pattern; presence of irregular mesh, stretch marks, spots, erythema, and blue-gray veil). The face-to-face assessment concluded that this one was pigmented basal cell carcinoma, where arboriform telangiectasia at the periphery of the lesion and leaf structures as well are identified. The anatomopathological study confirmed the diagnosis established in the face-to-face assessment.

Finally, the other case of benign melanocytic nevus was a 61-year-old female patient, who had a pigmented lesion in the dorsal median line, for unknown time, with atypical pigmentary network teledermoscopy and striae (lesion 39). In the face-to-face assessment, the dermoscopy was reassuring, in which a homogeneous pigment network was visualized. In this case, it was decided to perform the digital dermatoscopy, which showed a similar image to that of the teledermoscopy one. We suppose that the location of the lesion was the difficult point in the teledermoscopic and digital analysis, due to the difficulty in coupling the dermatoscope in maintaining the focus on the images capture.

There was one case where the palpation of the lesion was essential for the diagnostic conclusion, referring to the lesion 23, in which the telediagnostic hypotheses were of solar lentigo associated with blue nevus or melanocytic lesion with eccentric homogeneous pigmentation.

We also emphasize the case of lesion 21, which concerned a 22-year-old female patient, with a cystic fibrosis diagnosis, presenting a hyperpigmented macule, blackened in the center, and dark brown in the edges, present for 2 years, which evolved with the darkening of the lesion. The teledermoscopy identified an irregular network, striae, and gray-blue areas. The diagnostic hypotheses were atypical melanoma or melanocytic nevus and excisional biopsy as the conduct to be performed. In the face-to-face assessment, the same dermatoscopic structures were identified, maintaining the same dermatoscopic description, the same hypotheses, and the same conduct; however, the assistant dermatologist reported a more reassuring aspect after a global analysis of the case. The anatomopathological study revealed junctional melanocytic nevus associated with marked degree of melanin pigment incontinence

4. Discussion

The concern with confidence in the diagnosis of skin malignancy with teledermatology is reflected in the current orientation that all suspicion of malignancy of the skin should be seen face to face [6]. However, the incorporation of high-quality teledermoscopic images in addition to macroscopic images may challenge this premise. The comparisons showed that the face-to-face and teledermoscopic correlation of the pigmented lesions is high.

In 1999, the teledermoscopic study carried out by Piccolo et al. (Italy and Austria) analyzed pigmented lesions of 66 patients in two groups (face-to-face and asynchronous teledermoscopy) and found agreement in 60 cases (91%) [7]. All lesions were histopathologic and concordance between face-to-face diagnosis was 92% and 86% for teledermoscopy [7]. Although the number of correct diagnoses were lower in teledermoscopy, it was not statistically significant [7]. The

6 discordant cases between face-to-face and teledermoscopy were classified as high (4) and medium (2) degree of difficulty [7].

Massone et al., in Austria in 2008, carried out the first teledermoscopy study using cellular phones for image capture and the storage and referral system for two teledermoscopists, in which diagnostic correspondence was found between the face-to-face examination of pigmented lesions in 89% and 94 % [8]. In 2011, Kroemer also used cell phones to capture clinical and dermatoscopic images without a special mobile pocket dermatoscope adapter and analyzed clinical and dermatoscopic images of 80 patients (104 lesions) separately, finding a concordance of 85% and 79%, respectively, compared to face and /or anatomopathological one; the value of the clinical image evaluation combined with clinical information in the diagnosis of skin tumors was attributed as relevant [9]. A total of 322 clinical images and 278 dermatoscopic images were obtained, of which 1% and 6% were considered inadequate for decision-making. The quality reduction of the dermatoscopic image was grounded by the lack of a special dermatoscope mobile phone adapter [9].

In 2016, Arzberger et al. showed excellent agreement on recommendations ("self-monitoring", "short-term monitoring", and "excision") between dermatologists (face-to-face and teledermatology) in a cohort of 70 patients with moderate to high risk [1]. However, also in 2016, the study of dubious melanocytic lesions published by de Giorgi et al. highlighted the limitations of teledermoscopy when analyzing 10 challenging pigmented lesions by 10 different teledermatologists and demonstrated that the diagnostic concordance of the telediagnosis decreased after the observation of the (kappa statistical analysis between the histopathological diagnosis: face-to-face 0.6, clinical teledermatology 0.52 and teledermoscopy 0.38), which was justified by the complexity and dermatoscopic difficulty of the selected cases, including Spitzoid proliferation and atypical melanocytic nevus of the elderly, which can represent a pathological and a potential diagnostic failure due to its confusing dermatoscopic characteristics [1].

Another teledermoscopic challenge is the diagnosis of hypo- or nonpigmented lesions, as demonstrated by Fabbrocini in the study of pink-lesions (poor or absent pigmentation, absence of a regular network, and diameter less than 5mm), in which the clinical and dermatoscopic telediagnosis showed less diagnostic accuracy than the face-to-face one [1, 2]. In this same study, the dermoscopic structures were evaluated as for the best visualization, whether face-to-face or in dermatoscopic imaging [1, 2]. The conclusion drawn from this was that leaf structures, pseudocysts, comedolike openings, "blue-white structures", and "blotches" are detected with the same frequency in face-to-face analysis and in teledermoscopy [1, 2]. Other structures such as pigment network, regression structures, and diffuse pigmentation are more evident in teledermoscopic observation, whereas the vascular pattern, radiated streaks, and spots/globules are less frequently detected [1, 2].

An important factor that should be considered is the standardization of image and service equipment. There are still no universal imaging standards developed and implemented in teledermatology; however, there are systematic reviews that summarize the technology standards and image technique for acquiring digital dermatological images [2]. In 1997, it was concluded that a resolution of 768x512 pixels would be adequate for the purposes of teledermatology [1, 3]. In 2008, for instance, practical guidelines from the American Telemedicine Association advised at least 24 color bits and in 2012 it recommended a resolution of 800x600 pixels, but preferably 1024x768 ones [1, 4, 10]. The standards of such techniques include ambient conditions (illumination, background, and camera position), patient pose, patient consent, privacy, and confidentiality [2].

The study of basic notions of photography is very important to the training of dermatologists. In Brazil, there are few training centers that offer it in their programs; however, this is already a subject much addressed in the national congresses, where minicourses take place for the dermatologists.

In the present study, sending the images by the application generated a resolution reduction of 3264x2448 to 1280x960 pixels, which is still within the established technology standards for the purposes of teledermatology, allowing, along with the standards of the technique, the analysis of an image quality.

We selected the WhatsApp to perform the mobile teledermoscopy after the verification that, with the sending of the image, the reduction of the resolution would not compromise the image analysis, since it still remained within the established technology standards for the purposes of teledermatology. The other reasons for choosing were the practicality offered by the application and the greater ease of replication.

What the studies clearly demonstrate is that even though the diagnostic accuracy of the lesions may be slightly lower for teledermatology, it has the ability to screen clearly benign lesions, allowing obvious malignancy and suspicious lesions to be properly managed in secondary care facilities [4]. We boldly emphasize, however, that, in order to achieve excellence in such a method, a rigorous protocol, including good clinical history, high-quality photography, and the safety of the dermatological examination, is pivotally necessary to recognize other suspicious lesions.

5. Conclusion

Our study demonstrated a high concordance rate between the teledermoscopic and face-to-face diagnoses, comparable to those described in the medical literature, and it allows us to conclude that teledermoscopy, and in particular mobile teledermoscopy, is a promising method for the analysis of pigmented lesions and we firmly believe that it deserves attention for future applications, especially in our country, where the distribution of dermatologists is irregular and scarce in some regions, besides the nondominance of the dermatoscopic technique by a considerable portion of these ones. The latest medical census, for example, showed that the Southeast region concentrates 58.9% of the specialists, 15.8% throughout the South, 13.8% in the Northeast, 8% along the Midwest, and 3.5% throughout the North region. In absolute numbers, the variation ranges from 5 to 2183 dermatologists per state (Acre and São Paulo states, respectively) [1, 6].

We emphasize that the diagnosis did not influence the final decision making, which was based exclusively on face-to-face assessment, either in the diagnostic definition or in the established behavior; we also declare that there was no identification of the patients through the sent images, which contained only a numerical tag; we also affirm that the sharing of these ones was restricted to the two participating physicians; moreover, we emphasize that the data from anamnesis and physical examination are sometimes essential for this decision-making, especially when faced with doubtful lesions; we declare that the use of the dermoscopic adapter for image capture may have contributed positively to the quality of the images; and, lastly we affirm that the necessary infrastructure for the progress of this study was of minimal cost, with high practicality and functionality.

We conclude, hence, that prospective and randomized clinical studies, legal aspects, and systematized protocols are absolutely necessary for the advancement of mobile teledermoscopy in Brazil, once it stands out as a good diagnostic accuracy, practical, and low cost method.

References

[1] E. Arzberger, C. Curiel-Lewandrowski, A. Blum et al., "Teledermoscopy in high-risk melanoma patients: A comparative study of face-to-face and teledermatology visits," *Acta Dermato-Venereologica*, vol. 96, no. 6, pp. 779–783, 2016.

[2] E. Tensen, J. P. van der Heijden, M. W. Jaspers, and L. Witkamp, "Two Decades of Teledermatology: Current Status and Integration in National Healthcare Systems," *Current Dermatology Reports*, vol. 5, no. 2, pp. 96–104, 2016.

[3] G. Fabbrocini, A. Balato, O. Rescigno, M. Mariano, M. Scalvenzi, and B. Brunetti, "Telediagnosis and face-to-face diagnosis reliability for melanocytic and non-melanocytic 'pink' lesions," *Journal of the European Academy of Dermatology and Venereology*, vol. 22, no. 2, pp. 229–234, 2008.

[4] S. M. Halpern, "Does teledermoscopy validate teledermatology for triage of skin lesions?" *British Journal of Dermatology*, vol. 162, no. 4, pp. 709-710, 2010.

[5] C. Massone, R. Hofmann-Wellenhof, V. Ahlgrimm-Siess, G. Gabler, C. Ebner, and H. Peter Soyer, "Melanoma Screening with Cellular Phones," *PLoS ONE*, vol. 2, no. 5, 2007.

[6] Melanoma: assessment and management NICE guideline Published: 29 July 2015 nice.org.uk/guidance/ng14.

[7] D. Piccolo, J. Smolle, I. H. Wolf et al., "Face-to-face diagnosis vs telediagnosis of pigmented skin tumors: A teledermoscopic study," *JAMA Dermatology*, vol. 135, no. 12, pp. 1467–1471, 1999.

[8] C. Massone, E. M. T. Wurm, R. Hofmann-Wellenhof, and H. P. Soyer, "Teledermatology: An Update," *Seminars in Cutaneous Medicine and Surgery*, vol. 27, no. 1, pp. 101–105, 2008.

[9] S. Kroemer, J. Frühauf, T. M. Campbell et al., "Mobile teledermatology for skin tumour screening: Diagnostic accuracy of clinical and dermoscopic image tele-evaluation using cellular phones," *British Journal of Dermatology*, vol. 164, no. 5, pp. 973–979, 2011.

[10] K. McKoy, S. Norton, and C. Lappan, Quick guide to store-forward and live- interactive teledermatology for referring providers: American Telemedicine Association. 2012. Available from: http://www.americantelemed.org/docs/default-source/standards/quick-guideto-store-forward-and-live-interactive-teledermatology-forreferring-providers.pdf?sfvrsn=4.

13

The Anticipated Positive Psychosocial Impact of Present Web-Based E-Health Services and Future Mobile Health Applications: An Investigation among Older Swedes

S. Wiklund Axelsson, L. Nyberg, A. Näslund, and A. Melander Wikman

Department of Health Sciences, Luleå University of Technology, 971 87 Luleå, Sweden

Correspondence should be addressed to S. Wiklund Axelsson; sarwik@ltu.se

Academic Editor: Guy Pare

This study investigates the anticipated psychosocial impact of present web-based e-health services and future mobile health applications among older Swedes. Random sample's of Swedish citizens aged 55 years old and older were given a survey containing two different e-health scenarios which respondents rated according to their anticipated psychosocial impact by means of the PIADS instrument. Results consistently demonstrated the positive anticipation of psychosocial impacts for both scenarios. The future mobile health applications scored more positively than the present web-based e-health services. An increase in age correlated positively to lower impact scores. These findings indicate that from a psychosocial perspective, web-based e-health services and mobile health applications are likely to positively impact quality of life. This knowledge can be helpful when tailoring and implementing e-health services that are directed to older people.

1. Introduction

The world is facing an increasingly aging population which is presently placing heavy demand on health care services, and this continues into the future [1]. There are growing expectations that e-health will be the solution for these demands. E-health refers to "tools and services using information and communication technologies (ICTs) that can improve prevention, diagnosis, treatment, monitoring, and management and can benefit the entire community by improving access to care and quality of care and by making the health sector more efficient" [2]. The goal is to make e-health both more user-friendly and thus more widely accepted by involving patients in strategy, design, and implementation, as well as supporting the general increase in quality of life [2, 3].

European countries, such as Norway, Denmark, Germany, Greece, and Portugal, show steady development in using the Internet as a source for health information [4]. In Sweden, it is possible for citizens nationwide to use web-based e-health services offered by Swedish public health care providers to receive general e-health information online [5], receive personalized web-based e-health services (e.g., online e-prescription renewal), ask their doctors questions online, obtain medical devices, and reschedule doctor appointments [6, 7]. The next generation of e-health systems is mobile health applications that are "considered as the strongest contribution for the next generation e-health systems" [8]. These applications act closely with an individual and "focus on serving the needs of the user by providing widespread access to relevant information and/or remote data capture, thus eliminating the need for the user to be physically linked to a network or restricted to a specific geographic location" [9].

E-health has been recommended for supporting the health conditions of older adults [3]. For older adults, health is closely linked to aspects of quality of life, such as psychological well-being, independence, mobility, safety, and social involvement [10–13]. In turn, these aspects are impacted by personal and environmental factors that are equated with psychosocial factors [14] that are often challenged by health conditions which usually worsen with age [15]. Several self-reported evaluations of e-health services from the perspective of patients show a low effect on health related quality of life and psychological outcomes [16].

Clearly, investigating what impact e-health has on psychosocial issues among older adults matters to understanding how e-health can be supportive or counteractive to the health of older adults. In this sense, the full use and adoption of technology are related to its role, perceived usefulness, and meaning in an individualized context [17]. Benefits and lack of benefits affect the motivation for the introduction of new technology innovation among older adults [18]. In a previous study [19], we found a low degree of e-health service use among older adults in Sweden despite the extensive development of these services. The objective of this study was thus to investigate the anticipated psychosocial impact from present web-based-e-health services and future mobile health applications among older Swedes.

2. Methods

This study implemented a cross-sectional survey based on two scenarios, the Psychosocial Impact of Assistive Devices (PIADS) questionnaire and also background questions. The survey was distributed by post, and respondents answered the survey during telephone interviews or filled them in at home and returned by post. The study was approved by the Regional Ethical Review Board in Umeå, Sweden [Ref. no. 2594-10].

2.1. Sample. A total of 650 individuals aged 55–105 were randomly selected from the official identity and address registry for Swedish residents [20]. As shown in the flowchart of the inclusion process (Figure 1), a total of 154 persons responded to the survey, 368 declined, and 128 could not be reached. The age range for those who participated in the study was 55 to 91 years. A sample failure analysis showed that respondents differed from nonrespondents regarding age (mean respondent age was 71.9, while mean nonrespondent age was 74.1) ($P = 0.010$) but not with regard to gender ($P = 0.407$). The profile of the respondents is presented in Table 1.

2.2. Instrument. The two illustrated scenarios of this study's survey were based on focus group discussions from the research project MyHealth@Age (2008–2010) [21, 22] developed with a researcher focusing on pervasive and mobile computing at the Luleå University of Technology and ultimately, thereafter designed by a graphic designer. A scenario can be defined as a description of a possible set of events that might reasonably take place; for our survey, scenarios focus on use, what people can do with a system, and the consequences for users [23]. The present scenario illustrates existing web-based e-health services together with an explanatory text of how people are able to use web-based e-health services, if needed (see Figure 2). The future scenario illustrates mobile health applications under development together with an explanatory text of how people in the future will be able to use mobile health applications, if needed (see Figure 3).

2.2.1. Present Scenario. Presently and within the next few years, you can/are able to, if necessary,

(i) renew your prescriptions and book appointments at health care centers on the Internet,

(ii) receive SMS appointment reminders,

(iii) receive advice from the online medical counseling service,

(iv) contact health care staff by email,

(v) take your blood pressure, ECGs, and blood tests at home by yourself and send the results via the Internet to health care centers,

(vi) talk to health care staff about your test results using a web camera,

(vii) receive advice on how you should exercise and what you should eat to maintain or attain good health.

2.2.2. Future Scenario. In the future, you will be able to, if necessary,

(i) be in constant contact with a health professional via sensors that will alert your health care center if they detect any problems with a measured value,

(ii) track your fitness improvement by measuring walking distance, pulse, and blood pressure automatically,

(iii) recognize people and receive assistance in remembering their names with the help of special glasses,

(iv) wear a personal safety alarm that can determine your exact position in the event of you fall outdoors and need assistance,

(v) use a walking stick that shows you the way,

(vi) use sensors in your shoes to obtain better balance.

In responding to the illustrated scenarios (Figures 2 and 3) the Psychosocial Impact of Assistive Devices Scale (PIADS) questionnaire [24] was used to measure the anticipated impact on psychosocial factors of present web-based e-health services and future mobile health applications. The PIADS measures aspects related to quality of life that refer both to the person and the environment [14]. The scale is designed to assess the experienced or anticipated impact of assistive technological devices before using them, thus anticipating the successful use or rejection assistive technologies [25]. PIADS has good internal consistency as well as strong construct and predictive validity [25–27]. The questionnaire can be administered individually, in a group, or via a telephone interview [24]. It consists of 26 items based on the user's description of how devices impact quality of life. Each item is rated on a scale ranging from −3 (i.e., maximum negative impact) to +3 (i.e., maximum positive impact). Ratings are presented as three separate subscores that describe user perceptions along three dimensions (i.e., competence, adaptability, and self-esteem), as well as a total score. The competence dimension is evaluated by questions concerning topics such as competence, productivity, usefulness, performance, and independence. The adaptability dimension is evaluated by questions concerning topics such as the ability to participate, willingness to make changes, eagerness to try new things,

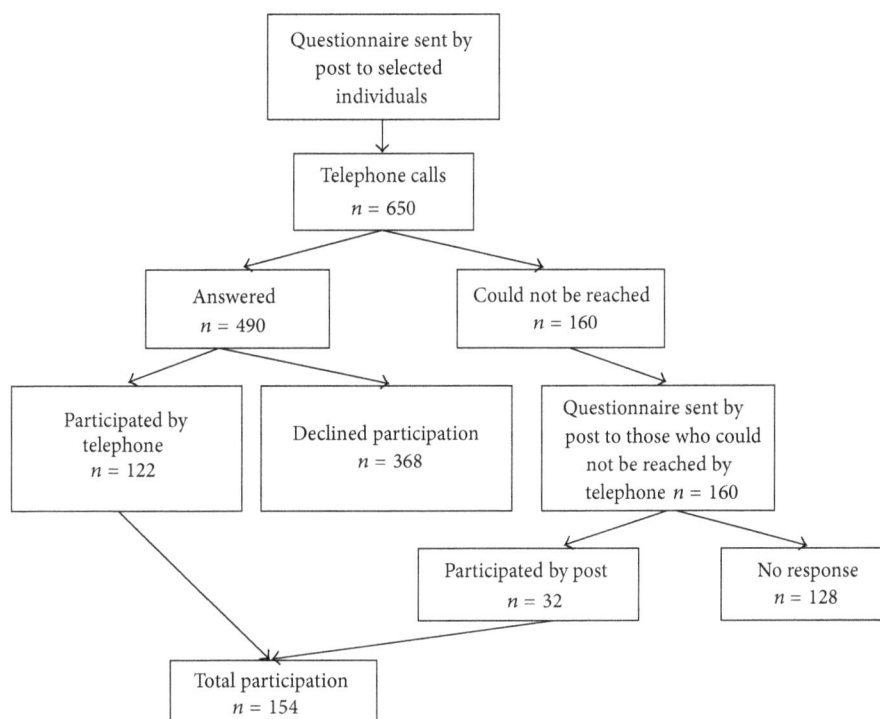

FIGURE 1: Flowchart of the inclusion process.

TABLE 1: Profile of respondents ($n = 154$).

	n (%)	Mean (SD)	n (no/yes)*	Md (q1, q3)***
Age		71.9 (±8.7)		
Female gender	80 (52)			
Living alone	49 (32)			
Education level				
Primary school	55 (36)			
College	50 (34)			
University	47 (31)			
Monthly income (SEK)				
<8,000	14 (9)			
8,000–18,000	71 (47)			
18,000–26,000	42 (28)			
>26,000	25 (16)			
Self-rated health (VAS 0–100)		72.5 (±18.0)		
Usage degree of mobile phone**				3.0 (2.0, 4.0)
Usage degree of SMS messaging**				1.0 (1.0, 2.0)
Usage degree of computer**				3.0 (1.0, 4.0)
Usage degree of e-mail**				2.0 (1.0, 3.0)
Usage degree of Internet**				3.0 (1.0, 4.0)
Used Internet for health information*			95/58	
Used Internet for information about physical activity*			130/23	
Used Internet for information about diet*			117/36	
Used mobile phone or advanced ICT in contacts with health care*			103/50	

*Self-reported usage of mobile phone, SMS, e-mail web, chat, blog, and audiovideo communication during a one-year period. **Self-rated ordinal scale for general ICT experience during a one year period: 1 = never; 2 = monthly; 3 = weekly; 4 = daily ***Md: median; q1: lowest quartile; q3: highest quartile.

TABLE 2: PIADS total score and subscores for web-based e-health services in present and mobile health applications in the future.

Variable	Present[*] Md (q1, q3)[***]	Future[**] Md (q1, q3)[***]	P value
Total score ($n = 147/150$)	0.81 (0.27, 1.23)	1.00 (0.46, 1.54)	<0.001
Competence sub-score ($n = 149/150$)	0.75 (0.29, 1.34)	1.00 (0.42, 1.52)	0.002
Adaptability sub-score ($n = 150/150$)	0.84 (0.34, 1.50)	1.17 (0.50, 1.83)	<0.001
Self-esteem sub-score ($n = 149/150$)	0.75 (0.13, 1.13)	0.88 (0.38, 1.50)	0.001

[*]Present = describing a scenario where web-based e-health services are able to be used in present. [**]Future = describing a scenario where mobile health applications will be able to be used in the future [***]Md: median; q1: lowest quartiles; q3: the highest quartiles.

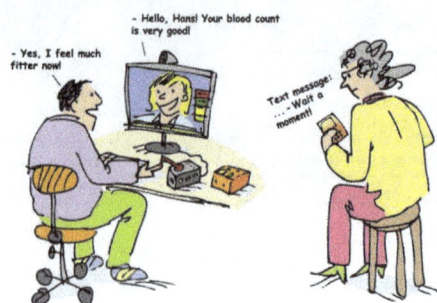

FIGURE 2: Web-based e-health services in the present.

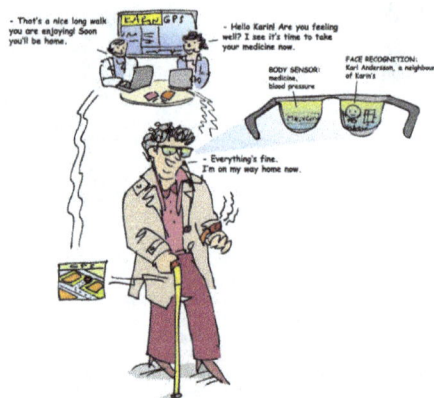

FIGURE 3: Mobile health applications in the future.

and ability to take advantage of opportunities. The self-esteem dimension is evaluated by questions concerning topics such as self-esteem, security, sense of power and control, and self-confidence [14].

The survey's background questions asked for respondents' age, gender, marital or cohabitation status, education level, income, self-rated health status according to a visual analog scale ranging from 0 to 100 and derived from the EQ-5D [28], and experience using ICT applications during a one-year period. Other questions inquired about use of the Internet for obtaining information about health, physical activity, and diet, while other questions asked respondents to report their experience using ICT for health care services (see Table 1). A pretest, with three older adults who responded to the survey and provided information including an information letter, background questions, and scenarios with PIADS, was conducted. The pretest clarified the importance of focusing

on anticipated events as opposed to experiences with web-based e-health services at the present and mobile health applications in the future when rating PIADS. A logbook was used by the telephone interviewers (i.e., the first author and an assistant) to collect spontaneous comments and feedback from respondents.

2.3. Procedure. The survey was distributed by post to 650 randomly selected individuals in batches of 100. After the expected delivery date, recipients were contacted by telephone. This process was repeated until all 650 surveys were distributed. Upon a recipient's consent to participate, a telephone interview was immediately conducted. First, a set of background questions were answered (see Table 1). Respondents were then asked to study the illustration of the web-based e-health services in the present scenario and read the written explanation in order to rate their anticipated psychosocial impact concerning the 26 items in the PIADS. The same procedure was repeated for the future scenario illustrating mobile health applications. During the telephone interviews, the comments of respondents were noted by the interviewers in a logbook. Recipients who declined to participate were asked to provide data regarding their gender and age. Recipients who could not be reached after five attempts by telephone were mailed a survey including a glossary to help them interpret the PIADS items (cf. [27]) and asked to complete and return the survey to researchers using prepaid, preaddressed envelopes.

2.4. Analyses. Parametric analyses were made for the variables age and self-rated health because they were ratio variables and normally distributed. All other variables were analyzed nonparametrically, as they were at either nominal or ordinal levels, or, as in the case of the PIADS scores, presented a skewed distribution. For analyses of the statistical inference of differences between two groups, a Student t-test was used for the parametric dependent variables, a Mann-Whitney U-test for ordinal variables, and the χ^2-test for nominal variables (see the description of sampling failure analysis on page 5 and Tables 3 and 4). When analyzing the differences in PIADS scores between the present and future scenarios (see Table 2), the Wilcoxon signed-rank test was used because of its dependent measurements. Correlations between PIADS total scores and parametric and ordinal scale variables were analyzed by the nonparametric Spearman's rank correlation (see Tables 3 and 4). All analyses followed standard procedures and considerations [29], and the significance level was set at 5%.

TABLE 3: Associations between PIADS total score for web-based e-health services in present scenario and respondents' profile variables (*n* = 147).

Independent variable	Mean rank difference	r_s	P value
Age		−0.217	**0.008**
Gender (female/male)	−4.5		0.520
Living alone/together with someone	−7.9		0.292
Education level		0.056	0.502
Income		0.113	0.174
Self-rated health (VAS 0–100)		0.110	0.184
Usage degree of a mobile phone**		0.167	**0.043**
Usage degree of SMS messaging**		0.270	**0.001**
Usage degree of a computer**		0.180	**0.029**
Usage degree of emails**		0.202	**0.014**
Usage degree of the Internet**		0.227	**0.006**
Used the Internet for health information (no/yes)*	−16.61		**0.021**
Used the Internet for information about physical activity (no/yes)*	−16.03		0.097
Used the Internet for information about diet (no/yes)*	−10.84		0.189
Used mobile phone or advanced ICT in contacts with health care*	−6.79		0.360

*Self-reported usage during a one-year period (no/yes). **Self-rated ordinal scale for ICT experience in a one-year period: 1 = never; 2 = monthly; 3 = weekly; 4 = daily; r_s: Spearman's rank correlation coefficient.
P value: statistical significance.
Bold: values below significance level 0.05.

TABLE 4: Associations between PIADS total score for the future mobile health applications scenario and respondents' profile variables (*n* = 150).

Independent variable	Mean rank difference	r_s	P value
Age		−0.212	**0.009**
Gender (female/male)	2.1		0.763
Living alone/together with someone	−4.0		0.600
Education level		0.002	0.984
Income		0.107	0.192
Self-rated health (VAS 0–100)		0.186	**0.022**
Usage degree of a mobile phone**		0.135	0.100
Usage degree of SMS messaging**		0.230	**0.005**
Usage degree of a computer**		0.124	0.132
Usage degree of emails**		0.202	0.165
Use degree of the Internet**		0.162	**0.048**
Used the Internet for health information (no/yes)*	−11.72.		0.107
Used the Internet for information about physical activity (no/yes)*	−19.16		0.052
Used the Internet for information about diet (no/yes)*	−15.51		0.064
Used mobile phone or advanced ICT in contacts with health care	−2.62		0.727

*Self-reported usage during a one-year period (no/yes). **Self-rated ordinal scale for ICT experience in a one year period: 1 = never; 2 = monthly; 3 = weekly; 4 = daily.
r_s: Spearman's rank correlation coefficient.
P value: statistical significance.
Bold: values below significance level 0.05.

3. Results

As shown in Table 2, data indicated that respondents anticipated positive psychosocial impacts for using web-based e-health services and mobile health applications regarding both present and future scenarios. Even first quartile values were consistently positive. Only 19 respondents (12%) reported negative total PIADS scores for the present scenario and 14 (9%) for the future scenario (data not shown). More importantly, both total PIADS score and sub-scores were significantly higher for the future scenario than those for the present. Among all scores, the adaptability sub-score showed the highest values.

Age was significantly related to the total PIADS scores regarding both web-based e-health service and mobile health application scenarios (see Tables 3 and 4), while gender, marital or cohabitation status, income, and educational levels were not. General ICT experience (mobile phone, SMS, computer use, email, and Internet use) was consistently and significantly associated with the psychosocial impact anticipated from the present scenario, but less consistently for the future scenario. At the same time, self-related health was associated with the anticipated psychosocial impact for the future scenario but not the present. Experience with health related ICT (SMS, email, web, chat, blog, and audiovideo communication) was not shown to be associated with the anticipated psychosocial outcome of either scenario except regarding using the Internet to retrieve health information in the present scenario.

4. Discussion

For both scenarios, a pattern of positive anticipation for the psychosocial impact of using web-based e-health services and mobile health applications is clear. Mobile health applications resulted in a higher anticipated psychosocial impact when compared to web-based e-health services. Contrary to our expectations, respondents did not rate more highly the anticipated psychosocial impact of the present scenario despite being familiar with its description of the services currently available in Sweden [6, 30, 31]. On the whole, it seems that older adults may find meaning from the perspective of the usefulness [17] of mobile health applications. The future scenario could be interpreted to suggest situations of independence and sociability for the mobile health application illustrate the transition of e-health services towards mobility and self-management.

Adaptability received the highest PIADS sub-score for both scenarios, particularly for mobile health applications in future scenario. Such a result suggests that these tools are more related to the environment in the sense that mobile health applications can serve as adapters that liberate users and enable them to pursue activities in daily life [14]. Independence was found to be imperative among older adults in order to avoid social exclusion [32] and is, in the sense of control and choice, of great importance when older adults use e-health services [33]. In one study [13], older adults with functional limitations reported that they were afraid of losing control and that control was strongly connected to feelings of independence. From the logbook, we read the following comments about scenario representing mobile health applications. "It would be fantastic if I could get that kind of help if I needed it;" "Do you really mean that this is being developed?," and "Yes, it would be helpful." This scenario painted respondents a picture of the technology being adapted to users instead of users being adapted to the technology and was perceived to be well integrated and will allow users autonomy without feeling intruded upon (cf. [9, 34–37]). These results could in turn reduce stigmatization (cf. [9, 38]). Mobile applications thus seem to be an important service that promotes mobility, which in turn positively impacts the quality of life of older adults [39].

The correlation between increased age and lower anticipated psychosocial impact may be expected, as previous research has shown a lower usage of ICT and a decreased interest in ICT communication with health care services at very old ages [31, 40]. The decreased psychosocial anticipations with increased age may be explained by the fact that the oldest adults perceive technical devices to be uninteresting because of low self-efficacy in relation to ICT use [41].

Results also showed a connection between general ICT use and the anticipation of web-based e-health services in the present scenario, as well as a connection between the use of SMS messaging and the Internet with the anticipation of mobile health applications in the future scenario. This result may confirm that web-based e-health services to some extent possess an image recognition factor similar to general usage. The mobile health applications in the future scenario, SMS messaging, and the Internet may be considered by the respondents to be more advanced, thus making the connection somewhat obvious.

Internal validity was strengthened by survey pretests, low internal data losses, a glossary explaining the PIADS items, and a standardized procedure during interviews. A few days after the first delivery of 100 surveys, all authors contacted five individuals by telephone for a total of 20 older adults in order to investigate the possibility that recipients needed clarification on the survey and interview procedures.

In the area of e-health, there are, to our knowledge, no instruments for evaluating psychosocial outcomes. We had to search in comparable areas and for assistive technology, there are a plethora of scales for assessing the impact and outcomes of devices. PIADS was developed and used in the context of assistive technology as wheelchairs, hearing aids, and so forth [42–44]. Quebec User Evaluation of Satisfaction with Assistive Technology (QUEST 2.0) assesses users' satisfaction of a device and assumes that an experience takes place with the device and that was not the case in our study [45]. Another one is Matching Person & Technology (MPT), an instrument that helps professionals together with the consumer, based on the person's goals, identify technologies which are desired and needed but not yet available [46]. MPT assesses the problems and barriers for use rather than anticipated psychosocial impact. We chose to use PIADS as an instrument because the design of this instrument fits our purpose, to evaluate the anticipated psychosocial impact of the e-health scenarios described. E-health means tools and services using information and communication technologies to assist the user, with it being important to measure the anticipated impact that these tools and services will have on the lives of older users and their environment. This study marks the first time that this instrument has been used to investigate the anticipated psychosocial impact of e-health services. We consider PIADS to be a valid instrument for this purpose, as it has been used to evaluate other technologies that support personal health [42–44].

We attempted to reduce the rate of nonresponses by making several telephone calls to recipients using a two-mode strategy (i.e., postal delivery and telephone interviews). Doing so may have positively affected the response rates. At the same time, it is possible that the number of questions negatively affected response rates. Other negative factors may include a lower interest level in the survey issues, health issues, and surveys in general [47]. Some recipients who declined to participate provided the following comments during telephone conversations: "I am too old to be answering this;" "I am not interested;" and "I am too sick." Other nonrespondents found the questions to be excessive in number or too difficult to answer.

Prestudy sample size calculations showed that in order to detect differences in PIADS scores between two unequally sized groups corresponding to at least moderate effect size, considering a significance level of 0.05 and a statistical power of 0.80, at least 319 respondents would be necessary. Considering an expected nonresponse rate of 50%, we therefore asked 650 persons to participate. Despite serious efforts to the contrary, the nonresponse rate was ultimately higher than expected (74%), which is an external validity threat for implying a potential nonresponse bias. This result also highlights possible type-II errors regarding P values bordering on statistical significance (see, e.g., Table 4). We nevertheless believe that our findings are of interest. First, the sample was derived from random selections of the official Swedish population registry. Second, we have reason to believe that the nonresponse bias may not have been too critical. Our data did not indicate large selection bias concerning gender and age, and the general ICT experience in our sample did not differ substantially from previously published results [31]. Although high response rates are preferred to ensure sample-to-population representativeness, empirical data seem to show that low response rates are not necessarily connected to large bias [48]. Third, as the PIADS scores were consistently positive to a high degree, we could expect that a possible overestimation resulting from sampling bias is less likely to distort the overall picture.

5. Conclusion

We found that the anticipated psychosocial impact was positive for web-based e-health applications in the present scenario and also for mobile health applications in the future scenario but was negatively correlated to an increase in age. Such findings may be interpreted to be especially interesting and unique since they concern an entire population of older adults and are not limited to specific diagnostic groups or samples participating in ICT trials. By contrast, our findings indicate that in a population of older people, e-health is likely to positively impact quality of life from a psychosocial perspective. Considering these aspects can serve as an important contribution to facilitating technology diffusion in health care among older adults. In the future, we can expect a continued increase in general ICT experiences among older adults, including the oldest, which will perhaps decrease the effects of advanced age on the anticipated impact. As long as differences persist, however, we must acknowledge the possible digital divide when implementing e-health. For the oldest members of the population, it is important to investigate their needs from a psychosocial perspective in order to tailor health care services that are meaningful in their particular context.

Acknowledgments

The authors would like to thank all of this study's participants. They would like to give special thanks to Kåre Synnes, Associate Professor in Pervasive and Mobile Computing at Luleå University of Technology, and Peter Sundström, artist and graphic designer in Luleå.

References

[1] European Commission, "The 2012 ageing report, " European Commission Directorate-General for Economic and Financial Affairs," http://ec.europa.eu/economy_finance/publications/european_economy/2012/pdf/ee-2012-2_en.pdf.

[2] European Commission, 2013, http://ec.europa.eu/health/ehealth/policy/index_en.htm.

[3] European Commission, *EHealth Action Plan 2012–2020—Innovative Healthcare For the 21st Century*, European Commission, Brussels, Belgium, 2012.

[4] P. E. Kummervold and R. Wynn, "Health information accessed on the internet: the development in 5 european countries," *International Journal of Telemedicine and Applications*, vol. 2012, Article ID 297416, 3 pages, 2012.

[5] The Swedish Parliament, "eHealth—benefits and business potential," Tech. Rep. 2011/12:RFR5, 2011/12, Riksdagstryckeriet, Stockholm, Sweden, 2012.

[6] Ministry of Health and Social Affairs, "National eHealth—the strategy for accessible and secure information in health and social care," Tech. Rep. S2011.023, Government offices of Sweden, 2010.

[7] M. L. Jung and K. Loria, "Acceptance of Swedish e-health services," *Journal of Multidisciplinary Healthcare*, vol. 3, pp. 55–63, 2010.

[8] B. M. C. Silva, J. J. P. C. Rodrigues, I. M. C. Lopes, T. M. F. Machado, and L. Zhou, "A Novel Cooperation Strategy for Mobile Health Applications," *IEEE Journal on Selected Areas in Communications/Supplement*, vol. 31, no. 9, pp. 28–36, 2013.

[9] G. Demiris, L. B. Afrin, S. Speedie et al., "Patient-centered applications: use of information technology to promote disease management and wellness. A white paper by the AMIA knowledge in motion working Group," *Journal of the American Medical Informatics Association*, vol. 15, no. 1, pp. 8–13, 2008.

[10] Z. Gabriel and A. Bowling, "Quality of life from the perspectives of older people," *Ageing and Society*, vol. 24, no. 5, pp. 675–691, 2004.

[11] R. Steele, A. Lo, C. Secombe, and Y. K. Wong, "Elderly persons' perception and acceptance of using wireless sensor networks to assist healthcare," *International Journal of Medical Informatics*, vol. 78, no. 12, pp. 788–801, 2009.

[12] A. Walker, "A European perspective on quality of life in old age," *European Journal of Ageing*, vol. 2, no. 1, pp. 2–12, 2005.

[13] A. Melander–Wikman, Y. Fältholm, and G. Gard, "Safety vs. privacy: elderly persons'experiences of a mobile safety alarm," *Health & Social Care in the Community*, vol. 16, pp. 337–346, 2008.

[14] J. Jutai and H. Day, "Psychosocial Impact of Assistive Devices Scale (PIADS)," *Technology and Disability*, vol. 14, no. 3, pp. 107–111, 2002.

[15] T. Obia, D. Ishmatovab, and N. Iwasakic, "Promoting ICT innovations for the ageing population in Japan," *International Journal of Medical Informatics*, vol. 82, pp. e47–e62, 2013.

[16] M. Cartwright, "Effect of telehealth on quality of life and psychological outcomes over 12 months (Whole Systems Demonstrator telehealth questionnaire study): nested study of patient reported outcomes in a pragmatic, cluster randomized controlled trial," *British Medical Journal*, vol. 346, no. 26, article f653, 2013.

[17] K. Renaud and J. Van Biljon, "Predicting technology acceptance and adoption by the elderly: a qualitative study," in *Proceedings of the Annual Research Conference of the South African Institute of Computer Scientists and Information Technologists on IT Research in Developing Countries: Riding the Wave of Technology*, pp. 210–219, October 2008.

[18] A.-S. Melenhorst, W. A. Rogers, and D. G. Bouwhuis, "Older adults' motivated choice for technological innovation: evidence for benefit-driven selectivity," *Psychology and Aging*, vol. 21, no. 1, pp. 190–195, 2006.

[19] S. Wiklund Axelsson, A. Melander Wikman, A. Näslund, and L. Nyberg, "Older people's health-related ICT-use in Sweden," *Gerontechnology*, vol. 12, no. 1, pp. 36–43, 2013.

[20] Swedish Population Register, SPAR, 2013, http://www.statenspersonadressregister.se/Om-SPAR/In-English.html.

[21] B. Bergvall-Kaareborn, D. Howcroft, A. Ståhlbröst, and A. Melander Wikman, "Participation in living lab: designing systems with users," in *Human Benefit Through the Diffusion of Information Systems Design Science Research*, J. Pries-Heje, J. J. Venable, D. Bunker, N. L. Russo, and J. I. DeGross, Eds., vol. 318, pp. 317–326, Springer, 2010.

[22] B. Bergvall-Kåreborn, T. Ghaye, and A. Melander Wikman, "A model for reflective participatory design. " The importance of participation, voice and space when designing systems with users," 2013.

[23] M. Jarke, X. Tung Bui, and J. M. Carroll, "Scenario management: an interdisciplinary approach," *Requirements Engineering*, vol. 3, no. 3-4, pp. 155–173, 1998.

[24] H. Day and J. Jutai, *Psychosocial Impact of Assistive Devices Scale (PIADS) Manual*, University of Western Ontario, Ontario, Canada, 2003.

[25] H. Day and J. Jutai, "Measuring the psychosocial impact of assistive devices: the PIADS," *Canadian Journal of Rehabilitation*, vol. 9, no. 3, pp. 159–168, 1996.

[26] J. Jutai, "Quality of life impact of assistive technology," *Rehabilitation Engineering*, vol. 14, pp. 2–6, 1999.

[27] H. Day, J. Jutai, and K. A. Campbell, "Development of a scale to measure the psychosocial impact of assistive devices: lessons learned and the road ahead," *Disability and Rehabilitation*, vol. 24, no. 1–3, pp. 31–37, 2002.

[28] R. Brooks, R. Rabin, and F. de Charro, *The Measurement and Valuation of Health Status Using EQ-5D: A European Perspective-Evidence From the EuroQol BIOMED Research Program*, Kluwer, Amsterdam, The Netherlands, 2003.

[29] B. Dawson, R. G. Trapp, and R. G. Trapp, *Basic & Clinical Biostatistics*, Lange Medical Books/McGraw-Hill, New York, NY, USA, 2004.

[30] Internet use in household and by individuals, 2012, http://epp rostat.ec.europa.eu/cache/ITY_OFFPUB/KS-SF-12-050/EN/ KS-SF-12-050-EN.PDF.

[31] O. Findahl, "Swedes and the internet 2012," Tech. Rep. 1, internetstatistik, Stockholm, Sweden, 2012.

[32] S. Bell and V. Menec, "You Don't Want to Ask for the Help' the imperative of independence is it related to social exclusion?," *Journal of Applied Gerontology*, 2013.

[33] A. Bowes and G. McColgan, "Telecare for older people promoting independence, participation, and identity," *Research on Aging*, vol. 35, pp. 32–49, 2013.

[34] K. Arning, A. Holzinger, and K. Miesenberger, "Different perspectives on technology acceptance: the role of technology type and age," *HCI and Usability for E-Inclusion*, vol. 5889, article 20, 2009.

[35] E. Hernández-Encuentra, M. Pousada, and B. Gómez-Zúniga, "ICT and older people: beyond usability," *Educational Gerontology*, vol. 35, no. 3, pp. 226–245, 2009.

[36] E. D. Mynatt, A.-S. Melenhorst, A. D. Fisk, and W. A. Rogers, "Aware technologies for aging in place: understanding user needs and attitudes," *IEEE Pervasive Computing*, vol. 3, no. 2, pp. 36–41, 2004.

[37] G. Demiris, M. J. Rantz, M. A. Aud et al., "Older adults attitudes towards and perceptions of 'smart home technologies: a pilot study," *Informatics for Health and Social Care*, vol. 29, no. 2, pp. 87–94, 2004.

[38] J. F. Coughlin, "Older adult perceptions of smart home technologies: implications for research, policy market innovations in healthcare," in *Proceedings of the 29th Annual International Conference of the IEEE EMB Cité Internationale*, pp. 1810–1815, Lyon, France, 2007.

[39] I. Plaza, L. Martín, S. Martin, and C. Medrano, "Mobile applications in an aging society: status and trends," *Journal of Systems and Software*, vol. 84, no. 11, pp. 1977–1988, 2011.

[40] H. Buysse, G. De Moor, P. Coorevits, G. Van Maele, J. Kaufman, and J. Ruige, "Main characteristics of type 1 and type 2 diabetic patients interested in the use of a telemonitoring platform," *Journal of Nursing and Healthcare of Chronic Illness*, vol. 3, pp. 456–468, 2011.

[41] K. V. Wild, N. C. Mattek, S. A. Maxwell, H. H. Dodge, H. B. Jimison, and J. A. Kaye, "Computer-related self-efficacy and anxiety in older adults with and without mild cognitive impairment," *Alzheimer's & Dementia*, vol. 8, pp. 544–552, 2012.

[42] I. Pettersson, G. Ahlström, and K. Törnquist, "The value of an outdoor powered wheelchair with regard to the quality of life

of persons with stroke: a follow-up study," *Assistive Technology*, vol. 19, no. 3, pp. 143–153, 2007.

[43] J. Jutai, P. Rigby, S. Ryan, and S. Stickel, "Psychosocial impact of electronic aids to daily living," *Assistive Technology*, vol. 12, no. 2, pp. 123–131, 2000.

[44] R. DeRosier and R. S. Farber, "Speech recognition software as an assistive device: a pilot study of user satisfaction and psychosocial impact," *Work*, vol. 25, no. 2, pp. 125–134, 2005.

[45] L. Demers, R. Weiss-Lambrou, and B. Ska, "The Quebec User Evaluation of Satisfaction with Assistive Technology (QUEST 2.0): an overview and recent progress," *Technology and Disability*, vol. 14, no. 3, pp. 101–105, 2002.

[46] M. J. Scherer and G. Craddock, "Matching Person & Technology (MPT) assessment process," *Technology and Disability*, vol. 14, no. 3, pp. 125–131, 2002.

[47] J. M. Brick and D. Williams, "Explaining rising nonresponse rates in cross-sectional surveys," *The Annals of the American Academy of Political and Social Science*, vol. 645, pp. 36–59, 2013.

[48] R. M. Groves, "Nonresponse rates and nonresponse bias in household surveys," *Public Opinion Quarterly*, vol. 70, no. 5, pp. 646–675, 2006.

14

A Wireless Emergency Telemedicine System for Patients Monitoring and Diagnosis

M. Abo-Zahhad, Sabah M. Ahmed, and O. Elnahas

Electrical and Electronic Engineering Department, Faculty of Engineering, Assiut University, Egypt

Correspondence should be addressed to M. Abo-Zahhad; zahhad@yahoo.com

Academic Editor: Sotiris A. Pavlopoulos

Recently, remote healthcare systems have received increasing attention in the last decade, explaining why intelligent systems with physiology signal monitoring for e-health care are an emerging area of development. Therefore, this study adopts a system which includes continuous collection and evaluation of multiple vital signs, long-term healthcare, and a cellular connection to a medical center in emergency case and it transfers all acquired raw data by the internet in normal case. The proposed system can continuously acquire four different physiological signs, for example, ECG, SpO2, temperature, and blood pressure and further relayed them to an intelligent data analysis scheme to diagnose abnormal pulses for exploring potential chronic diseases. The proposed system also has a friendly web-based interface for medical staff to observe immediate pulse signals for remote treatment. Once abnormal event happened or the request to real-time display vital signs is confirmed, all physiological signs will be immediately transmitted to remote medical server through both cellular networks and internet. Also data can be transmitted to a family member's mobile phone or doctor's phone through GPRS. A prototype of such system has been successfully developed and implemented, which will offer high standard of healthcare with a major reduction in cost for our society.

1. Introduction

A healthcare system in the last decade was made possible due to the recent advances in wireless and network technologies, linked with recent advances in nanotechnologies and ubiquitous computing systems. The term telemedicine refers to the utilization of telecommunication technology for medical diagnosis, treatment, and patient care [1]. The aim of telemedicine is to provide expert-based healthcare to understaffed remote sites through modern telecommunication (wireless communications) and information technologies. One of the benefits of telemedicine is cost savings, because information is less expensive to transport than are people. Advances in medical technologies have led to accelerated growth of the elderly population in many countries, resulting in an increasing requirement for home health monitoring to ensure that elderly patients can lead independent lives [2]. Many physiological signals can be measured from individuals in their living environments during daily activities and are potentially applied to observe the deviations of health status in the early phase or to alert paramedics automatically in

emergency cases [3]. Especially for remote monitoring of physiological parameters, all the studies developed and currently used in this area can be categorized by several aspects: type of sensors, type of data communication, monitoring device, and signal processing/medical algorithms [4]. So these aspects along with recent studies will be discussed in this section. As shown in Figure 1 the main telemedicine system components in recent years include biosignal sensors, processing units, data communication networks, and medical service center.

The biosignal sensors are responsible for acquiring the physiological data (patient's vital signs) and transmitting it to the signal processing unit. Several studies are made focusing only on designing these sensors to be tiny in size [5], maintain patient mobility [6], and consume low operating power to reduce battery size which can last for longer durations [7]. A collection of wearable medical sensors could communicate using personal area network or body network [8], which can be even integrated into user's clothes [9]. At the next stage, sensor layer of every remote monitoring system is typically connected to the processing device for

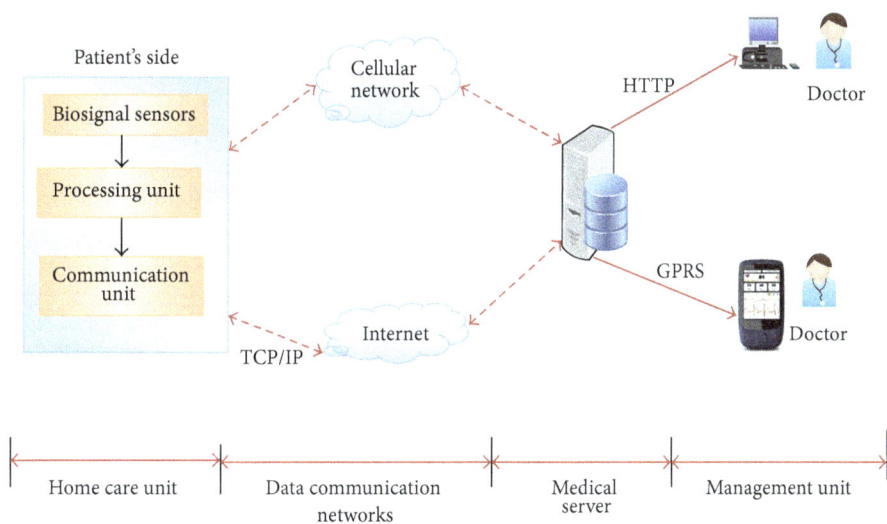

FIGURE 1: Main components of telemedicine system.

signal acquisition, processing, analysis, and formatting data to be sent to the communication layer. The processing unit may evaluate patient status and trends in patient's medical condition. Processing unit can be PC [10], mobile phone [11], or embedded system (microcontroller, DSP processor, and FPGA) [12]. Many medical algorithms were developed in recent telemedicine studies to help in patient diagnosis [13] and early detection of cardiovascular diseases [14]. Among human vital signals, pulse assessment has long been a research area of interest in the physiology field, because the pulse reflects a person's state of health [15]. Many investigations have proposed monitoring systems that can measure various biosignals and provide QRS detection and arrhythmia classification [14], real-time ECG classification algorithm [13], and heart rate variability measurement [14]. Also recent advances in wireless and network technologies make it possible to develop a wireless telemedicine system which offers an effective means of bringing healthcare services to patients. Telemedicine systems can be divided into two modes of operations: real-time mode, in which patient data are available at the server end immediately after acquisition, and store-and-forward mode, which involves accessing the data at a later time. In both modes, the vital signs are transmitted via computer networks [16], cellular networks [17], public telephone networks [18], or cable TV networks [19] to the server. In these system models, an expert is expected at places where he/she can use a PC to access the server for analyzing the vital signs data, and the patient is bounded at a fixed place like home or healthcare center where a PC is equipped for transmitting these data. The use of wired network connected PCs limits the degree of freedom of both doctors and patients to move around.

To improve the mobility of the doctor, the global system for mobile (GSM) communication mobile telephony network was used for connecting the server [20]. In [21], Hung and Zhang implemented a wireless application protocol (WAP) based telemonitoring system. It utilized WAP devices as mobile access terminals and allowed doctors to browse the monitored data on WAP devices in store-and-forward mode [22]. In such systems the improvement on the mobility of the patient is much less, compared to the doctor. In many previous telemedicine systems, the sensor unit consisted of an ECG data acquisition circuit, an A/D converter, and a storage unit. To provide a very limited mobility of the patient, this unit was equipped with an indoor, wireless transmitter for feeding the monitored data to a network connected PC [18, 21]. A GSM modem was equipped with a PC for real-time transmission of ECG data from a moving ambulance vehicle in [23]. In [24], Rasid and Woodward suggested a mobile telemonitoring system using a Bluetooth enabled processor unit, which transmits the monitored data to a Bluetooth mobile phone and subsequently via the GSM/GPRS (general packet radio services) network to the server. On the other hand, Engin et al. [25] used a mobile phone to transmit the measured ECG signal in real-time mode. In these designs [24, 25], the mobility of the patient is improved. However, the analysis of ECG is not performed in the place where the ECG is acquired; for example, the ECG is analyzed at the server end. In fact, there is a loss of efficiency in the use of the GSM/GPRS network because normal ECGs are also transferred, which implies a high cost. Lin et al. [26] developed a mobile patient monitoring system that integrates PDA technology and wireless local area network (WLAN) technology to transmit a patient's vital signs in real-time to a remote central management unit. The system was based on a small-sized mobile ECG recording device which sends measurement data wirelessly to the mobile phone [27]. In the mobile phone, the received data is analyzed and in cases of any abnormalities found among parts of the measurement data, it will be sent to a server. However, because of the limits of processing units within the mobile phone, the overall performance was hardly operated in an ideal condition [28]. Delay in the data transmission might also disrupt the data analysis and measurement. According to the discussed components of the telemedicine system, all systems developed can be categorized by several

TABLE 1: Set of telemedicine studies along with aspects which each study concerns.

Reference number	Biosignal sensors	Communication technology		Medical algorithm	Comments
		GSM/GPRS	Internet		
[29]	ECG, BP, HR TEMP.	√	√		WSN, type of localization method for patients and an energy efficient transmission strategy, video streaming.
[3]	HR, SPO2, TEMP., RESP.	√			Implement a prototype of telemedicine system based on wireless technology using GSM and GPS.
[4]	Weight, activity, BP	√	√		Android application for monitoring and using Bluetooth enabled sensors.
[5]	BP, HR, TEMP.	√	√		Design of sensors to reduce power consumption using VLSI and FPGA.
[6]	ECG, HR, SPO2, TEMP., RESP.		√		Wearable belt; high quality and flexible modules for signal conditioning are designed and assembled together.
[9]	ECG, BP, HR TEMP., PPG		√	√	Small rang RF transmission, smart wearable vest, deriving BP and HR from ECG.
[14]	ECG		√	√	QRS detection algorithm, extraction of heart rate variability, implemented in the PDA and GPS.
[13]	ECG	√	√	√	A real-time ECG classification algorithm, GPS, and a real-time R wave detection algorithm.
[15]	Pulse signal		√	√	Intelligent data analysis scheme to diagnose abnormal pulses for exploring potential chronic diseases.
[22]	ECG, HR, SPO2, TEMP., RESP.		√		Vital signals are acquired from the monitor using the RS232 interface and transmitted through the internet.
[23]	ECG, BP, HR TEMP.	√	√	√	Commercial monitors are used for the acquisition of biosignals and Huffman algorithm for ECG signal compression, GSM, GPRS, POTS, or satellite.

aspects: type of sensors, type of connection between sensors, monitoring/processing device, data communication technology, and signal processing algorithms. Table 1 summarizes a set of telemedicine studies in the last decades along with aspects which each study concern.

In this paper, we propose a wireless telemedicine system which integrates sensor unit, processing unit, and communication unit in one chip bounded to patient's body called mobile-care unit. This will improve patient's mobility and will not affect active daily life during monitoring. To lower the cost of using GPRS network, only abnormal readings are transmitted so the proposed system operates in two modes, store-and-forward mode and real-time mode. In store-and-forward mode the care unit records and transmits patient's vital signs to the server through the internet. When an abnormal heartbeat that the doctor concerns is detected, the care unit transmits it to the server via GPRS network in real-time. The doctor at the server side could communicate with the patient also by using SMS if necessary. The proposed system also has a friendly web-based interface for medical staff to observe immediate vital signs for remote treatment which will give more mobility for medical staff. The remainder of this paper is organized as follows. The system is described in Section 2. The proposed system consists of a mobile-care unit and a server. The hardware and software designs of the mobile-care unit are described in Section 2.2. The system has been implemented and tested. Finally, Section 3 contains some discussions and conclusions.

2. System Design

This section describes in detail the system design based on physiological sensor, signal processing, embedded system, and wireless communication and World Wide Web technologies. Figure 2 illustrates the architecture of the proposed system. Section 2.1 presents an overview of the system architecture. Section 2.2 describes the system components and the detail of the system operation.

2.1. System Architecture. The aim of this study is to design and implement a telemedicine system with intelligent data analysis based on physiological sensors, embedded system,

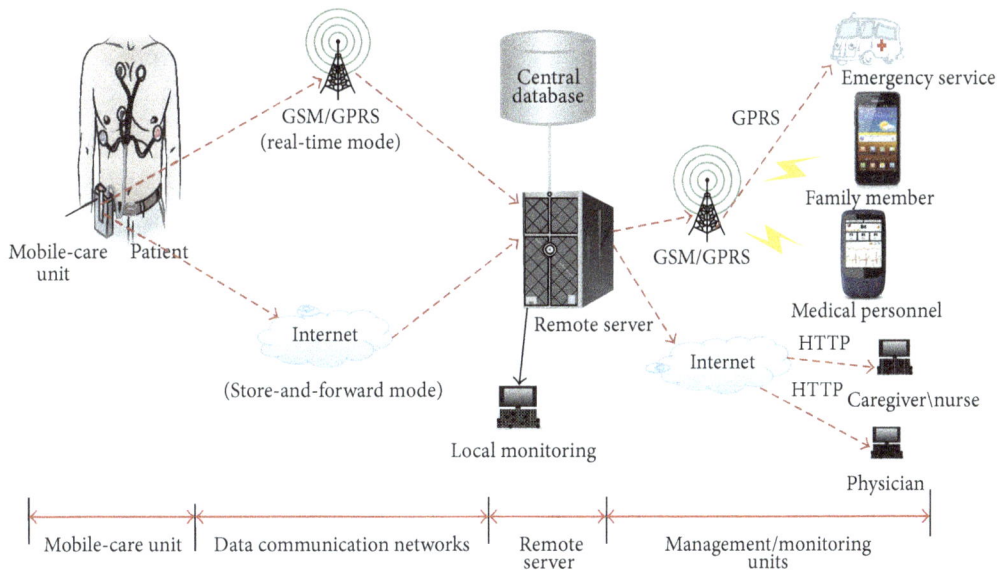

FIGURE 2: The architecture of the proposed system.

wireless communication, and World Wide Web for vital signs monitoring, patient diagnosis, and home care. Architecture of the proposed system is shown in Figure 2. It mainly comprises the following parts.

(1) Mobile-care unit: it could be bound to patient's body and could acquire real-time or periodical vital signs information without affecting their normal activities. Then an intelligent data analysis scheme is applied to identify abnormal pulses and transmits these data to the remote server by wireless communication through either internet in store-and-forward mode for normal case or cellular networks in real-time mode for abnormal case. The transmission of patient data in real-time mode can also be operated manually. Whenever the user feels uncomfortable, he can transfer his current vital signs to the management unit for advice or a checkup. By this way, the cost for using the GPRS network is lowered because only abnormal signals are transmitted. For possible long-term store-and-forward mode, the raw data can be stored in the extended secure digital flash memory contained in the mobile-care unit.

(2) The remote server: it stores the received vital signs in a human physiology database and displays the physiology signals to the medical personnel through application program for diagnosis. Also, it enables remote access for caregivers and physicians to obtain vital signs through web-based interface over internet to monitor these data on their pervasive devices. After examining the vital signs data, the doctor can send a feedback MMS message to the user. The message

may contain medical advice and/or a list of control commands to the mobile-care device for resending the abnormal case's vital signs data. Also remote server may alarm family member in abnormal case and call emergency service to transport patient to nearest medical center.

(3) Pervasive devices: pervasive devices include laptop, personal digital assistant (PDA), and mobile phone. Through these terminal devices family members or doctors can acquire abundant information about the healthcare recipients anywhere and at any time.

2.2. System Components. This section details the system components of the proposed emergency telemedicine system for patient monitoring and diagnosis.

2.2.1. Mobile-Care Unit. In the proposed system the mobile-care unit was designed to be portable and lightweight which means it is easy to carry and easy to use making patients do nothing. The mobile-care unit consists mainly of three modules. These are mainly vital-sign signals acquisition module, data control and processing module (MCU), and data communication module. Thus it can collect critical biosignals, including three-lead ECG, HR, blood pressure, and SpO2 which are vital signs. Also, it may evaluate patient status and trends in patient's medical condition and it may generate emergency alert if the patient's condition is critical. Moreover, it should support wireless communication and be compatible with global positioning information system to locate the patient position for emergency help. Figure 3

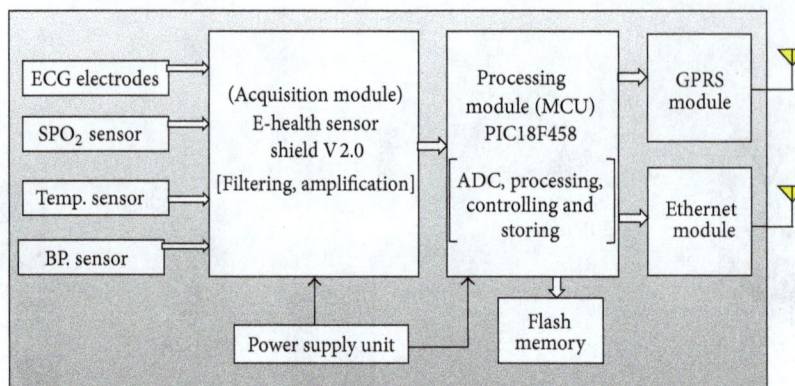

FIGURE 3: Mobile-care unit.

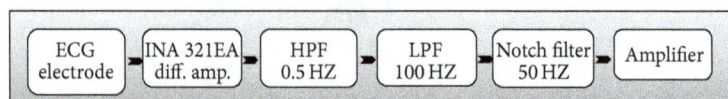

FIGURE 4: Block diagram of ECG acquisition hardware.

illustrates a block diagram of mobile-care unit. Also mobile-care unit includes local data storage which is used for raw data recording together with signals processing results.

(1) Vital-Sign Signals Acquisition Module. Vital-sign signals acquisition module is responsible for collecting vital signs and then sends it to processing module for ADC, processing, and abnormal detection. E-health sensor shield V2.0 is selected to work as vital-sign signals acquisition module. This module can continuously acquire physiological signs like ECG, SpO2, body temperature, and blood pressure as shown in Figure 3. All of vital signs measurements will be non-invasive measurement. Noninvasive measurement of vital signs certainly has an advantage over its invasive counterpart due to the ease of use and lack of risks involved in such measurements.

ECG Sensor. An ECG is a bioelectric signal which records the heart's electrical activity versus time. The electrocardiogram is obtained by measuring electrical potential between two points of the body using specific conditioning circuit. In the proposed mobile-care unit ECG signals from the electrodes are amplified with a gain of 300 and filtered with the cut-off frequencies of 0.5 Hz in the high pass filter and 100 Hz in the low pass filter.

The ECG signals are typically 1mV peak-to-peak; an amplification of 300 is necessary to render this signal usable for heart rate detection and realizing a clean morphological reproduction. A differential amplifier with gain of 20 avoids the noises overriding the ECG signals; this is achieved by an instrumentation amplifier (INA321EA), CMRR of 100 dB, and at the end an operational amplifier (Analog AD8625) is used to amplify the signal with a gain of 15. The ECG signals are restricted in bandwidth of 0.5–100 Hz using second order Butterworth high pass and low pass filters after the first stages of amplification. The power line interference in the ECG

signal is filtered by a 50 Hz notch filter, which is user selectable to avoid loss of 50 Hz component of the ECG signals. Then the ECG signal is fed to the analog input of processing unit for digitizing and analysis. Figure 4 illustrates the block diagram of ECG signal acquisition hardware.

Temperature Sensor. The temperature of a healthy person is about $37°C$; it may slightly or temporarily increase in hot environment or in physical activity; in extreme effort, the increase may be very high. It is of great medical importance to measure body temperature. The reason is that a number of diseases are accompanied by characteristic changes in body temperature. Likewise, the course of certain diseases can be monitored by measuring body temperature, and the efficiency of a treatment initiated can be evaluated by the physician. An industrial CMOS integrated-circuit temperature sensor shown in Figure 5(a) was chosen and connected to signal conditioning circuit shown in Figure 5(b) to calibrate and amplify the signal before feeding it to processing unit.

Blood Oxygenation Measurement (SpO2) and Heart Rate. SpO2 or pulse oximetry is the measure of oxygen saturation in the blood, which is related to the heart pulse when the blood is pumped from the heart to other parts of the human body. When the heart pumps and relaxes, there will be a differential in absorption of light at a thin point of a human body. Oxygenated hemoglobin absorbs more infrared light waves and allows more red light waves to pass through. However, deoxygenated (or reduced) hemoglobin absorbs more red light waves and allows more infrared light waves to pass through. This unique property of hemoglobin with respect to red and infrared light wave allows oxygen saturation to be detected noninvasively. Pulse oximetry is a simple yet reliable method to measure oxygen saturation that otherwise would have to be measured by invasive methods. Red (660 nm) and

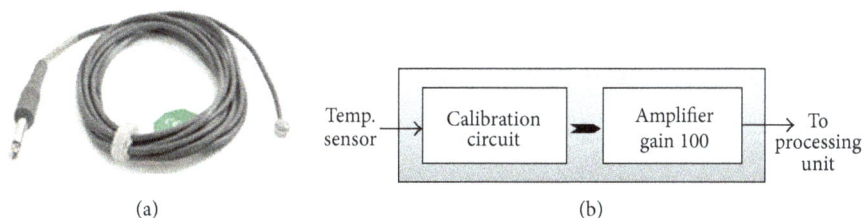

FIGURE 5: (a) Temperature sensor. (b) Signal conditioning circuit.

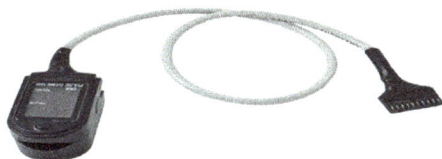

FIGURE 6: SpO2/HR sensor.

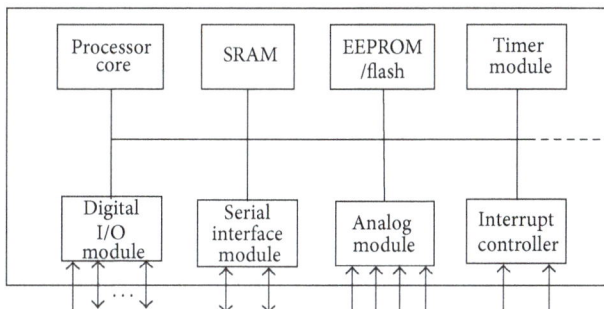

FIGURE 7: Architecture of microcontroller.

infrared (940 nm) LEDs were chosen and populated onto a custom-made sensor shown in Figure 6. Besides oxygen saturation in the blood the used sensor also provides heart rate. The output of the SpO2/HR sensor is fed to processing unit through acquisition module. Specifications of various physiological parameters monitored in the proposed system are listed in Table 2.

(2) Data Control and Processing Module. Data control and processing module is the heart of the medical care unit. The main function of this module can be divided into two parts: in the first part the developed algorithm synchronizes, controls, and maintains the accurate operation and communication of all the other modules. In the second part the developed algorithm digitizes and processes the acquired vital-sign signals to determine if their respective values are above the preset limit or not. If any or all of these values are above their respective critical values then triggering alarm is made. After that all processed data is transmitted to communication layer. This module mainly consists of a microcontroller which is chosen to verify certain specifications. Microcontrol unit (MCU) with powerful processing and control capability is needed to adapt a large amount of data acquiring and processing. Moreover, this module also possesses a high degree of system integration as well as more extension interfaces. We select 8 bit PIC18F458 microcontroller as the MCU of medical care unit. It has input-output circuitry and peripherals built-in, allowing it to interface more or less directly with real-world devices such as sensors. Modern microcontrollers often need little external circuitry. Among the most accessible are the PIC microcontrollers. A microcontroller already contains all components which allow it to operate stand alone and it has been designed in particular for monitoring and/or control tasks. In consequence, in addition to the processor it includes RAM, ROM, and EEPROM memory units, SPI, I2C, CAN, ADC, and UASRT interface controllers, one or more timers, an interrupt controller, and general purpose I/O pins. Figure 7 shows the architecture of the MCU.

We can summarize the main functions of MCU in the proposed system as follows.

(1) It receives and digitizes the signals acquired from vital sign sensors.

(2) It controls the operation of all connected modules as shown in Figure 8.

(3) It processes the received signals using different sorts of processing techniques and algorithms.

(4) It sets up a connection with the remote server and transmits to it the analysis results and raw data using communication techniques.

(5) It stores analysis results and raw data to flash memory.

(3) Software Components of the Processing Unit. The MCU controls and coordinates all activities of mobile-care unit. Figure 9 shows the workflow about the mobile-care unit. Software has been written in C language to simulate MCU and its components. It is based on the following concepts.

(1) Sensor and module initialization component: it is in charge of starting, initializing, and configuring the medical care unit.

(2) Vital signs perception component: it acquires the values of vital signs from sensor nodes.

(3) Vital signs processing component: it realizes data conversion and processing and carries out patient diagnosis by determining the health status of patient.

(4) Information transmission component: data exchange between mobile-care unit and server is realized with the help of this component.

TABLE 2: Specification of various physiological parameters monitored.

Physiological parameter	Specifications	Typical values for average healthy person
ECG	Frequency: 0.5 HZ–100 HZ Amplitude: 0.25–100 mv	R-WAVE amplitude: >4.5 mv QRS complex: (0.04–0.12) msec
Heart rate (HR)	40–220 beats per minute	60–100 beats/minute
Body temperature	32°C–40°C	About 37.5°C
Blood pressure	Systolic: 50–300 mmHg Diastolic: 40–140 mmHg	Systolic: less than 120 mmHg Diastolic: less than 80 mmHg
Blood oxygenation (SpO2)	Measurement range: 70–100%	Around 94% to 99%
Respiratory rate	2–50 breath/min.	Adults: 12–24 breaths per minute

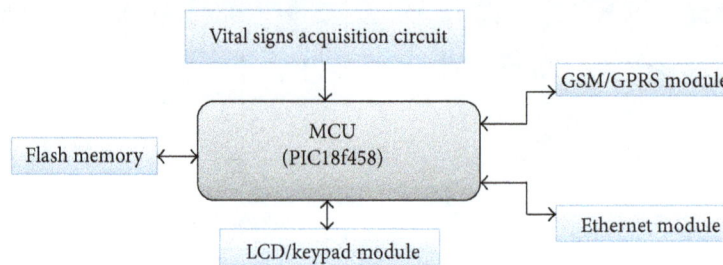

FIGURE 8: Functions of MCU.

(5) Information receiving component: it helps the node to receive the controlling or inquiring requests from the server.

(6) Exception notification component: when the abnormal sensing information appears, it sends a message to the server immediately and sends out the alarm as soon as possible.

(4) Data Communication Module. Data communication module helps the medical staff to get patient's physiological data by connecting medical care unit to other networks such as cellular network or internet. It is responsible for uploading the received vital signs data to the remote care server through cellular network to carry out the patient's health condition monitoring and diagnosis. This module operates in two modes: store-and-forward mode in which mobile-care device records patient's vital signs continuously up to specified period and transmits it to the remote server and real-time mode which operates when an abnormal heartbeat is detected. Mobile-care unit transmits all vital signs to the remote server via GSM/GPRS network in real-time. In the proposed system, medical care unit can send data through internet network either by UDP or TCP protocols using ENC28J60 Ethernet module shown in Figure 10(a). For real-time connection in emergency cases vital signs are transmitted through GSM/GPRS networks using sim900 GSM/GPRS module shown in Figure 10(b). The GSM/GPRS module used operates at Quad-Band 850/900/1800/1900 MHz and is controlled via AT commands.

2.2.2. Remote Server Unit. In the application of telemedicine, the medical information usually needs to be distributed among medical doctors and display, archival, and analysis devices. Therefore, the remote server unit is developed with the purpose of receiving, storing, and distributing the vital sign data from patients. The server is composed of presentation tier, web tier, and database tier. A multitier architecture allows for separation of concerns where any tier in the system can be expanded and updated with minimal or no effect on the client tiers. The following subsections discuss the three tiers further.

(1) Presentation Tier. The presentation tier allows the authorized user to interact with the received patient's data through application program developed using C# language. The interface design provides most of the general as well as functional requirements as follows.

(i) Access constraints are applied all the time based on the authorized user registered in the database.

(ii) It includes lists of patients and personal information about patients.

(iii) It displays patients' vital signals and sets thresholds for each measurable parameter.

(iv) It alerts healthcare providers in abnormal cases.

(v) It adds new patient, new consultation, and drug prescription.

(vi) It shows past medical records for all patients including diseases, past surgeries, clinical findings, past medication, allergies, and images.

(vii) It provides search for all registered patients by patient's ID or patient's name.

(viii) It shows notations (patient experience) while taking measurements.

(ix) It sends messages including instructions for patients and drug prescription.

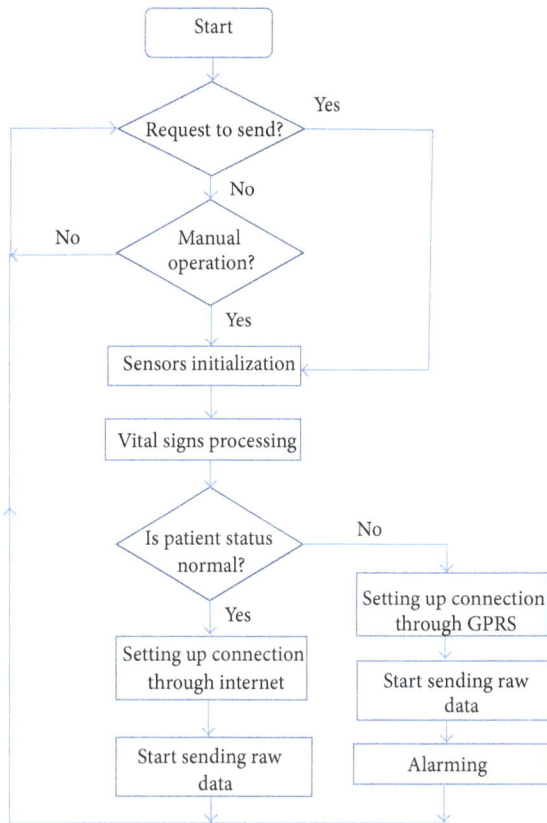

FIGURE 9: Work flow about mobile-care unit.

(x) Sensor data will be automatically reloaded at predefined time intervals to keep the view updated.

Screen shots of the developed software are shown in Figures 11, 12 and 13.

(2) Web Tier. Web tier allows different users such as physicians, doctors, and medical center to interact with the server through a web interface. Remote web user will have real-time and continuous access to patients' vital signs through the internet. The web user interfaces with the web components using HTTP protocol over TCP/IP connection. The information and content are presented to the user using an internet browser through webpage designed using Microsoft visual studio 2010. The designed webpage provides the most general functions of developed application in the presentation tier discussed previously. Screen shots of the designed webpage are shown in Figures 14 and 15.

(3) Database Tier. The database tier is responsible for storage, retrieval, update, and integrity of the data to and from the presentation and web tiers. The most common way to access the database is by using drivers that allow accessing a relational database management (RDBMS) to query or update the data records. The driver used in the implementation of the proposed system is JDBC drivers and the database is deployed on a SQL database server. The database tier provides the ability to do the following:

(i) store, retrieve, and update patient's record including his/her medical personnel's contact information and other details;

(ii) store and retrieve the received physiological sensor data transmitted by medical care unit;

(iii) store, retrieve, and update patient's consultations and drug prescriptions;

(iv) store and retrieve patient's notation during sessions;

(v) store, retrieve, and update registered doctors, physicians, and nurses;

(vi) store, retrieve, and update the ECG data, record time, location of the R wave, and estimated ECG beat type.

Figure 16 shows screen shot for how to search.

2.2.3. Monitoring Units. Web tier in the remote server is designed to allow remote user to acquire abundant information about the healthcare recipients anywhere and at any time using pervasive devices such as laptop, PDA, and mobile phone. Finally we can say that the proposed system can operate in the following three situations.

(1) Time-based connection: all data needed by the remote caregivers or specialists should be uploaded. Data compression is essential to limit the upload time. In this situation the remote caregiver should determine time schedule for uploading all patient data to remote server. The time schedule is stored in the mobile-care unit so it will upload data according to this time schedule.

(2) Emergency connection: to lower the cost of using GSM/GPRS network we develop algorithm which detects abnormal heartbeats. So during sensor monitoring, if the mobile-care unit detects an abnormal condition it sends the collected data to the remote server in order to receive clinical assessment and treatment planning.

(3) (Event awareness) connection on demand: the mobile-care unit uploads the amount of data requested by the remote caregivers or specialists to monitor the health status of the patient.

3. Conclusion and Future Scope

This paper proposes the design and implementation of a wireless telemedicine system, in which all physiological vital signs are transmitted to remote medical server through both cellular networks in emergency case and internet in normal case for long-term monitoring. By this, the cost of using GSM/GPRS network is reduced as only abnormal cases will be transmitted through cellular network. Also the proposed system presents friendly web-based interface for medical staff to observe immediate vital signs for remote treatment. Comparing this system with other systems which are mentioned in the introduction [18–28], the proposed system integrates sensor unit, processing unit, and communication

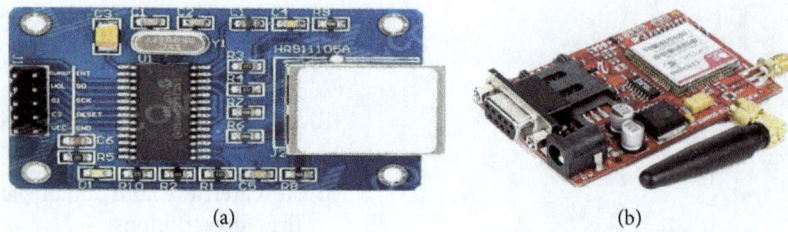

FIGURE 10: (a) ENC28J60 Ethernet module and (b) Sim900 GSM/GPRS module.

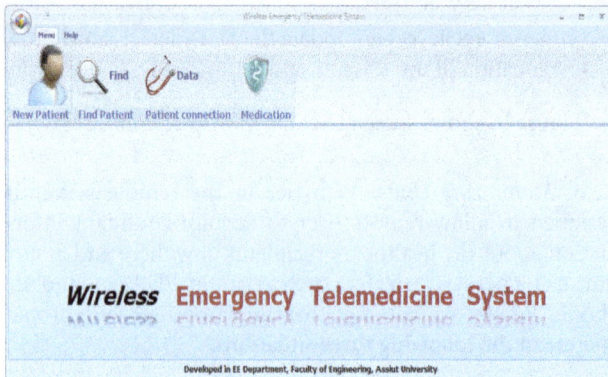

FIGURE 11: Screen shot of the developed interface main page.

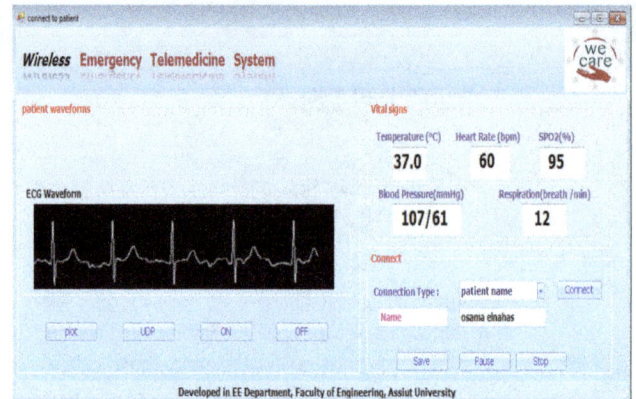

FIGURE 13: Displaying patient's vital signs.

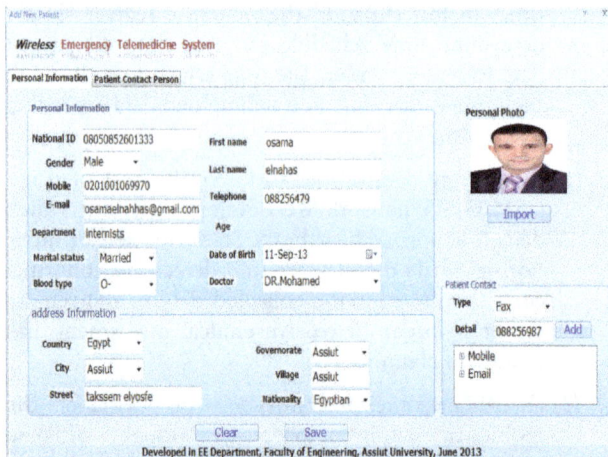

FIGURE 12: Add new patient screen shot.

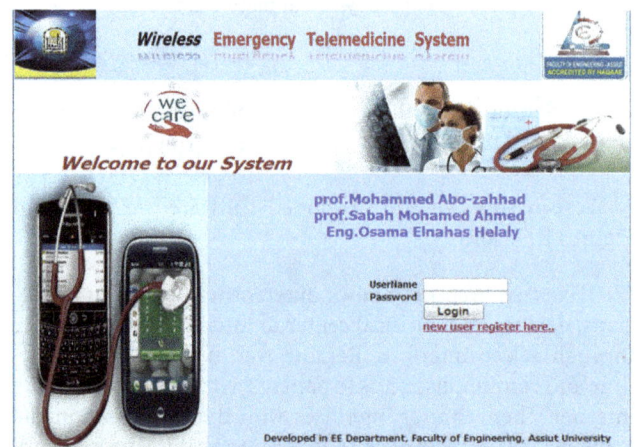

FIGURE 14: User authentication page.

unit in one chip bound to patient's body called mobile-care unit, so patient could do his/her daily activities during monitoring. In other words, this will improve the mobility of patient. Also the proposed system provides an ability to continuously monitor patient's vital health conditions instead of the discrete measurements.

In the future, a lot of work could be done in the three main aspects of telemedicine systems to enhance the healthcare services. The three main aspects are type of sensors, signal processing algorithms, and data communication technology. In the sensor layer wireless sensor network of wearable noninvasive sensor units can be designed. Fabrication of sensors can be improved to obtain small size and low power

sensors to improve patient's mobility and prolong network lifetime. Also we can increase the number of transmitted vital signs to have a complete picture of patient's case. For more improvement in telemedicine systems, many medical algorithms can be developed to help in patient diagnosis and early detection of cardiovascular diseases and real-time analysis of vital signs can be performed in the place where the vital signs are acquired. The latest achievement on a smart phone market provided an opportunity to integrate smart phones in telemedicine systems. For example, android based mobile phones patient monitoring application could be developed which allows doctors to monitor the health

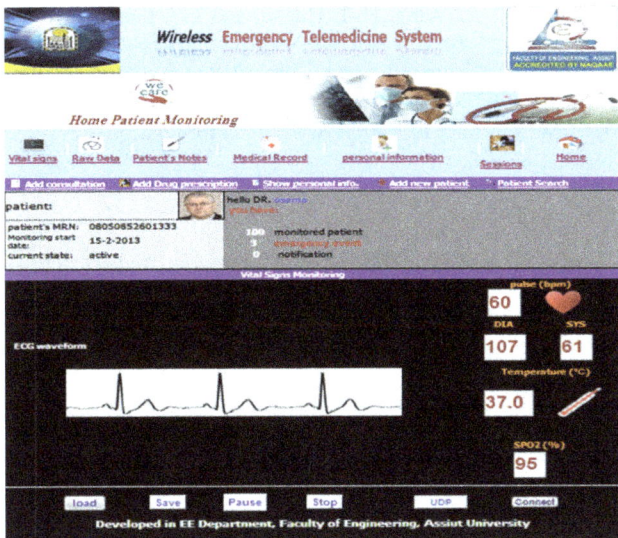

FIGURE 15: Displaying patient's vital signs.

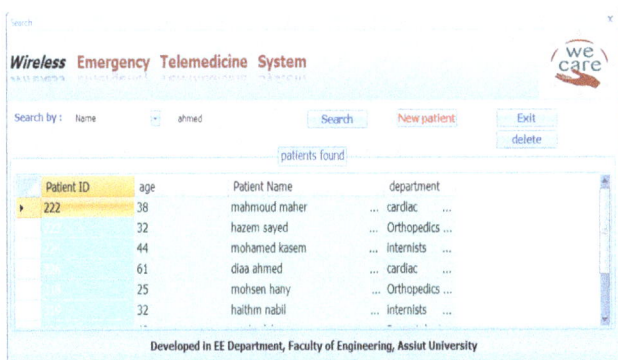

FIGURE 16: Screen shot for how to search.

status of a patient using the easy to understand user interface (UI). This application also provides alerts, reminders, and emergency notifications for vital measurements to help doctors to take timely decisions in emergency situations. Finally for data communication technologies, in many countries, 3G mobile networks like the UMTS are currently installed and operating, which provide bandwidth up to 2 Mbps maximum (typically hundreds of kbps) [30]. This will enable the transmission of more information like continuous 12 leads of ECG when monitoring cardiac patients from a moving ambulance vehicle. Furthermore, the current introduction of new services like video telephony through wireless networks is an addition that can help with communications between a healthcare provider (nurse, paramedics) and an expert doctor. The current activities in what is termed as the 4G mobile networks promise ubiquitous access to differing radio network technologies, thus offering, beyond extended coverage, also the most effective connection mode at the point of contact, even using simultaneously more than one wireless access technologies and seamlessly moving between them.

The use of locating systems such as the global positioning system (GPS), the geographical information systems (GIS), and intelligent traffic control systems also has the potential to improve healthcare services, for example, when a moving ambulance vehicle is trying to reach a patient using the fastest route or when an ambulance vehicle carrying a patient is trying to get to the base hospital.

References

[1] S. Pavlopoulos, R. H. Istepanian, S. Laxminarayan, and C. S. Pattichis, "Emergency health care systems and services: section overview," in *Proceedings of the 5th International IEEE EMBS Special Topic Conference on Information Technology Applications in Biomedicine*, pp. 371–374, 2006.

[2] R. Anta, S. El-Wahab, and A. Giuffrida, *Mobile Health: The potential of Mobile Telephony to Bring Health Care to the Majority*, Inter-American Development Bank, 2009.

[3] M. F. Wyne, V. K. Vitla, P. R. Raougari, and A. G. Syed, "Remote patient monitoring using GSM and GPS technologies," *Journal of Computing Sciences in Colleges*, vol. 24, no. 4, pp. 189–195, 2009.

[4] M.-K. Suh, C.-A. Chen, J. Woodbridge et al., "A remote patient monitoring system for congestive heart failure," *Journal of Medical Systems*, vol. 35, no. 5, pp. 1165–1179, 2011.

[5] A. Hande, T. Polk, W. Walker, and D. Bhatia, "Self-powered wireless sensor networks for remote patient monitoring in hospitals," *Sensors*, vol. 6, no. 9, pp. 1102–1117, 2006.

[6] E. Sardini and M. Serpelloni, "Instrumented wearable belt for wireless health monitoring," *Procedia Engineering*, vol. 5, pp. 580–583, 2010.

[7] F. E. H. Tay, D. G. Guo, L. Xu, M. N. Nyan, and K. L. Yap, "MEMSWear-biomonitoring system for remote vital signs monitoring," *Journal of the Franklin Institute*, vol. 346, no. 6, pp. 531–542, 2009.

[8] H. Alemdar and C. Ersoy, "Wireless sensor networks for healthcare: a survey," *Computer Networks*, vol. 54, no. 15, pp. 2688–2710, 2010.

[9] P. S. Pandian, K. Mohanavelu, K. P. Safeer et al., "Smart Vest: wearable multi-parameter remote physiological monitoring system," *Medical Engineering & Physics*, vol. 30, no. 4, pp. 466–477, 2008.

[10] B. Mehta, D. Rengarajan, and A. Prasad, "Real time patient tele-monitoring system using LabVIEW," *International Journal of Scientific and Engineering Research*, vol. 3, no. 4, pp. 435–445, 2012.

[11] A. Loutfi, G. Akner, and P. Dahl, *An android based monitoring and alarm system for patients with chronic obtrusive disease [M.S. thesis]*, Department of Technology at Orebro University, 2011.

[12] V. K. Sambaraju, *Design of a Wireless Cardiogram System for Acute and Long-Term Health Care Monitoring*, ProQuest, 2011.

[13] C. Wen, M.-F. Yeh, K.-C. Chang, and R.-G. Lee, "Real-time ECG telemonitoring system design with mobile phone platform," *Measurement*, vol. 41, no. 4, pp. 463–470, 2008.

[14] G. Tartarisco, G. Baldus, D. Corda et al., "Personal Health System architecture for stress monitoring and support to clinical

decisions," *Computer Communications*, vol. 35, no. 11, pp. 1296–1305, 2012.

[15] C.-M. Chen, "Web-based remote human pulse monitoring system with intelligent data analysis for home health care," *Expert Systems with Applications*, vol. 38, no. 3, pp. 2011–2019, 2011.

[16] E. Dolatabadi and S. Primak, "Ubiquitous WBAN-based electrocardiogram monitoring system," in *Proceedings of the 13th IEEE International Conference on e-Health Networking, Applications and Services (HEALTHCOM '11)*, pp. 110–113, Columbia, Mo, USA, June 2011.

[17] R. Sukanesh, S. P. Rajan, S. Vijayprasath, S. J. Prabhu, and P. Subathra, "GSM based ECG tele-alert system," *International Journal of Computer Science and Application*, pp. 112–116, 2010.

[18] J. Bai, Y. Zhang, D. Shen et al., "A portable ECG and blood pressure telemonitoring system," *IEEE Engineering in Medicine and Biology Magazine*, vol. 18, no. 4, pp. 63–70, 1999.

[19] R.-G. Lee, H.-S. Chen, C.-C. Lin, K.-C. Chang, and J.-H. Chen, "Home telecare system using cable television plants—an experimental field trial," *IEEE Transactions on Information Technology in Biomedicine*, vol. 4, no. 1, pp. 37–44, 2000.

[20] R. Sukanesh, P. Gautham, P. T. Arunmozhivarman, S. P. Rajan, and S. Vijayprasath, "Cellular phone based biomedical system for health care," in *Proceedings of the IEEE International Conference on Communication Control and Computing Technologies (ICCCCT '10)*, pp. 550–553, Ramanathapuram, India, October 2010.

[21] K. Hung and Y.-T. Zhang, "Implementation of a WAP-based telemedicine system for patient monitoring," *IEEE Transactions on Information Technology in Biomedicine*, vol. 7, no. 2, pp. 101–107, 2003.

[22] M. V. M. Figueredo and J. S. Dias, "Mobile telemedicine system for home care and patient monitoring," in *Proceedings of the 26th Annual International Conference of the IEEE Engineering in Medicine and Biology Society (EMBC '04)*, vol. 2, pp. 3387–3390, September 2004.

[23] E. Kyriacou, S. Pavlopoulos, and D. Koutsouris, "An emergency telemedicine system based on wireless communication technology: a case study," in *M-Health: Emerging Mobile Health Systems*, pp. 401–416, Springer, New York, NY, USA, 2006.

[24] M. F. A. Rasid and B. Woodward, "Bluetooth telemedicine processor for multichannel biomedical signal transmission via mobile cellular networks," *IEEE Transactions on Information Technology in Biomedicine*, vol. 9, no. 1, pp. 35–43, 2005.

[25] M. Engin, E. Çağlav, and E. Z. Engin, "Real-time ECG signal transmission via telephone network," *Measurement*, vol. 37, no. 2, pp. 167–171, 2005.

[26] Y.-H. Lin, I.-C. Jan, P. C.-I. Ko, Y.-Y. Chen, J.-M. Wong, and G.-J. Jan, "A wireless PDA-based physiological monitoring system for patient transport," *IEEE Transactions on Information Technology in Biomedicine*, vol. 8, no. 4, pp. 439–447, 2004.

[27] S. Khoór, J. Nieberl, K. Fügedi, and E. Kail, "Internet-based, GPRS, long-term ECG monitoring and non-linear heart-rate analysis for cardiovascular telemedicine management," in *Proceedings of the Computers in Cardiology*, vol. 28, pp. 209–212, Thessaloniki, Greece, September 2003.

[28] L. Zievski, B. Bojovic, V. Cevic et al., "A novel mobile transtelephonic system with synthesized 12-lead ECG," *IEEE Transaction on Information Technology in Biomedicine*, vol. 8, no. 4, pp. 428–438, 2004.

[29] C. Sha, R.-C. Wang, H.-P. Huang, and L.-J. Sun, "A type of healthcare system based on intelligent wireless sensor networks," *The Journal of China Universities of Posts and Telecommunications*, vol. 17, supplement 1, pp. 30–39, 2010.

[30] "UMTS forum," 2013, http://www.umts-forum.org.

15

Nurses' Experience of Using an Application to Support New Parents after Early Discharge

Dorthe Boe Danbjørg,[1,2] **Lis Wagner,**[1] **Bjarne Rønde Kristensen,**[2] **and Jane Clemensen**[3]

[1]*Research Unit of Nursing, Institute of Clinical Research, University of Southern Denmark, Campusvej 55, 5230 Odense M, Denmark*
[2]*Odense University Hospital, Department of Gynaecology and Obstetrics, Søndre Boulevard 29, 5000 Odense C, Denmark*
[3]*Odense University Hospital, CIMT, University of Southern Denmark, Søndre Boulevard 29, 5000 Odense C, Denmark*

Correspondence should be addressed to Dorthe Boe Danbjørg; dortheboe@gmail.com

Academic Editor: Malcolm Clarke

Background. A development towards earlier postnatal discharge presents a challenge to find new ways to provide information and support to families. A possibility is the use of telemedicine. *Objective.* To explore how using an app in nursing practice affects the nurses' ability to offer support and information to postnatal mothers who are discharged early and their families. *Design.* Participatory design. An app with a chat, a knowledgebase, and automated messages was tried out between hospital and parents at home. *Settings.* The intervention took place on a postnatal ward with approximately 1,000 births a year. *Participants.* At the onset of the intervention, 17 nurses, all women, were working on the ward. At the end of the intervention, 16 nurses were employed, all women. *Methods.* Participant observation and two focus group interviews. The data analysis was inspired by systematic text condensation. *Results.* The nurses on the postnatal ward consider that the use of the app gives families easier access to timely information and support. *Conclusions.* The app gives the nurses the possibility to offer support and information to the parents being early discharged. The app is experienced as a lifeline that connects the homes of the new parents with the hospital.

1. Background

Since the 1990s, the average length of postnatal hospital stay has declined, both in Denmark and internationally. The most prominent reasons are a renewed focus on the fact that giving birth is not a disease and the general need for cost savings in the healthcare system [1–4]. In Denmark, the average length of postnatal hospitalization has decreased from 92 hours in 2007 to 77 hours in 2012 [3].

A Danish questionnaire study (N = 1,507 women) identified that 44.3% of the women who were discharged early (within 24 hours) from postnatal care experienced a lack of follow-up support; that is, they felt that they did not receive the support needed to care for the newborn; 37.5% did not receive support for postnatal self-care, and 46.1% did not receive adequate support around breastfeeding [5]. These findings concur with results in international research [2, 6, 7]. Studies show that new parents experience concerns, uncertainty, doubts, and feelings of insecurity during the

postnatal period and are in need of follow-up support after early discharge [2, 6, 8–10]. Support is important when becoming a parent—Barclay et al. underline that one of the mediating factors in becoming a mother is "the nature of social support available," which includes partner, family, friends, and health professionals [11].

A sense of security is a central element to support as it might influence a parent's journey towards becoming a successful parent. Persson et al. have developed the concept "parents' postnatal sense of security." They identified the following dimensions as important for both parents' postnatal sense of security: empowerment from staff, affinity within the family, and the health and wellbeing of the family. An empowering organisation was fundamental for strengthening this [9, 12–15].

If the parents feel insecure it can have a negative effect on parental self-efficacy (PSE). The definition of PSE is as follows: "beliefs or judgments a parent holds of their capabilities to organize and execute a set of tasks related to parenting a child" [16]. For parents to employ parenting behavior positively, they must have confidence in performing the specific behavior. Parents with high self-efficacy are likely to make a greater effort than parents with low self-efficacy. Bandura has clarified what it is that enables an individual to build self-efficacy beliefs. Important aspects are mastery learning, where you can gain positive experiences, when you are doing things yourselves, vicarious experiences, that is, seeing others perform, and verbal persuasion, where others assure you that you hold the ability to perform a certain task [17, 18].

The new trend towards shorter hospital stays has affected healthcare professionals' practice. They experience that they have too little time to support new parents and to give individualised and timely information [6, 19].

In 2011, The Region of Southern Denmark issued a new policy regarding the postnatal period, in which early postnatal discharge (i.e., from four to six hours; max. 24 hours) was to become general practice following uncomplicated delivery for first-time and multiparous mothers. This shift in the postnatal care presents a challenge in terms of finding new ways to provide the sufficient support that meet the needs of the new parents with a postnatal follow-up that can enhance PSE and a sense of postnatal security.

One possibility is the use of telemedicine, which can provide an innovative solution [20–22].

Telemedicine has also been developed within obstetrics practice [23–27]. It seems that telemedicine has the potential to provide appropriate support to early discharged mothers and their families, because it offers the possibility for new parents to be guided by healthcare professionals in their transition into parenthood. Findings by Lindberg show that both parents and healthcare professionals find that telemedicine has the potential to provide appropriate support because it presents new ways to communicate that can substitute for face-to-face contact and it can be a valuable and functional complement to usual practice [25, 26].

We wanted to explore this potential and therefore designed and developed a software application (app), which was tested in a pilot study prior to the intervention [28].

1.1. Aim.
The aim is to explore how nurses experience using an app in nursing practice and how it impacts their ability to offer support and information to postnatal mothers who are discharged early and their families, in a way that will enhance the families' sense of security and self-efficacy.

2. Methods, Participants, and Data Collection

2.1. Design.
This study applied a participatory design (PD). It combines the use of qualitative methods and intervention, based on collaboration with users. The PD approach involves defining problems and indicating solutions in designing sustainable IT solutions for practice together with the users. An essential aspect of designing and developing a new technology is the intervention phase, where the actual technology is tried out in practice and concrete experiences with the use of the new technology are gained. Participatory design

can be viewed as hermeneutics, where new understanding is developed through a circular collaboration between the researcher's understanding and an attempt to interpret a certain phenomenon in collaboration with the participants [29].

PD has its origins in action research [29–32]. Action research spans a wide landscape of differentiated, but primarily qualitative, research strategies for bringing about change through action, developing and improving practice [33].

2.2. Intervention.
This study was an intervention study where an app was tested between hospital staff and new parents at home following early postnatal discharge. The content, format, and style of the app were designed on the basis of the parents' identified needs, in close cooperation with the nurses on the postnatal ward, and with the assistance of a team of computer programmers. The identified needs have previously been reported in depth [6].

In brief, new families requested an individualised postnatal follow-up, timely information and guidance, and accessibility to, and new ways to communicate with, healthcare professionals. This reflected the professional concern that the nurses had as to how they can ensure a postnatal care, which will ensure a sense of security, wellbeing, and parental self-efficacy, when the new parents are being early discharged. The app was designed with the following functionalities that should accommodate the needs of the early discharged parents.

(1) Asynchronous communication, online chat, where the families could send text messages to the healthcare professionals as well as photos and videos and receive an answer within four hours. This method of communication may diminish the barrier in accessing healthcare professionals after hospital discharge.

(2) A knowledgebase consisting of information material with a search function for easier access to information. The information material was evidence-based and written and compiled by the nurses on the ward. The information material consisted of written material about the postnatal period, for instance, information about breastfeeding, skin-to-skin contact, the mother's restitution after giving birth, and practical advice about baby care. The knowledgebase also contained instructions videos with guidance about breastfeeding, skin-to-skin contact, the wellbeing of the baby, baby clues, and how to bathe the baby.

(3) Messages sent out automatically every 12 hours from the time of birth. The messages relate to the age of the baby and should be relevant to the new parents providing them with information about breastfeeding, the baby's first bowel movement, and so on. The nurses had written down what they would normally inform and instruct the new parents about in the first postnatal days. It was rewritten into short messages that the new families would receive every 12th hour for the first 4 days after their baby was born. In

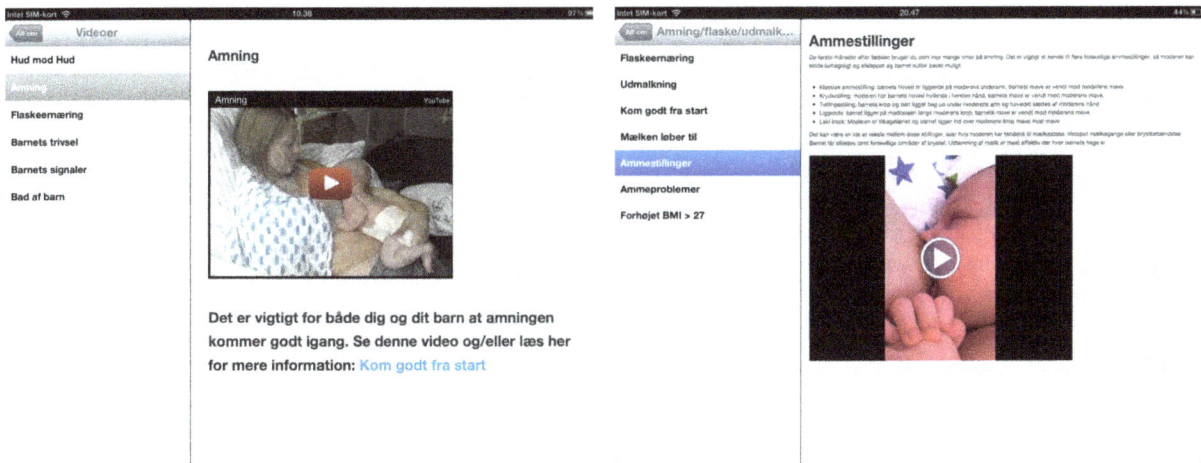

FIGURE 1

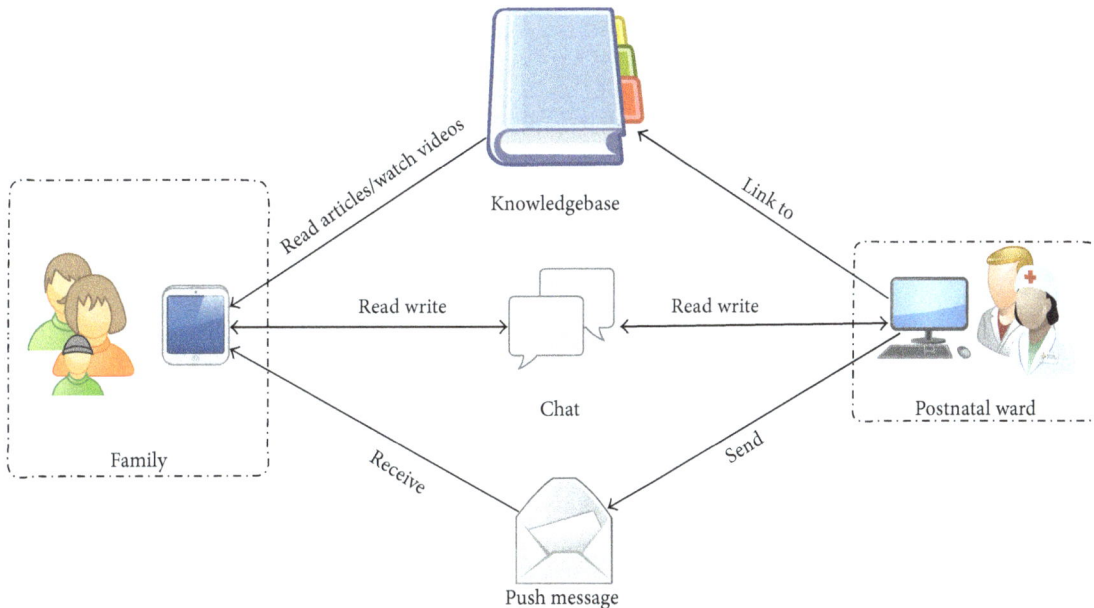

FIGURE 2

the messages there are relevant links to the knowledgebase with more thorough information. The following is an excerpt of a message.

24 hours after giving birth. Your boy has to suck efficiently at least 6–8 times a day. Your baby will often wake up and show signs of hunger, if not you [sic] have to wake him up, read more about that here: "Get a good beginning" and "Breastfeeding." (Figures 1 and 2).

The parents were given an iPad to take home on loan on which the app was installed. They had access to the app for seven days. They were to return the iPad to the hospital after seven days in a prestamped package.

Prior to the intervention, we tested the app in a pilot study [28], where the nurses were instructed in the use of the app and the accompanying website. The nurses registered the new parents on the website and used it to check for messages. The nurses were responsible for the online chat, which in practice meant that they had to check it every four hours and send replies to the families. Two of the nurses were responsible for updating the knowledgebase. These responsibilities were additional to the nurses' assigned duties involving caring for the patients admitted to the postnatal ward. No extra time was allocated in their shift for the additional work involved in answering messages.

2.3. Sample and Context. The study took place on a postnatal ward that handles approximately 1,000 births a year and included nurses employed on the ward. The management at the ward had initiated the project after the implementation of the new postnatal policy in The Region of Southern

Denmark. The nurses at the ward were all involved in the project and willing to participate in the intervention.

During the course of the study, four nurses moved job and three were employed. The newly employed nurses were introduced to the intervention. At the onset of the intervention, 17 nurses, all women, were working on the ward. Their professional postnatal experience varied from less than one year to 30 years, with a mean of 10.2 years. At the end of the intervention, there were 16 nurses employed, all women. Their professional postnatal experience varied from under one year to 30 years, with a mean of 7.1 years.

2.4. Data Collection. Participant observation was carried out on the postnatal ward from March to August 2013, on average one day a week, in all 20 days. The data were primarily collected during day shifts, though five times were also during evening shifts. The nurses were not followed through an entire shift, because the focus was how they experienced using the app in nursing practice and how it affected their ability to offer support and information to postnatal mothers who are discharged early.

The data from the participant observation are based on informal conversations with the nurses. The informal conversations took place during the nurses' coffee or lunch breaks or in the nurses' office. Sometimes they spontaneously started talking about the app, and other times we would ask a question to initiate a talk. Occasionally we were also assisting them with practical advice or help concerning the iPads or the webpage, which automatically led to conversations about the app and how they experienced using it.

Field notes were taken concurrently with a focus on place, participants, and activity. The following served as a guideline for the observations: what happens at the time of observation and what intentions and feelings occur in the situation [34].

We also conducted two focus group interviews [35, 36]. All the nurses on the ward who had taken part in the study were invited to a focus group interview. Nine out of a possible 13 nurses attended. The other nurses could not attend on the given dates, due to either work or personal matters. The number of participants who could attend on the chosen dates determined the size of each group, which ended up being four and five. The focus group interviews were held in the employee staff-room on the postnatal ward.

Before each focus group interview commenced, the moderator (the first author) introduced the purpose of the interview and clarified the guidelines and the focus: experiences using the app in nursing practice and how it affects their ability to offer support and information to postnatal mothers who are discharged early.

An interview guide was compiled. The overall theme focused on the nurses' experiences, which formed the basis of the discussion [37, 38]. Some additional questions were asked during the discussion. The development nurse on the ward participated as a comoderator, made notes during the interviews, and evaluated the atmosphere and interaction. The focus group interviews lasted 44 and 55 minutes, respectively, and were audio-recorded and transcribed verbatim.

3. Ethical Considerations

The participants received oral and written information about the study and were included after providing their informed consent, in compliance with the Helsinki Declaration [39]. The first author asked the nurses if they would like to participate in a focus group interview, and they were given time to think it over. They were told that participation was voluntary and that the focus group interviews would be held during working hours.

The study was submitted to the Scientific Ethics Committee. The committee decided that approval from an ethics committee was unnecessary according to the national legislation in Denmark (S-20110171). The Danish Data Protection Agency registered and approved the study (2008-58-0035).

4. Data Analysis

The data analysis was inspired by Malterud's systematic text condensation (STC) [40] and organised according to the steps taken in the analysis, as shown in Table 1. STC is a descriptive and explorative method used in the analysis of qualitative data, such as interview studies, observational studies, and in the analysis of written texts [41]. Giorgi's psychological phenomenological analysis was the starting point for STC. He developed the descriptive phenomenological method in psychology [38, 41, 42]. STC is a development of Giorgi's principles, including four comparable steps of analysis. It is pragmatic in the sense that it is easy to both follow and share due to the elaborated steps of the analysis.

Firstly, we captured an overall impression of the data and extracted a preliminary set of main themes.

Secondly, the data was divided into meaningful topics, which were relevant to the study question. Next, the meaningful topics were condensed and coded. Finally, the findings were synthesized, involving a shift from condensation to descriptions and categories. The codes were developed based on the preliminary themes identified in the first step and the theoretical framework.

In order to optimise validation, three researchers from the research team were involved in the analysis process. Our findings were subsequently discussed in relation to relevant literature and theory.

5. Results

The categories that emerged from the data analysis were as follows:

(1) an app as a means of providing support,

(2) an app as a means of conveying timely and accessible information.

The categories are presented below and are illustrated by quotations from the two focus group interviews (FGI) and from conversations that took place during the participant observation (PO).

Step 1: from medley to themes: superior themes extracted after the first open reading of the text	Step 2: from themes to codes. Identifying the meaningful units. The meaningful units are coded based on the superior themes as well as the preunderstanding and the theoretical frame		Step 3: from codes to meaning. The meaningful units are sorted into groups with respect to the codes; hereby overall categories arise from the coding process, which then are divided into subcategories
	Quotations	[Code]	
No tears	"I answer their questions… (…). I look at the photo of the umbilicus for instance or whatever it is. But I do not have the mother's tears. It creates a distance"	[Lack of senses] [one sided dialoque] [sic]	Telemedicine as a means of providing support
Open door	"And I think that it is a help. They feel that it is ok that they take contact"	[help available]	
Repetition	"Then they get the pop-up messages which means they get the information one more time, that's great"	[timely information]	Telemedicine as a means for timely and accessible information.
A lot of information in a short time	"You are just talking, talking, talking… And how much do they really remember?"	[Too much information]	

5.1. An App as a Means of Providing Support

5.1.1. Adjustment to New Ways of Communicating.
The nurses were hesitant at first when they had to chat online with the families, that is, using written instead of verbal communication. The following example occurred during a lunch break on the ward at the very beginning of the intervention.

> One of the nurses (nurse T) related that she had answered a message: "Well, I think it was very time consuming. It was all new to me and normally I would just talk on the phone, but I really had to think twice before sending the message". One of the other nurses (nurse K) supplemented this with: "Yes, it does take quite some time and the mother who wrote, well, how would I put it, the message wasn't well articulated". Nurse T continued: "It wasn't that it was difficult, but it just felt so different to write to a family instead of just talking". Nurse K then said: "It is probably also a matter of time—we have to get used to it." (Field note, March 2013, PO)

Another concern was that when communicating in writing, one uses fewer of the senses.

> I answer their questions (…) I look at the photo of the umbilicus, for instance, or whatever it is. But I do not have the mother's tears. It creates a distance. (Nurse I, FGI)

Though, after a period of time using the app, the nurses no longer felt that it was such a big challenge or that it involved changes to their work.

> Maybe you have to have some ping-pong, to ask the right questions, like you would have asked, if you were in the room [i.e. face to face]. But it hasn't been difficult. (Nurse D, FGI)

However, they did state that a lot depended on the type of questions that they had to answer on the online chat. Messages that were accompanied by, for example, a photo of an umbilicus were considered "easy" to answer, whereas questions about breastfeeding were more difficult, since more information and dialogue were required in order to make a judgment and give the appropriate support.

> But, that's also the point. Well, they can get answers to something very specific, but it is also the intention that where it is very complicated, and there are a lot of problems, we need to see them. (Nurse A, FGI)

The nurses stressed that the written communication cannot "stand alone," but they emphasized that there was always the option to invite the parents to come to the ward for more guidance face-to-face and that this occurred on occasion.

The nurses had to check the chat for messages every 4 hours, which showed to be a constant challenge. Explanations given for forgetting to check the online chat were that the nurses were too busy and there were challenges to adjust to the new procedures; the nurses had to go to the office to check the chat, and they usually spend most of their time in the patients' rooms or the nursery room.

> We do delegate who is responsible for the chat during the shift, but then oh no we have forgotten it. I have responded to one that was 14 hours old. (Nurse A, FGI)

5.1.2. Connecting Hospital and Home.
The app gave the parents the option to stay at home, while, for instance, having the baby's umbilicus assessed, because they could send a photo. The nurses found that the possibility to send photos was an advantage instead of the parents having to explain how the umbilicus looked like, over the phone. It provided

the nurses with a more accurate impression of the umbilicus, and they experienced that it increased their possibility to provide the appropriate advice and support.

The following example shows the differences between the distinctive forms of contact the nurses used. It took place during a coffee break on the ward.

> *One of the nurses had assessed an umbilicus based on a photo sent using the online chat. She could see that the baby was red in the groin, so she also wrote a note on that to the family. One of the nurses said: "well, that would not be possible over the phone". To which another replied: "but, if they had been here [on the ward], you could have seen the whole baby, not just the groin, and then you could also check the armpits, for instance." (Field note, March 2013, PO)*

The nurses agreed that families often found it difficult to contact healthcare professionals, because they did not want to disturb, which they ascribed to cultural factors or general expectations in society.

> *I also think it is just a cultural thing. Nowadays, people with kids—they want to take care of themselves. (Nurse D, FGI)*

The nurses also discussed that the new parents were reluctant to call the ward for help, even though the nurses told them that they should always call, if they had any doubt when they had been discharged. They thought that it was because the parents had experienced that the nurses were busy, and then they did not want to disturb.

> *They find it difficult to take contact. They feel it is inconvenient, because they have experienced that we were busy. (Nurse V, FGI)*

The nurses experienced that the app gave the families an opportunity to make contact with them after discharge, where they did not feel that they were intruding.

> *And I think that's a help. They feel that it is ok that they make contact. (Nurse V, FGI)*

5.2. An App as a Means of Conveying Timely and Accessible Information

5.2.1. Accessible Information. The nurses emphasized that one of the advantages of the app was that the information material for the parents was in digital instead of paper form.

> *Paper, it is all over, a mess, whereas the iPad—they know where that is. It suits them. Paper doesn't. (Nurse I, FGI)*

The nurses expressed that there was a lot of information material handed out at the hospital, and they questioned how much of it the families actually read. They considered it an advantage that it was now in digital form, as it seemed to appeal more to the families, because they could easily access

it on the iPad and they could also search within the material in the same way as using "Google" or other search engines.

Another possibility was watching the instruction videos. The nurses experienced that this was a suitable way for the new parents to be guided. For instance, the nurses at the ward showed the admitted parents how to bathe the baby, but this was at a fixed time during the day, and if the parents watched the video, they could watch it whenever they wanted.

> *When they are admitted for such a short time, it becomes very hectic to tell and show them everything. This way they can do it, when they want to and also when they are at home. (Nurse K, FGI)*

They also found that it was easy for them to refer to a video or a written instruction.

> *Well she wrote me a question, and I answer her back, but I also wrote that I thought she should read the information, it was easy to do, because I knew that she could find it easily on the app. (Nurse S, June 2013, PO)*

The nurses told that the parents reported that they felt secure with the app. They knew where to look for the information, and at the same time they knew that they could easily get in contact with the nurses at the ward.

> *And then she [a mother] told me that she was so secure, because it was just like having a nurse standing outside the door. (Nurse B, August 2013, PO)*

5.2.2. Timely Information. The nurses had to adjust to the new policy with the early discharge. It stressed them because they had shorter time with the individual family.

> *Well they come from the delivery ward, and then they are here for such a short period of time. And they sometimes just fall asleep, when I talk to them. They need something differently. (Nurse V, FGI)*

The nurses expressed that it was reassuring to know that when the families were discharged with the app they were drip-fed information in the form of automated messages. It relieved some the pressure they might feel when discharging mothers early, in terms of the duty to "have informed thoroughly enough."

> *I think that there is so much information that they need in such a short time. Then you are just talking and talking, while you think, how much do they remember, when they come home. (Nurse A, FGI)*

The nurses often had a feeling that the families could not retain all the general information. The nurses considered that the automated messages seemed to meet this challenge by providing families with timely information.

> *Knowing that, if there is something that I have forgotten, they get the pop-up messages, which*

TABLE 2

Functions of the app	Aspects supported	Supports
Knowledgebase, videos & information	Possibility for consistent relevant information	PPSS
	Acting independently (mastery experiences)	PSE/PPSS
	Seeing others perform, for instance, videos about breastfeeding (vicarious experiences)	PSE
Automated messages	Timely information	PPSS
	Being reassured (verbal persuasion)	PSE/PPSS
Online chat, asynchronous communication	Access to healthcare	PPSS
	Being reassured (verbal persuasion)	PSE
	Support (verbal persuasion)	PSE/PPSS

means they get the information one more time, that's great. (Nurse A, FGI)

The nurses regarded the automated messages that the families received as a tool to stimulate the families' curiosity and also their capacity to take control of their situation. The nurses believed that because of the interactive links in the automated messages, when the parents read the messages, they could easily read additional information material in the knowledgebase or they could address a question to the nurses on the postnatal ward. The nurses experienced that the parents took control of their situation and the messages made the parents feel well prepared for the postnatal period. The messages served either to reassure them or to allow them to react, if they required more information or support.

It is like a pat on the shoulder. Everything is ok. (Nurse D, FGI)

6. Discussion

In this study, we found that the nurses consider that the app gives them the possibility to offer support to the families discharged early, as it provided easier access to timely information and support, and it enhanced opportunities for families to initiate contact after discharge. They nurses find that the app connects the homes and the hospital.

The nurses state that the written asynchronous environment offers an easy way to offer families support. They feel that it connects the hospital setting with the home and goes some way towards reducing the gap, which families can experience as a barrier, in the fact that they are reluctant to contact the hospital staff for support after discharge [2, 6, 43]. Other studies have also found that when new families are discharged, it is essential that they are able to get professional support whenever they need it [25, 44, 45]. Persson et al. have identified that accessibility to support from healthcare professionals is an essential part of experiencing a postnatal sense of security [9, 14, 15, 46] (Table 2).

The nurses regard the app as a lifeline for families because it increases access to professional support. The app constitutes a new way of making support available. This is in line with the conclusions from a study by Bjoernes et al. in 2012 that explored the possibilities involved in online contact between nurses and men with prostate cancer (*n* = 34).

The patients experienced a feeling of partnership in dialogue (via e-mail) that supported their ability to be active and it gave them a feeling of freedom and security. They saw the written asynchronous contact as providing a flexible and calm communication environment and as a way to substitute for the reduction in face-to-face contact at the hospital [47].

Yet an important aspect is that the new parents are depending on the fact that the nurses do check the chat every 4 hours in order to have access to support, and the study showed that it was a constant challenge. Even though the nurses thought they just had to get used to the new routine, we discussed new ways of remembering the chat, because it was critical for the parents' sense of security that they could rely on it.

The nurses in our study also found that when the face-to-face contact was reduced due to the early discharge the automated messages and the use of instructions videos were a suitable way for informing the new parents. This relates to Bandura's viewpoints on interactive computer-assisted feedback as a convenient means to inform, enable, motivate, and offer support [48]. It offers a way to reassure parents that their newborn is healthy and to help parents to feel in control of their new situation, which are factors that enhance a postnatal sense of security [12] as well as PSE [17, 18, 48] (Table 2).

Another aspect of the instruction videos is the potential of enhancing PSE through vicarious experiences, where the parents can see others perform, for instance, breastfeeding positions and bathing the child (Table 2).

The results revealed that the nurses feel the app enhances patients' curiosity and, to some extent, it encourages parents to act more independently, because they can easily search for information themselves. The nurses experienced that the new parents are more likely to seek for information themselves, when it is digitalized than in a paper pamphlet. According to Bandura, acting independently and thereby gaining one's own experience are a way of achieving mastery experiences, which strengthen PSE [18] (Table 2).

The nurses found that the automated messages serve to reassure parents, and this suggests that the messages could potentially have the effect of encouragement. According to Bandura, verbal persuasion contributes to PSE because the parents are convinced that they can cope successfully [18]. This can contribute to the achievement of a feeling of success.

Also personal messages with encouraging feedback from healthcare professionals could to some extent substitute for the verbal persuasion that the families would receive if they were admitted for a longer duration after childbirth.

Bandura also states that because it is readily accessible and convenient, there are advantages in offering internet-delivered guidance. This is reflected in our study, where the nurses point out that the asynchronous communication is essential to their view of the app as a lifeline. It is easy to seek help; the families do not encounter a barrier in contacting the nurses for advice. This is because they do not feel that they are disturbing the nurses, as opposed to making a synchronous phone call. This is described in the literature as an issue in healthcare, because patients are often reluctant to contact healthcare professionals, even when they have something important to ask or discuss [2, 49]. It seems that the app has potential to be more efficient in ensuring access to healthcare than a phone.

Other studies have tested videoconferencing in the postnatal period [23, 24, 26]; it was valued as a supplement to traditional practice. The midwives saw that communicating via videoconferencing was almost equivalent to having a face-to-face meeting. The same was found in other studies that involved videoconferencing; the healthcare professionals experienced that it is possible to create an intimate relationship and proximity in technology-mediated care and that it provides a tool for patients to develop a sense of security at home [50, 51].

The transmission of photos gives new options compared to phone-mediated contact. A photo can "say more than a 1000 words" [52], where the nurses can actually see and observe instead of both families and nurses having to rely on written or oral descriptions over the phone. Other studies have pointed out further advantages for patients in staying at home instead of going to the hospital, in terms of time saved on travelling and waiting for a consultation [53].

The use of online communication such as e-mail or text messaging involves a language-analogue mediation—it is a dialogue, but not like a dialogue that two people have face-to-face or mediated by the phone [52]. The nurses addressed that the online chat function changed their way of communicating with the families, which they experienced to change their support to the new parents. This can be explained by applying Ihde's postphenomenological theory, where he underlines that the technological mediation of human practice shapes our experiences of the situations in which we are engaged. Technology is not a neutral tool; it provides a framework and invites us to employ certain use-patterns [52, 54–56]. When communicating face-to-face or on the phone, they felt they could use more of their senses to assess the patient's expressions or voice and evaluate their emotional or mental state as when communicating online. In this situation, as compared to when conducting a written dialogue, they felt it would be more natural for them to extend the dialogue to issues other than the one initially addressed.

However a report from the Institute for Healthcare Informatics [57] on the use of social media shows that patients also use social media for emotional support, which indicates that it is no longer only through face-to-face dialogue that people feel they can get emotional support. The report concludes that there have been essential changes in the way people communicate, and as a consequence the new technologies will change how healthcare operates on a global scale [57]. This development is also underpinned by a review by Plantin and Daneback [58] that showed the majority of today's parents search for not only information, but also social support on the internet. As a result of this development and because of the reduction in face-to-face contact, it has become more common for hospital staff to both communicate online [27, 59] and offer telephone support [60] following early discharge.

The limitation of our study is that it was a small-scale study. However the participatory design process with involving the participants in the design of the technologies was valuable. We could use the concrete experiences with the use of the app in the intervention in the further design process, where there had to be adjustments to the chat function. The new adjustments mean that the nurses do not have to check the computer for new messages, but they got an iPhone, where they receive a notification, whenever there is a new message.

There is a potential to assess the app in a randomized controlled trial for a more generalizable knowledge.

The development nurse on the ward was chosen to be the comoderator. She was newly employed and had not been a part of the intervention. Yet some of the nurses at the ward were familiar with her, which could contribute to a comfortable and safe atmosphere during the interview [35, 61].

7. Conclusion

The app gives the nurses the possibility to offer support and information to the parents being early discharged, as the app is experienced as a lifeline that connects the homes of the new parents with the hospital.

The written asynchronous communication provides an easy way for the nurses to offer the new parents support, when they are being early discharged, because the parents find it easier to contact the nurses through the app than the phone. This provides access to the healthcare professionals, which is essential in order to ensure parents' postnatal sense of security.

The automated messages are a suitable way for informing the new parents and it encourages them to act independently, which can enhance parental self-efficacy because the parents are inspired to take action thereby gaining mastery experiences.

The nurses experience that the app offers an efficient way to provide information to the parents as compared to pamphlets, because the parents were more likely to seek information when it was digitalized.

The nurses generally tend to focus their actions around providing information, and they do not consider that written communication lends itself to a more open and extended dialogue. This could be a question of needing more time to adapt to this new way of communicating. With more time, they could possibly use the asynchronous communication not only to convey information and for observation purposes, but also to offer emotional support.

Acknowledgments

The authors would like to thank the participants in the study; their participation, engagement, and sharing of experiences have allowed this study to be conducted. The Region of Southern Denmark, the University of Southern Denmark, the Danish Nurses' Organization, and The Novo Nordisk Foundation funded the project.

References

[1] S. Brown, R. Small, B. Faber, A. Krastev, and P. Davis, "Early postnatal discharge from hospital for healthy mothers and term infants," *Cochrane Database of Systematic Reviews*, no. 3, Article ID CD002958, 2002.

[2] K. Johansson, C. Aarts, and E. Darj, "First-time parents' experiences of home-based postnatal care in Sweden," *Upsala Journal of Medical Sciences*, vol. 115, no. 2, pp. 131–137, 2010.

[3] L. Sørensen, "Readmission among newborn infants 2007–2012," 2013.

[4] L. Sørensen, "Barselperioden efter ukompliceret fødsel : en kvalitativ'undersøgelse af hvilke ressourcer barselkvinden har, hvordan hun bruger sine ressourcer, samt hvordan barselgangens indsats matcher disse," MPH 2001:13, Nordiska hälsovårdshögskolan. 60s, Göteborg, Sweden.

[5] Unit of Patient Perceived Quality, *Women's Experience of Pregnancy, Birth and the Postnatal Period in the Capital Region of Denmark*, 2010.

[6] D. B. Danbjørg, L. Wagner, and J. Clemensen, "Do families after early postnatal discharge need new ways to communicate with the hospital? A feasibility study," *Midwifery*, vol. 30, no. 6, pp. 725–732, 2014.

[7] S. Kanotra, D. D'Angelo, T. M. Phares, B. Morrow, W. D. Barfield, and A. Lansky, "Challenges faced by new mothers in the early postpartum period: an analysis of comment data from the 2000 Pregnancy Risk Assessment Monitoring System (PRAMS) survey," *Maternal and Child Health Journal*, vol. 11, no. 6, pp. 549–558, 2007.

[8] H. L. McLachlan, L. Gold, D. A. Forster, J. Yelland, J. Rayner, and S. Rayner, "Women's views of postnatal care in the context of the increasing pressure on postnatal beds in Australia," *Women & Birth*, vol. 22, no. 4, pp. 128–133, 2009.

[9] E. K. Persson, B. Fridlund, L. J. Kvist, and A.-K. Dykes, "Mothers' sense of security in the first postnatal week: interview study," *Journal of Advanced Nursing*, vol. 67, no. 1, pp. 105–116, 2011.

[10] A. M. Fink, "Early hospital discharge in maternal and newborn care," *Journal of Obstetric, Gynecologic, and Neonatal Nursing*, vol. 40, no. 2, pp. 149–156, 2011.

[11] L. Barclay, L. Everitt, F. Rogan, V. Schmied, and A. Wyllie, "Becoming a mother—an analysis of women's experience of early motherhood," *Journal of Advanced Nursing*, vol. 25, no. 4, pp. 719–728, 1997.

[12] E. K. Persson and A. K. Dykes, "Parents' experience of early discharge from hospital after birth in Sweden," *Midwifery*, vol. 18, no. 1, pp. 53–60, 2002.

[13] E. K. Persson and A.-K. Dykes, "Important variables for parents' postnatal sense of security: evaluating a new Swedish instrument (the PPSS instrument)," *Midwifery*, vol. 25, no. 4, pp. 449–460, 2009.

[14] E. K. Persson, B. Fridlund, and A.-K. Dykes, "Parents' postnatal sense of security (PPSS): development of the PPSS instrument," *Scandinavian Journal of Caring Sciences*, vol. 21, no. 1, pp. 118–125, 2007.

[15] E. K. Persson, B. Fridlund, L. J. Kvist, and A.-K. Dykes, "Fathers' sense of security during the first postnatal week—a qualitative interview study in Sweden," *Midwifery*, vol. 28, no. 5, pp. e697–e704, 2012.

[16] F. de Montigny and C. Lacharité, "Perceived parental efficacy: concept analysis," *Journal of Advanced Nursing*, vol. 49, no. 4, pp. 387–396, 2005.

[17] A. Bandura, "Self-efficacy: toward a unifying theory of behavioral change," *Psychological Review*, vol. 84, no. 2, pp. 191–215, 1977.

[18] A. Bandura, *Self-Efficacy. The Exercise of Control*, W. H. Freeman, 1997.

[19] I. Lindberg, K. Christensson, and K. Öhrling, "Midwives' experience of organisational and professional change," *Midwifery*, vol. 21, no. 4, pp. 355–364, 2005.

[20] J. Clemensen, S. B. Larsen, M. Kirkevold, and N. Ejskjaer, "Treatment of diabetic foot ulcers in the home: video consultations as an alternative to outpatient hospital care," *International Journal of Telemedicine and Applications*, vol. 2008, Article ID 132890, 6 pages, 2008.

[21] J. Craig and V. Patterson, "Introduction to the practice of telemedicine," *Journal of Telemedicine and Telecare*, vol. 11, no. 1, pp. 3–9, 2005.

[22] N. M. Hjelm, "Benefits and drawbacks of telemedicine," *Journal of Telemedicine and Telecare*, vol. 11, no. 2, pp. 60–70, 2005.

[23] E. F. Magann, S. S. McKelvey, W. C. Hitt, M. V. Smith, G. A. Azam, and C. L. Lowery, "The use of telemedicine in obstetrics: a review of the literature," *Obstetrical and Gynecological Survey*, vol. 66, no. 3, pp. 170–178, 2011.

[24] I. N. Odibo, P. J. Wendel, and E. F. Magann, "Telemedicine in obstetrics," *Clinical Obstetrics and Gynecology*, vol. 56, no. 3, pp. 422–433, 2013.

[25] I. Lindberg, K. Christensson, and K. Öhrling, "Parents' experiences of using videoconferencing as a support in early discharge after childbirth," *Midwifery*, vol. 25, no. 4, pp. 357–365, 2009.

[26] I. Lindberg, K. Öhrling, and K. Christensson, "Midwives' experience of using videoconferencing to support parents who were discharged early after childbirth," *Journal of Telemedicine and Telecare*, vol. 13, no. 4, pp. 202–205, 2007.

[27] A. H. Salonen, M. Kaunonen, P. Åstedt-Kurki, A.-L. Järvenpää, H. Isoaho, and M.-T. Tarkka, "Effectiveness of an internet-based intervention enhancing Finnish parents' parenting satisfaction and parenting self-efficacy during the postpartum period," *Midwifery*, vol. 27, no. 6, pp. 832–841, 2011.

[28] D. B. Danbjorg, L. Wagner, and J. Clemensen, "Designing, developing and testing an app for parents being discharged early postnatal," *The Journal for Nurse Practitioners*, vol. 10, no. 10, pp. 794–802, 2014.

[29] F. Kensing, *Methods and Practices in Participartory Design*, ITU Press, 2003.

[30] K. Bødker, F. Kensing, and J. Simonsen, *Participatory IT Design: Designing for Business and Workplace Realities*, The MIT Press, 2004.

[31] L. Wagner, "Two decades of integrated health care in Denmark," *Tidsskrift for Sygeplejeforskning*, vol. 2, pp. 13–20, 2006.

[32] J. Clemensen, S. B. Larsen, M. Kyng, and M. Kirkevold, "Participatory design in health sciences: using cooperative experimental methods in developing health services and computer technology," *Qualitative Health Research*, vol. 17, no. 1, pp. 122–130, 2007.

[33] A. Titchen and A. Binnie, "Action research: a strategy for theory generation and testing," *International Journal of Nursing Studies*, vol. 31, no. 1, pp. 1–12, 1994.

[34] J. P. Spradley, *Participant Observation*, Holt, Rinehart & Winston, New York, NY, USA, 1980.

[35] K. Malterud, *Focusgroups as a Research Method in Medicine and Health*, Universitetsforlaget, Oslo, Norway, 2012.

[36] B. Halkier, *Focus Groups*, Samfundslitteratur & Roskilde Universitetsforlag, Frederiksberg, Denmark, 2002.

[37] J. P. Spradley, *The Etnographic Interview*, Wadswoth Group, 1979.

[38] S. Kvale, *Interviews: An Introduction to Qualitative Research Interviewing*, Sage Publications, Thousand Oaks, Calif, USA, 1998.

[39] WMA, "WMA declaration of Helsinki—ethical principles for medical research involving human subjects," in *55th WMA General Assembly*, Tokyo, Japan, October 2004, http://www.wma.net/en/30publications/10policies/b3/.

[40] K. Malterud, *Qualitative Methods in Medical Research*, Universitetsforlaget, 2nd edition, 2003.

[41] K. Malterud, "Systematic text condensation: a strategy for qualitative analysis," *Scandinavian Journal of Public Health*, vol. 40, no. 8, pp. 795–805, 2012.

[42] A. Giorgi, "Sketch of a psychological phenomenological method," in *Phenomenology and Psychological Research*, A. Giorgi, Ed., Duquesne University Press, Pittsburgh, Pa, USA, 1985.

[43] C. Wilkins, "A qualitative study exploring the support needs of first-time mothers on their journey towards intuitive parenting," *Midwifery*, vol. 22, no. 2, pp. 169–180, 2006.

[44] M. Löf, E. C. Svalenius, and E. K. Persson, "Factors that influence first-time mothers' choice and experience of early discharge," *Scandinavian Journal of Caring Sciences*, vol. 20, no. 3, pp. 323–330, 2006.

[45] L. Sørensen and E. O. C. Hall, "Resources among new mothers—early discharged multiparous women," *Nordic Journal of Nursing Research & Clinical Studies*, vol. 24, no. 1, pp. 20–24, 2004.

[46] L. J. Kvist and E. K. Persson, "Evaluation of changes in postnatal care using the 'Parents' Postnatal Sense of Security' instrument and an assessment of the instrument's reliability and validity," *BMC Pregnancy and Childbirth*, vol. 9, article 35, 2009.

[47] C. D. Bjoernes, B. S. Laursen, C. Delmar, E. Cummings, and C. Nohr, "A dialogue-based web application enhances personalized access to healthcare professionals—an intervention study," *BMC Medical Informatics and Decision Making*, vol. 12, no. 1, article 96, 2012.

[48] A. Bandura, "Health promotion by social cognitive means," *Health Education and Behavior*, vol. 31, no. 2, pp. 143–164, 2004.

[49] D. B. Danbjørg, L. Wagner, and J. Clemensen, "Do families after early postnatal discharge need new ways to communicate with the hospital? A feasibility study," *Midwifery*, vol. 30, no. 6, pp. 725–732, 2014.

[50] B. Lindberg, K. Axelsson, and K. Öhrling, "Experience with videoconferencing between a neonatal unit and the families' home from the perspective of certified paediatric nurses," *Journal of Telemedicine and Telecare*, vol. 15, no. 6, pp. 275–280, 2009.

[51] A. Sorknæs, *The Effects of Real-Time Telemedicine Video Consultations between Nurses and Patients with Severe Chronic Obstructive Pulmonary Disease (COPD)*, University of Southern Denmark, Odense, Denmark, 2013.

[52] D. Ihde, *Bodies in Technology*, University of Minnesota Press, Minneapolis, Minn, USA, 2002.

[53] J. Clemensen, S. B. Larsen, and N. Ejskjaer, "Telemedical treatment at home of diabetic foot ulcers," *Journal of Telemedicine and Telecare*, vol. 11, supplement 2, pp. S14–S16, 2005.

[54] D. Ihde, *Heidegger's Technologies Postphenomenological Perspectives*, Fordham University Press, Bronx, NY, USA, 2010.

[55] D. Ihde, *Technology and the Lifeworld from Garden to Earth*, Indiana University Press, Bloomington, Ind, USA, 1990.

[56] L. Hunniche and F. Olesen, *Technologi in Health Practice*, Munksgaard, 2014.

[57] The IMS Institute for Healthcare Informatics, *Engaging Patients through Social Media*, The IMS Institute for Healthcare Informatics, 2014.

[58] L. Plantin and K. Daneback, "Parenthood, information and support on the internet. A literature review of research on parents and professionals online," *BMC Family Practice*, vol. 10, article 34, 2009.

[59] A. H. Salonen, K. F. Pridham, R. L. Brown, and M. Kaunonen, "Impact of an internet-based intervention on Finnish mothers' perceptions of parenting satisfaction, infant centrality and depressive symptoms during the postpartum year," *Midwifery*, vol. 30, no. 1, pp. 112–122, 2014.

[60] T. Lavender, Y. Richens, S. J. Milan, R. M. D. Smyth, and T. Dowswell, "Telephone support for women during pregnancy and the first six weeks postpartum," *Cochrane Database of Systematic Reviews*, no. 7, Article ID CD009338, 2013.

[61] R. Krueger, "Ouality control in focus group research," in *Succesful Focus Groups*, D. Morgan, Ed., pp. 65–88, Sage, Newbury Park, Calif, USA, 1993.

16

Feasibility and Acceptability of Utilizing a Smartphone Based Application to Monitor Outpatient Discharge Instruction Compliance in Cardiac Disease Patients around Discharge from Hospitalization

Aimee M. Layton,[1] James Whitworth,[2] James Peacock,[3] Matthew N. Bartels,[4] Patricia A. Jellen,[5] and Byron M. Thomashow[1]

[1]Division of Pulmonary, Allergy and Critical Care Medicine, Department of Medicine, Columbia University Medical Center, VC3-365 Center for Chest Disease NYPH-CUMC, 622 W. 168th Street, New York, NY 10032, USA
[2]Department of Biobehavioral Sciences, Teachers College, Columbia University, 522 W. 120th Street, New York, NY 10027, USA
[3]Division of Cardiology, Department of Medicine, Columbia University Medical Center, 622 W. 168th Street, New York, NY 10032, USA
[4]Department of Physical Medicine and Rehabilitation, Montefiore Medical Center, 111 E. 210th Street, Bronx, NY 10467, USA
[5]Center for Chest Disease, New York Presbyterian Hospital, 622 W. 168th Street, New York, NY 10032, USA

Correspondence should be addressed to Aimee M. Layton; aml2135@columbia.edu

Academic Editor: Manolis Tsiknakis

The purpose of this study was to determine the feasibility and acceptability of utilizing a smartphone based application to monitor compliance in patients with cardiac disease around discharge. For 60 days after discharge, patients' medication compliance, physical activity, follow-up care, symptoms, and reading of education material were monitored daily with the application. 16 patients were enrolled in the study (12 males, 4 females, age 55 ± 18 years) during their hospital stay. Five participants were rehospitalized during the study and did not use the application once discharged. Seven participants completed 1–30 days and four patients completed >31 days. For those 11 patients, medication reminders were utilized 37% (1–30-day group) and 53% (>31-day group) of the time, education material was read 44% (1–30) and 53% (>31) of the time, and physical activity was reported 25% (1–30) and 42% (>31) of the time. Findings demonstrated that patients with stable health utilized the application, even if only minimally. Patients with decreased breath sounds by physical exam and who reported their health as fair to poor on the day of discharge were less likely to utilize the application. Acceptability of the application to report health status varied among the stable patients.

1. Introduction

In order to improve healthcare quality for patients with several chronic conditions, the Patient Protection and Affordable Care Act of 2010 instituted penalties for hospital reimbursement if a patient admitted for myocardial infarction, congestive heart failure, or pneumonia was readmitted to the institution within 30 days of the original discharge (Patient Protection Affordable Care Act 2010). As such, hospitals have been faced with identifying patients in these cohorts who may be at high risk for hospital readmission and implementing interventions in hopes of improving patient care and reducing penalties that may be incurred by early readmission [1, 2].

Multicomponent interventions that feature early assessment of discharge needs have been found to be beneficial in reducing readmission rates [3]. These multicomponent interventions have made use of education, timely transfer to primary care teams, post-acute followup between 24 and 72 hrs by nurse of physician, and appropriate referrals to support services such as rehabilitation programs [3] and the use of home exercise programs [4]. Although these programs may be effective, the extensive time and staffing needed for their implementation and success can limit their feasibility [5]. Alternatives to one-on-one patient to healthcare provider interaction have begun to be developed to potentially allow for a greater implementation of such interventions [6]. Various telemedicine approaches, such as smartphone applications, are being considered as potential tools for allowing healthcare professionals to implement and monitor patients remotely.

Smartphone applications are inexpensive and, unlike other forms of telemedicine, do not require home installation [7]. Smartphone applications can be utilized not just for accessing and tracking health information but also as a tool allowing practitioners and the patient's social support system to become more involved in his/her care without being physically present and in educational content delivery [8].

Areas where wireless health monitoring has been found to have succeeded in monitoring and tracking patients' health have been in patients with heart failure [9]. Patient's weight, blood pressure, and symptoms have been successfully monitored remotely by several telemedicine or structured telephone support systems [10]. However, these studies utilized multifaceted systems that provided and received information by more than just a smartphone application. Also the adoption of patients to utilize telemedicine systems has been an issue [11]. Chaudhry et al. found that recently discharged patients with heart failure had poor adherence of using the telemedicine system given to them after discharge. Given the age and demographics of heart failure patients, it is not clear whether a strictly smartphone application would be well adopted or demonstrate similar adoption problems as other telemedicine systems. Although there are potential benefits of utilizing smartphone technology for monitoring patients who are at high risk for being readmitted, the feasibility of monitoring heart failure patients or postmyocardial infarction patients via a strictly smartphone application has not yet been well documented. To our knowledge, there has been no report on the frequency of application use or potential barriers these patients may have in utilizing such technology after hospitalization.

The purpose of this study was to investigate the feasibility and acceptability of a smartphone iOS application to monitor and assist with patient medication compliance, education, home exercise, symptom changes, and transition to outpatient care team after hospitalization. The aim of this study was to determine the frequency of application use, potential barriers of use, and potential dropout rate in collecting this type of data in such population.

2. Methods

This study was a qualitative study discussing the home-based feasibility and acceptability of utilizing a smartphone application to collect health information and interact with patients with CHF or CAD around discharge.

The iOS application administered daily educational material, medication reminders, doctor appointment reminders,

and monitored activity level. Process measurements, such as user engagement, daily task completion, and perceived value of the application to the patient, were recorded. Secondary outcome measures were activity level, medication compliance, follow-up care, enrollment into support programs such as cardiac or pulmonary rehabilitation program when applicable, and 30–60 day readmission rates in our population. Patients were given the usual standard of care throughout the study and the iOS application was only used to supplement outpatient discharge instructions and compliance, not to be used in place of the usual standard of care. Patients were instructed to follow all of their doctors' and nurses instructions and if there were any questions or confusion to contact their physician. All treating physicians were notified of their patient's participation in the study.

2.1. Participants. Hospitalized patients with a diagnosis of coronary artery disease (CAD) or congestive heart failure (CHF) were recruited. Patients were not considered for enrollment until clinical staff informed the study personnel that the patient would be eligible for discharge within the next 3 days. Study exclusion criteria consisted of a lack of described diagnosis, inability to perform physical activity, unstable angina, neurological deficit that makes the individual unable to understand and follow directions, being illiterate, non-English-speaking, and no home WiFi connection.

Physicians and nurses working on the inpatient cardiac units identified 180 patients for the study team who were admitted with a primary diagnosis of CAD or CHF and were eligible for discharge. The study team then approached the patients and screened them for patient interest and eligibility. The study staff made it clear that participation was completely voluntary and all usual care would continue regardless of study participation. If the patient demonstrated interest in participation, the study staff informed the patient of what study participation would involve and received his/her consent to participate. This study was approved by the Columbia University Medical Center's Institutional Review Board. All participants signed informed consent prior to participating.

2.2. Protocol. Once patients consented to participating in the study, either the iOS application (Wellframe Application by Wellframe, Cambridge, MA) was uploaded to their smartphone or, if the patient did not own a device that could operate an iOS application, an iPod touch (iPod touch model A1367, Apple Inc., Cupertino, CA) was lent to the participant for the duration of the study. Patients were then given an orientation to how to use the device. A one-page instruction sheet was also given to the patient and the patient was instructed to practice using the application during their hospital stay. Study staff then followed up with the patient prior to discharge to ensure that there were no further questions regarding the use of the application. Figure 1 demonstrates the study personnel follow-up phone call protocol to collect information on rehospitalization, symptoms, and connection with outpatient care team.

Each day the participants received reminders to take their medication at self-selected times, brief condition

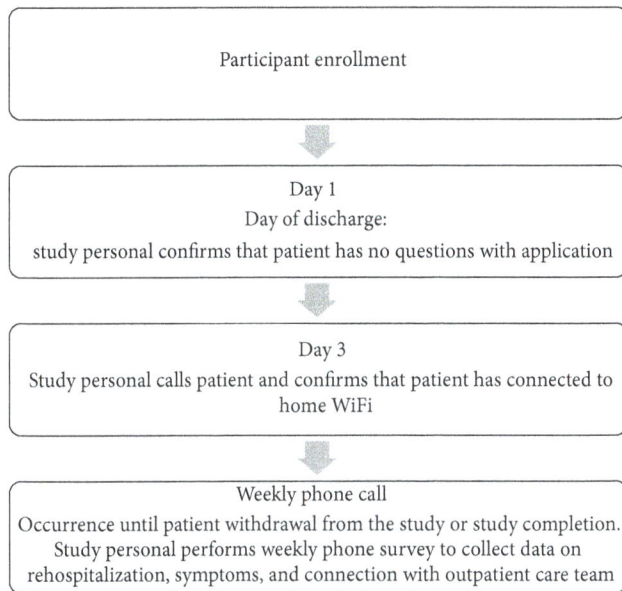

FIGURE 1: Study protocol.

TABLE 1: Educational content topics.

Topic	General description of the following was included:
Coronary heart disease	Pathology, management, and symptoms
Medications	The value of medications, instructions for taking medications, and potential side-effects
Exercise	The benefits of exercise and guidance for exercising safely
Nutrition	General nutritional recommendations and benefits
Smoking	Benefits of smoking cessation/reduction and resources for quitting
Alcohol	General guidance and recommendations around alcohol consumption for cardiovascular health and recovery
Psychosocial	Information and resources around mood disorders
Biometric risk factors	Supporting patients to "know their numbers" (ie., blood pressure, weight/BMI, lipids, or oxygen when applicable)

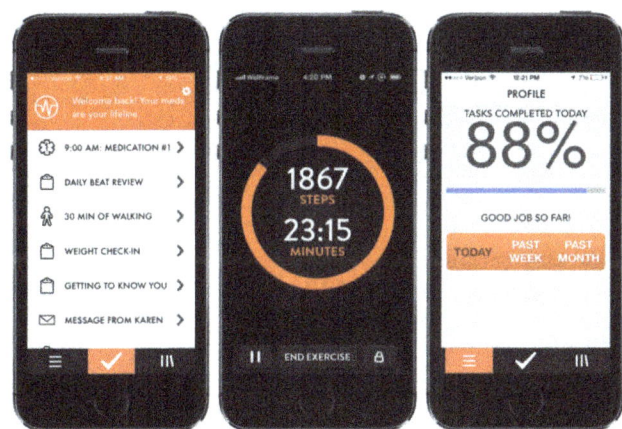

FIGURE 2: Example of application interface and content.

specific educational videos, and readings, and when relevant participants received reminders for upcoming appointments with healthcare providers. Additionally, participants could report changes in symptoms (e.g., dyspnea) and biometric measurements (e.g., heart rate) and track their physical activity through the iOS application's pedometer. Patients were considered "compliant" if greater than 50% of the "Daily To-Do Tasks" were completed. Figure 2 depicts an example of the application's "Daily To-Do Tasks."

2.3. Measurements

2.3.1. iOS Application Content. The Wellframe application recorded medication compliance by self-report. The time of day the patient takes his or her medication was programmed into the application. Each day, at the programmed time, a medication reminder would appear on the patient's smart phone or iPod touch. The patient would then have to confirm

by touching "yes" or "no" if he or she took their medication. If the patient selected "no," an option to be reminded again in an hour would appear. If the patient selected "yes," then a second reminder would appear on the phone or iPod touch an hour later.

Educational material was given to the patient daily via the patient's "Daily To-Do's." The patient would be prompted to click on the educational reading material or video. Once the patient viewed the educational material, a check would appear on his or her "To-Do List" to demonstrate that task had been completed. The educational material consisted of disease management, smoking sensation, importance of attending cardiac or pulmonary rehab programs, and potential psychosocial issues associated with heart disease. Every day the patient received one of the "education topics" to read. Full list of topics can be seen in Table 1.

The patients were also sent daily messages encouraging him or her to perform daily walking, stretches, and light strengthening exercises (home based cardiac rehabilitation program) [12, 13].

When the patient tapped the prompt on his/her "To-Do" list to perform his/her daily exercises, he/she was then taken to a second screen that included instructions for the exercises, videos for the stretches and light strengthening exercises, and a pedometer for walking. At the end of the exercise regimen, the patient was asked to enter his/her level of breathlessness based on a modified Borg scale of perceived exertion [14]. For safety, the research team monitored the patient's exercises remotely and if a patient reported a level of breathlessness higher than 4 (somewhat severe), reported a heart rate exceeding 150 bpm, or had any adverse symptoms (e.g., dizziness, nausea, headache, chest discomfort, lightheadedness, drop in blood pressure, unusual heartbeat, or palpitations) the Medical Director of the Cardiac and Pulmonary Rehabilitation Program here at New York Presbyterian Hospital was alerted and a plan was in place to contact the patient. Patients were instructed to forgo the exercise program if they began a cardiac rehabilitation program.

Daily survey questions were asked regarding breathlessness, overall control of health, ease of using the application, medication side effects, and biometric measurements. Biometric measurements included weight, blood pressure, and heart rate.

During the weekly phone calls, the study staff would ask the patient if he or she had been enrolled in a cardiac rehabilitation program or had any upcoming doctor appointments. If the patient responded in the affirmative, then the staff would ask for the dates and times and enter the appointments into the patient's application via the dashboard. Staff also surveyed the patient to if he or she found the application useful and how is it most helpful. Lastly, the staff would inquire if the patient has seen his/her physician during the past week and if he or she has been recently hospitalized (if yes, then why). If the patient could not be reached after three attempts (over the course of 3 days), then a person the patient had designated as an acceptable emergency contact person for the study was contacted to confirm the patient's safety and if he or she had been hospitalized.

2.3.2. The Dashboard. Patient data was uploaded to a remote dashboard for the study staff to view and send messages to the patient via a secure server (approved by Columbia University Information Technology Department as a HIPPA compliant and secure server approval forms attached). Data was uploaded real time and the study staff would contact the patient via the application 1-2 times per week to provide encouragement. The study team could also request a response from a patient via the messaging system on the dashboard and modify a patient's medication reminders or exercise protocol if necessary via the dashboard or by contacting Wellframe.

2.3.3. Chart Review. Demographics, anthropometry, and ejection fraction and information about the patient's hospital stay were obtained by reviewing the electronic hospital chart. Information about any complications during the patient's stay, breath sounds by physical exam, and medications were retrieved from the physicians and/or nursing notes. For "day of discharge" information, notes within 24 hrs of discharged were considered acceptable and data from that note were retrieved. The pain scale and resting dyspnea scores were collected from the physical therapist's note on the day of discharge or the day prior to discharge if there was no physical therapy note provided at the day of discharge. Sleep quality and self-report description of healthy values were obtained via the Wellframe application at the day of discharge. All patients were asked to respond to the "daily beat questions" on the day of discharge so that the study team could ensure that the application was working properly.

2.4. Data Analysis. We tested the feasibility of using this application in patients with CHF or CAD after hospitalization by collecting data on the frequency of application use, usage barriers described by the patient population, study dropout rate, and type of data patients were more or less likely to provide.

Based on previous behavior usage research, investigating the usage of smartphone applications [15], we selected to analyze standard ethnographic and user data. Application usage was described by analyzing the frequency of response to symptom and biometric data survey questions, medication reminders, clicks on educational content, pedometer readings, and clicks of stretches and strengthening exercise videos. The logging in of system usage to detect adherence has been utilized in other telemedicine studies [11, 16, 17]. Study population size is similar to previous feasibility studies [17, 18]. Acceptability was tested by collecting data on application usage and types of questions patients choose to respond to about their health. To better define the type of patients that may be more or less likely to utilize the application, objective health parameters and self-described health status were collected. Patient's responses and usage were graphed to determine behavioral trends. Statistical analysis was performed using SPSS version 21 (IBM Corp., Armonk, NY, 10504). Nonnumeric variables (insurance, dyspnea, breath sounds, and description of health) were coded by severity. A linear regression test was used to determine whether any of the variables collected had a relationship with the amount with which a patient utilized the application. Significance was set a priori at $P < 0.05$.

3. Results

3.1. Participant Characteristics. Between July 2013 and December 2013, 158 patients were approached for the study. Twenty-two patients who were identified as eligible for the study were not approached because they were asleep or with a treating physician when study personnel attempted recruitment. In all of these occurrences the study personnel attempted to return to the patient's room for recruitment; however, the patient had been discharged. Figure 3 depicts the breakdown of patients approached, declined participation, met exclusion criteria, and included. Of the 158 patients approached, 16 were enrolled in the study (12 M, 4 F, age 55 ± 18 years). Of the 16 patients, two were African American, one was Asian, one was Hispanic, and twelve were Caucasian. The largest barriers to enrollment were language and access to home WiFi.

Table 2 describes each patient's demographics, diagnosis, and socioeconomic status based on insurance provider. Ten of the patients who participated in the study had a diagnosis of CAD and were hospitalized for a cardiac intervention. Five of the patients were hospitalized with a primary admitting diagnosis of CHF. Most of our patients had private insurance providers.

3.2. Acceptability Analysis. The number of days patients interacted with the application after discharge and the characteristics of the patient's health are described in Table 3. The five patients who were readmitted to the hospital during

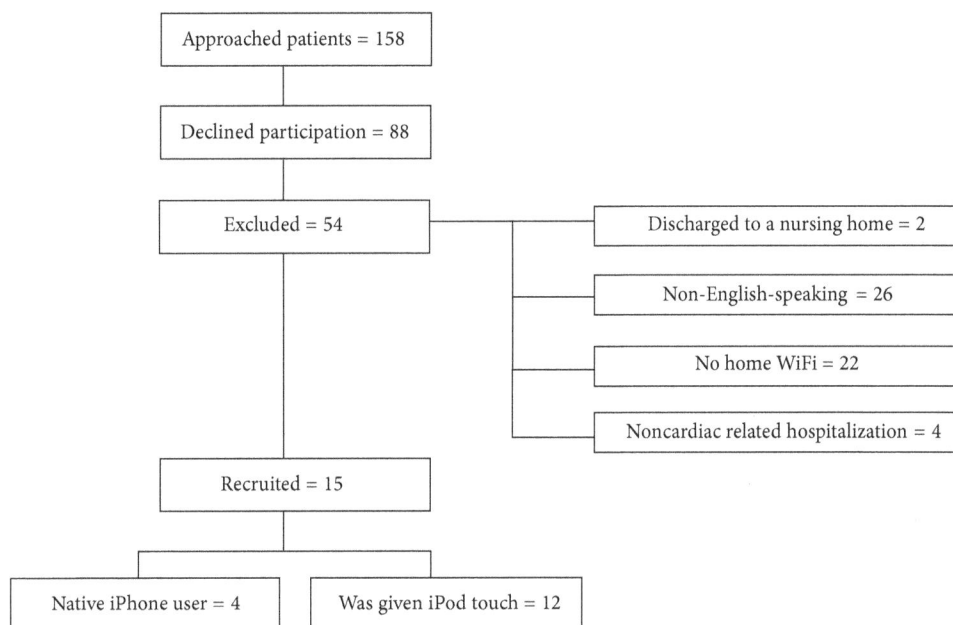

FIGURE 3: Participant recruitment and study population diagram.

TABLE 2: Demographics.

Subject	Age	Dx	Gender	Socioeconomic status by insurance provider
1	54	CAD	M	Private Ins
2	50	CHF	M	Medicare
3	84	CAD	M	Medicare
4	40	CHF	M	None
5	81	CHF	M	Medicare
6	49	CHF	F	Private Ins
7	37	CAD	F	Medicaid
8	40	CAD	M	Private Ins
9	69	CAD	M	Private Ins
10	60	CAD	M	Private Ins
11	26	CAD	F	Private Ins
12	72	CAD	F	Medicare
13	28	CHF	M	Medicaid
14	70	CAD	M	Medicare
15	71	CAD	M	Medicaid
16	46	CHF	M	Private Ins
Avg	55	CAD = 10, CHF = 6	M = 12, F = 4	7 = Private Ins, 4 = Medicare, 3 = Medicaid, 1 = none
SD	18			

Dx: diagnosis, CAD: coronary artery disease, CHF: congestive heart failure, BMI: body mass index, Private Ins: private insurance company provider, EF: ejection fraction, M: male, and F: female.

the study duration (average of 7 days after discharge) did not utilize the application once discharged from the hospital. Of the remaining patients, all who were not readmitted, the application was utilized between 1 day and the complete 60 days. The average amount of days with which a patient utilized the application was 17. The average body mass index revealed that our patients were on average obese. The reported estimated ejection fractions by ECHO (EF) (taken after intervention when applicable) revealed that the majority of our patients had an EF of >55% except for 4 patients who

had EFs of <45%. Of note, the patients who did not interact with the application were also the patients with more severe complications and complaints during their hospital stay, with the exception of one. This may reflect that sicker patients were less likely to utilize the application.

During the study, five patients (31%) were readmitted to the hospital, with the average readmission time of 7 days. Of note, all five patients only interacted with the application while being in the hospital and did not interact with the application once discharged. Of the 11 other patients, who were not

TABLE 3: Days interacted with the application after discharge, anthropometric measurement, severity of heart disease measurements, and hospital stay information.

Subject	Number of days patient interacted with app after discharge	EF	BMI (kg/m^2)	Length of hospital stay	Readmitted to hospital within 60 days		Complications or complaints post-op
1	0	65%	28.9	19	SOB	7 days	Afib, R diaphragm paralysis
2	0	20%	39.4	6	Infection	24 hrs	Day of discharge, complained of chills
3	0	65%	29.4	19	Thrombo-cytopenia	3 days	Volume overload, Afib, knee pain
4	0	60%	54.0	8	SOB chest pressure	3 days	SOB
5	0	10%	23.8	3	Cardiac arrest	~3 wks	None
6	1	63%	29.1	2	No		None
7	1	25%	44.6	12	No		None
8	1	55%	21.0	5	No		L foot pain
9	5	60%	26.4	5	No		None
10	13	55%	24.8	4	No		None
11	26	55%	21.3	5	No		Post-op anemia
12	30	60%	38.4	9	No		Back pain
13	40	55%	25.0	8	No		None
14	48	60%	27.1	9	No		None
15	52	55%	27.4	13	No		Post-op anemia
16	58	45%	24.1	13	No		None
Mean	17	51%	30.3	9	5 = Yes, 11 = No		
Std	21	17%	9.2	5			

App: application, SOB: shortness of breath, Afib: atrial fibrillation, R: right, L: left, post-op: postoperative, R/O: rule out, and std: standard deviation.

readmitted during the course of the study, 8 interacted with the application within the first day after discharge, 1 interacted with the application 3 days after discharge, and 2 interacted with the application greater than 1 week after discharge (Table 1). Ten patients withdrew from the study prior to day 60; however, of these ten patients, five agreed to participate in the 60-day follow-up survey to verify if he or she had been hospitalized within 60 days after discharge. Four of the ten patients declined any further participation in the study. Retrospective chart review confirmed that all four patients were not readmitted to the hospital within 60 days of discharge.

3.2.1. Correlates of Application Use.
Results demonstrated that patients with unstable health after discharge had a lack of application use. All patients who were readmitted during the study did not utilize the application once discharged. These results are not suggesting a causational relationship but a correlative relationship, where application use may be a good indicator of overall health status.

Other correlatives of application use were breath sounds by physical exam within 24 hrs of discharge and the patient's self-report of health status at the day of discharge (Table 4). Analysis revealed that decreased breath sounds or crackles by physical exam within 24 hrs of discharge had a significant relationship with application use ($R^2 = 0.370$, $P = 0.021$). The patient's self-report of his or her health status at the day of discharge also had a significant relationship with application

use ($R^2 = 0.335$, $P = 0.038$). Breath sounds and self-report of health were independent predictors of application use and could explain 79% of the variability in application use when modeled together ($R^2 = 0.625$, $P = 0.02$).

3.2.2. Usage Barriers.
The patients that found the application helpful also utilized the application the most and remained in the study the longest. Reasons patients gave to why the application was not helpful were the inability to change medication reminder times, the inability to enter doctor's appointments or other reminders themselves (the study team would have to enter these reminders into the dashboard and then the patient would receive the reminder), the pedometer would stop counting if another application on the device was opened (this is a limitation of iOS software design), and the general inconvenience of being asked to use the application on a regular basis. Upgrades to the application software and user interface have resolved many of these issues. Unfortunately, the inconvenience of entering data for a research study is a common limitation to participant compliance. Positive responses to application use were the usefulness of the medication reminders, the educational information provided in the "Daily Beat," and the stretching and exercise videos.

3.3. Feasibility Analysis.
Seven patients completed 1–30 days of the trial. Figure 4 demonstrates the overall compliance

TABLE 4: Day of discharge information.

Subject	Pain scale	Resting HR	Dyspnea	BS on exam DOD	Day of discharge described health as	Discharged with pain medication
1	0	107	Moderate	Decreased, wheeze	Fair	Oxycodone, Tylenol
2	5	99	Mild	Decreased	Fair	Tylenol
3	0	74	Moderate	Decreased/crackles	Good	Oxycodone, Percocet
4	0	85	Very mild	N/A	Poor	None
5	0	93	None	Crackles	Good	Aspirin
6	N/A	96	None	Clear	Fair	Toradol, Tylenol
7	0	72	Mild	Decreased	N/A	None
8	5	95	None	Clear	N/A	Hydromorphone
9	0.5	71	None	Trace crackles	Good	Aspirin
10	2	88	None	Clear	N/A	Oxycodone, Tylenol
11	6	94	Moderate	Clear	Good	Tylenol w/Codeine
12	10	68	Moderate	Trace crackles	Fair	Aspirin, Vicodin
13	0	99	None	N/A	Excellent	Aspirin
14	4	86	Very mild	Clear	Good	Tylenol
15	0	100	Very mild	Clear	Good	Oxycodone
16	0	100	None	Clear	Very good	Tylenol, Morphine
Mean	2	89				
Std	3	12				

HR: heart rate, BS: breath sounds, DOD: day of discharge, std: standard deviation.

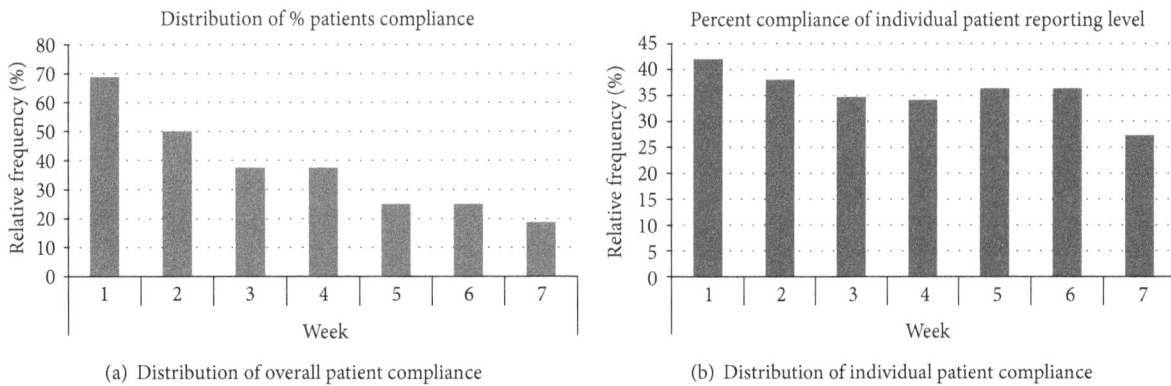

(a) Distribution of overall patient compliance

(b) Distribution of individual patient compliance

FIGURE 4: Distribution of compliance frequency.

of application usage. Sixty-nine percent of the patient population utilized the application during week one; however, the percent of relative frequency of use diminished to only 19% by week 7, demonstrating poor adherence over time (Figure 4(a)). During week 1, the patients answered the application questions with a median of 42% of the time. Over time, compliance diminished to a nadir of 27% (Figure 4(b)). On average, those patients utilized the medication reminders 37% of the time, read education material 44% of the time, answered survey questions through the application 55% of the time, and performed the recommended physical activity 25% of the time. Four patients completed

31–60 days of the trial and utilized medication reminders 53% of the time, read education material 53% of the time, answered survey questions through the application 93% of the time, and performed the recommended physical activity 42% of the time. The data reveals that the patients who completed 31–60 days of the trial utilized the application more than those who withdrew prior to day 31. Patients who answered most of the survey questions continued to answer most of the survey questions throughout the study protocol. Patients who answered fewer than half of the survey questions in the first week proceeded to drop out to the study the following week. A common theme of patients who completed

TABLE 5: Synopsis of survey questions and answers by patients after discharge.

Survey questions	Days after discharge						
	1–7 ($N = 11$)	8–14 ($N = 8$)	15–21 ($N = 6$)	22–28 ($N = 6$)	29–35 ($N = 4$)	36–42 ($N = 4$)	43–58 ($N = 3$)
How breathless do you feel?	54%	75%	100%	83%	100%	100%	100%
Weight (lbs)	50%	83%	40%	50%	100%	100%	100%
How easy do you find using this app?	22%	33%	Question no longer asked				
Please count your pulse for 20 seconds	31%	63%	83%	67%	100%	100%	100%
How would you describe your health today?	73%	33%	83%	100%	100%	100%	100%
I am in control of my own health	33%	67%	75%	75%	100%	100%	100%
Do you like the exercises on the app?	29%	67%	Question no longer asked				

greater than 31 days was the presence of a family member during study recruitment. It appeared that when the patient's family support valued the patient utilizing the application, the patient was more likely to utilize the application for >31 days and be more compliant with the use of the application.

Both groups participated with the survey tool that requested the patient to rate his or her breathlessness, take his or her pulse, enter his or her weight, describe his or her health that day, and respond to the ease of using the application's feature (Table 4). The patients who remained in the study the longest were the most compliant in answering these survey questions. Patients were more likely to answer the questions about shortness of breath, entering their weight and describing their health, and least likely to answer the questions regarding the ease of using the application or how in control of their health they felt they were (Table 4). In the patients who withdrew prior to day 31, they utilized the educational material the most and the physical activity aspect of the application the least. The patients who completed 31–60 days of the trial utilized the medication reminders and educational material equally.

4. Discussion

4.1. Principal Findings. This study has shown that collecting information regarding postdischarge compliance and patients' health status via smartphone application in patients with heart failure or coronary artery disease may be feasible but not without limitation. Our results indicate that patients who were medically stable were more likely to utilize the application than patients who are unstable. Results also demonstrated that patients were more likely to respond to medication compliance questions, read education content, and respond to a few survey questions but not all and were less likely to report physical activity through the application (Table 5).

Acceptability of the application was low but similar to that of other studies. Min et al. [18] reported a smart phone application median compliance rating of 41% in their population of women undergoing treatment for breast cancer. Chaudhry et al. [11] reported a 90% adherence in telemonitoring use

in a population of patients with heart failure during the first week of the study but adherence decreased to ~55% by week 26. The low application compliance reported by this and other studies may reflect that although remote monitoring is convenient, the sample sizes needed for such research may be larger than those of other forms of survey tools or interventions. Therefore, future research in the field of remote monitoring may want to consider this low compliance rate when calculating desired sample sizes.

Compliance results also revealed higher acceptability rate in patients who remained in the study for greater than 31 days versus those who withdrew prior to 31 days. This relationship revealed a subset of patients who were more likely to utilize smart phone applications than others. Application usage is difficult to predict; however, work by Shin et al. [19] found that cellular network, time of day, and previous app use are all highly related to application usage. Hospitals that are seeking to utilize this kind of technology to track and interact with high risk patients may want to take into account these factors to optimize usage. Companies seeking to design applications for this use may also want to take into account these factors when designing their application.

Factors that impacted acceptability or barriers for usage were reported to be the inability to interact with the application as much as the individual required. As the patient's health and needs evolved, the application needed to be able to evolve. Also in patients whose health status was deteriorating, the application usage was decreased. These findings demonstrated a utility with smartphone applications to identify patients that need a care team to intervene rather than relying on technological remote monitoring. As highlighted by Pandor et al. [10], remote monitoring of patient's with HF health does not appear to impact the course of the patient's health unless monitoring dictates an action. Even when the remote monitoring dictates an action, study results have not always been positive [11]. Telemonitoring did not appear to provide a benefit over usual care when used to decrease rehospitalization [11]. Therefore, remote monitoring appears to be most useful in highlighting changes in behavior, rather than eliciting changes in outcomes. Thus, data collected by remote monitoring may be most useful for hospitals that are looking to allocate resources towards the patients who are most likely to be readmitted, rather than replacing usual care [11]. These results are not suggesting a causational relationship but an associative relationship between health status and application use. It is important to stress that smartphone applications may be most successful in helping to bridge the communication between care team and patient rather than be used to replace the need for one-to-one in-person interaction.

A novelty of this application to the growing "telemedicine" market was the immediate feedback mechanism via the application to a dashboard the clinician can log into, rather than other immediate feedback systems such as phone or video conference. Additionally, the telemedicine systems that involve home setup can cause a delay in information being received by the hospital. The average readmission time in our patient population was 7 days and mode was 3 days, and thus there was value in the ability to follow patients' status upon immediate discharge. For the above reasons, more of the remote monitoring market is moving to application use. The results from this study can help guide researchers, administrators, and companies in what aspect of the application appeared to be valued by the patient, such as medication reminder and educational content, and what aspects were underutilized, such as the pedometer and ability to communicate with the study team via the application.

A barrier to utilizing certain telemedicine devices discussed in prior research has been the barrier of training staff and patients on how to use the technology appropriately and in a timely fashion [20]. Some physicians expressed frustration with the time and level of technological sophistication needed to utilize certain technology [20]. A benefit to this particular application was the intuitive and simple user interface that took almost no training. However, this application was very limited in the information the clinician can gain from it. Perhaps future versions or application will include interfacing with diagnostic equipment that can provide a pulse rate, distinguish an arrhythmia, and allow for photographs to be uploaded to the dashboard. This would expand the use of the application beyond distinguishing the patient's general health state. However the cost-benefit ratio must be considered. Gurné et al. [21] described the incremental costs of using some telemedicine systems as being greater than the benefit in some settings. With each interface that an application builds, the cost increases. Also the ethics of attempting to replace in-person interaction with a multidisciplinary team in high risk patient populations, such as the one studied, should be considered [21]. However, the use of such applications as a tool to extend the reach of the care team, rather than a replacement, may allow for an inexpensive and manageable technique to identify patients who are in need of such in-person care.

There were limitations to this pilot study. Our patient population was not representative of the average patient here at New York Presbyterian as our initial version of the application was only in English. Since the completion of the study a Spanish version has been developed. Further research is needed to determine if these findings can be extrapolated to the Spanish speaking population. The WiFi requirement also limited recruitment. It is our suggestion that future

work should consider a data plan that allows the patient to utilize the device with or without WiFi, although this feature does add a further expense. Future work in a larger and more diverse population may be beneficial to confirm the relationships reported in these findings and allow for findings to be extrapolated to other patient populations. Lastly, the use of such application as a survey tool was useful however limited. A validated health questionnaire was not utilized for this study. This made the interpretation of the survey data limited. As a test of feasibility, the survey tool demonstrated that patients would respond to the daily questions and what questions the patients preferred; however, the applicability of these responses was limited.

5. Conclusion

This study demonstrated the feasibility and acceptability of utilizing an iOS application to monitor outpatient behavior in a group of patients considered to be at "high risk for readmission." Findings demonstrated that patients with stable health utilized the application more than patients with unstable health. The acceptability of the application varied greatly. There remains a need to better define aspects of smart phone applications that will result in optimal patient compliance; however, these results demonstrated that usage alone may be a useful tool to highlight patients in need of closer monitoring.

Acknowledgment

Wellframe Inc. supplied the smart phone applications and iPod touches for this study.

References

[1] G. Giamouzis, A. Kalogeropoulos, V. Georgiopoulou et al., "Hospitalization epidemic in patients with heart failure: risk factors, risk prediction, knowledge gaps, and future directions," *Journal of Cardiac Failure*, vol. 17, no. 1, pp. 54–75, 2011.

[2] H. M. Krumholz, Y.-T. Chen, Y. Wang, V. Vaccarino, M. J. Radford, and R. I. Horwitz, "Predictors of readmission among elderly survivors of admission with heart failure," *American Heart Journal*, vol. 139, no. 1, pp. 72–77, 2000.

[3] I. A. Scott, "Preventing the rebound: improving care transition in hospital discharge processes," *Australian Health Review*, vol. 34, no. 4, pp. 445–451, 2010.

[4] D. Seidel, A. Cheung, E.-S. Suh, Y. Raste, M. Atakhorrami, and M. A. Spruit, "Physical inactivity and risk of hospitalisation for chronic obstructive pulmonary disease," *International Journal of Tuberculosis and Lung Disease*, vol. 16, no. 8, pp. 1015–1019, 2012.

[5] S. Manning, "Bridging the gap between hospital and home: A new model of care for reducing readmission rates in chronic heart failure," *Journal of Cardiovascular Nursing*, vol. 26, no. 5, pp. 368–376, 2011.

[6] S. D. Anker, F. Koehler, and W. T. Abraham, "Telemedicine and remote management of patients with heart failure," *The Lancet*, vol. 378, no. 9792, pp. 731–739, 2011.

[7] N. M. Hjelm, "Benefits and drawbacks of telemedicine," *Journal of Telemedicine and Telecare*, vol. 11, no. 2, pp. 60–70, 2005.

[8] P. Klasnja and W. Pratt, "Healthcare in the pocket: mapping the space of mobile-phone health interventions," *Journal of Biomedical Informatics*, vol. 45, no. 1, pp. 184–198, 2012.

[9] M.-K. Suh, C.-A. Chen, J. Woodbridge et al., "A remote patient monitoring system for congestive heart failure," *Journal of Medical Systems*, vol. 35, no. 5, pp. 1165–1179, 2011.

[10] A. Pandor, T. Gomersall, J. W. Stevens et al., "Remote monitoring after recent hospital discharge in patients with heart failure: a systematic review and network meta-analysis," *Heart*, vol. 99, no. 23, pp. 1717–1726, 2013.

[11] S. I. Chaudhry, J. A. Mattera, J. P. Curtis et al., "Telemonitoring in patients with heart failure," *The New England Journal of Medicine*, vol. 363, no. 24, pp. 2301–2309, 2010.

[12] K. Jolly, R. S. Tayor, G. Y. H. Lip et al., "Home-based exercise rehabilitation in addition to specialist heart failure nurse care: design, rationale and recruitment to the Birmingham rehabilitation uptake maximisation study for patients with congestive heart failure (BRUM-CHF): a randomised controlled trial," *BMC Cardiovascular Disorders*, vol. 7, article 9, 2007.

[13] H. M. Dalal, P. H. Evans, J. L. Campbell et al., "Home-based versus hospital-based rehabilitation after myocardial infarction: a randomized trial with preference arms—Cornwall Heart Attack Rehabilitation Management Study (CHARMS)," *International Journal of Cardiology*, vol. 119, no. 2, pp. 202–211, 2007.

[14] G. Borg, "Ratings of perceived exertion and heart rates during short-term cycle exercise and their use in a new cycling srength test," *International Journal of Sports Medicine*, vol. 3, no. 3, pp. 153–158, 1982.

[15] T. M. T. Do, J. Blom, and D. Gatica-Perez, "Smartphone usage in the wild: a large-scale analysis of applications and context," in *Proceedings of the ACM International Conference on Multimodal Interaction (ICMI '11)*, pp. 353–360, November 2011.

[16] D. Scherr, P. Kastner, A. Kollmann et al., "Effect of home-based telemonitoring using mobile phone technology on the outcome of heart failure patients after an episode of acute decompensation: randomized controlled trial," *Journal of Medical Internet Research*, vol. 11, no. 3, p. e34, 2009.

[17] S. Winkler, M. Schieber, S. Lücke et al., "A new telemonitoring system intended for chronic heart failure patients using mobile telephone technology—feasibility study," *International Journal of Cardiology*, vol. 153, no. 1, pp. 55–58, 2011.

[18] Y. H. Min, J. W. Lee, Y. W. Shin et al., "Daily collection of self-reporting sleep disturbance data via a smartphone app in breast cancer patients receiving chemotherapy: a feasibility study," *Journal of Medical Internet Research*, vol. 16, no. 5, p. e135, 2014.

[19] C. Shin, J. H. Hong, and A. K. Dey, "Understanding and prediction of mobile application usage for smart phones," in *Proceedings of the 14th International Conference on Ubiquitous Computing (UbiComp '12)*, pp. 173–182, September 2012.

[20] D. L. Paul, K. E. Pearlson, and R. R. McDaniel Jr., "Assessing technological barriers to telemedicine: technology-management implications," *IEEE Transactions on Engineering Management*, vol. 46, no. 3, pp. 279–288, 1999.

[21] O. Gurné, V. Conraads, L. Missault et al., "A critical review on telemonitoring in heart failure," *Acta Cardiologica*, vol. 67, no. 4, pp. 439–444, 2012.

17

The Internet Use for Health Information Seeking among Ghanaian University Students

Benedict Osei Asibey,[1] **Seth Agyemang,**[1] **and Augustina Boakye Dankwah**[2]

[1]*Department of Geography and Rural Development, Faculty of Humanities and Social Sciences,*
 Kwame Nkrumah University of Science and Technology, Kumasi, Ghana
[2]*Department of Geography and Resource Development, Faculty of Social Sciences, University of Ghana, Legon, Accra, Ghana*

Correspondence should be addressed to Benedict Osei Asibey; benedictofall@gmail.com

Academic Editor: Malcolm Clarke

The aim of the study was to investigate university students' use of the Internet for health purpose in the Ghanaian context. The study employed a quantitative cross-sectional design. A total of 650 out of 740 students selected from 3 different universities participated, giving a response rate of 87.7% (650/740). Data were obtained using questionnaires and frequency and percentages were used to analyze data. The results show that university students are active users of the Internet as 78.3% (509/650) used Internet daily and 67.7% (440/650) use Internet for health purposes, for reasons including availability and ease of accessing information, privacy, confidentiality, and affordability. Use of Internet was constrained by unreliable and slow connection, high cost of Internet, and unreliable power supply. Also, 72.4% (315/435) used the online health information obtained as a basis for lifestyle change and only 39.5% (170/430) consulted health professionals after obtaining online information. The study concludes that students use Internet to seek online health support. The use of Internet to communicate with young people in relation to their health must therefore be explored. There is the need to be aware of online safety issues for young adults, including the need to provide information on privacy options.

1. Introduction

The Internet is a global network "information superhighway" that enables computers and other communication gadgets to communicate directly and transparently [1]. Internet is defined as a global broadcasting capability, a system for information broadcasting, and a means for interaction and collaboration between individuals and their communication devices irrespective of their geographical location [2].

The Internet, given its availability, affordability, and versatility, is used for different purposes, including increasing health-related purposes. The Internet is a very popular and important source of health information for both healthcare professionals and patients, as it offers the formal access to high quality, huge volume, current, and relevant healthcare information [3]. Thus, it has become increasingly common for people to locate health information and support with the use of Internet worldwide [4, 5]. For instance, the

Pew Internet and American Life Project in 2000 and 2009, respectively, reported that 55% and 80% of adults in the United States of America who had access to Internet used it to obtain medical or health information and support [4, 6, 7]. In Europe, the Health Service Executive in 2007 reported that 18% of Irish people used Internet for health information [8, 9].

In spite of the benefits of using Internet for health purpose, the existing literatures have mainly focused on developed countries, with little research work done in developing countries, particularly Africa. In order to bridge this knowledge gap there is the need to examine the use of the Internet for health purposes among the youth in sub-Saharan Africa. This study focused on university students in Ghana.

2. Background to Ghana's Healthcare Services

Access to basic healthcare services in Ghana still remains a huge challenge, and average life expectancy is about 10 years below the global average [10]. Preventable diseases such cholera and malaria continue to exert a heavy toll on the population. Other issues such as HIV AIDS, tuberculosis, and infant, child, and maternal mortality are still a force to reckon with, in spite of the giant strides made so far. Health professionals and healthcare services are being overwhelmed by the increasingly huge demand for healthcare. Though gradually improving, Ghana's doctor-to-patient ratio is still alarming. It was 1 : 10,341 in 2010, 1 : 10,170 in 2013, and stood at 1 : 9,043 in 2014. This is below the WHO standard of 1 : 600. The nurse-to-population ratios of 1 : 1,516 in 2010, 1 : 1,084 in 2013, and 1 : 959 in 2014 still fall below the WHO standard. The picture painted is that of inadequate number of health professionals against a population of 25.90 million [10]. The challenge of access is compounded by inadequate funds to finance health operations, poor and inadequate health infrastructure, and shortage of qualified health professionals.

It becomes imperative therefore to find alternative means of seeking healthcare that meet the minimum qualifications. One emerging innovation is to make health information accessible to all on a platform which can be reached by all irrespective of location and socioeconomic background, which is the Internet. Previous studies in Ghana have revealed that several Ghanaians use the Internet for different purposes [11–15]. The liberalization of the telecommunications sector allowing the market to be inundated with so many companies offering attractive packages and bonuses has certainly contributed to this boost. Statistics from the National Communication Authority (NCA) reveals that about 24.4 million Ghanaians use mobile phone [12]. The number of Internet users in Ghana in 2009 was 1.3 million, 93rd in the world, and reached 4.2 million in 2012, 69th in the world [13]. Also, NCA's mobile voice and mobile data market share trends for December 2015 reported that the number of mobile data subscribers in Ghana rose from about 17.73 million to 18.03 million, representing an access rate of 65.74 percent [14]. By the second quarter of 2016, mobile data subscription in Ghana according to the National Communications Authority had reached 18.8 million [15] This means that smart phone users in the country can have access to the Internet, the only other requirement being the availability of data. With the consequent exposure to ICT through the educational system, the potential for use of the Internet as a health seeking channel both is wide and should therefore be taken advantage of.

3. Justifying the Need for the Research

In spite of the evident infiltration of ICT accompanied by use of the Internet in sub-Saharan Africa, especially among the youth, not many studies have explored the use of Internet for health purposes. Studies in this area are largely concentrated on the developed world [6, 8, 9, 16–19]. There is a scarcity of research in Ghana done in this domain. The few works on Ghana have narrowly focused on teens in the junior high schools and other out-of-school youths [20–22]. It is thus not clear how university students, an important and recognizable segment of the population, with necessarily wide access to modern information technologies (mobile phones, desktop computers, laptops, and tablets) use the Internet for seeking health information and support.

Therefore, the aim of this study is to investigate the use of Internet among university students in Ghana for seeking online health information and support. The study specifically focuses on (1) access and use of Internet by students and (2) students' use of Internet for health purposes.

4. Methods

4.1. Study Design and Sampling. The study used a quantitative cross-sectional design and concentrated on 3 Ghanaian universities including 2 public universities (University of Ghana, Accra, and Kwame Nkrumah University of Science and Technology, Kumasi) and 1 private one (Central University, Accra). The study purposively focused on recruiting students at all levels (undergraduate, master's, and doctoral).

Convenient sampling was used to select a total of 740 students from the three universities. Of the 740 originally sampled university students, 650 participated by responding to the questionnaire, giving a response rate of 87.7%. These consisted of 250 each from University of Ghana and Kwame Nkrumah University of Science and Technology and 150 from the Central University. By the study protocol, only students from departments with inadequate health knowledge and information were included in the study. Students from departments more exposed to programmes or modules with adequate health-related information such as medicine, community health, nursing, public health, optometry, pharmacy, allied health, and other related faculties were not included. The sample also included undergraduate, master's, and doctoral students. Participation in the study was voluntary.

4.2. Research Instrument. Data were collected using the questionnaire. The researchers designed the questionnaire based on themes identified during the extensive review of literature. The questionnaire contained a mixture of different items ranging from multiple-choice to Likert-type scales and in some cases provided respondents with the opportunity for free expression.

The questionnaire consisted of 45 items grouped under 8 different headings labeled from A to H. Section A comprised 6 items and elicited demographic and background information of respondents including age, gender, level/year of study, type of accommodation, subject of study, and type of institution (whether public or private). The next 9 questions in Section B sought information on students' access and use of the Internet including questions on whether or not they use Internet, number of hours of Internet use per day, means of Internet access, type of Internet used on campus, and place of primary Internet access. Students were also asked to indicate their level of experience in using the Internet and also the challenges that they face in their access and use of the Internet.

Section C focused on the students' use of Internet for health purpose and covered issues like whether or not students have used the Internet for health purpose. Section D focused on how participants used the Internet, including frequency for specific health purposes. Frequency of use of

Internet for specific a health purpose was measured using a 4-point Likert scale as follows: 1, always; 2, often; 3, occasionally; 4, never. The last item under this section was about the frequency of finding the health information sought by students using the Internet, and this was measured using a 5-point Likert scale as follows: 1, always; 2, most of the time; 3, only sometimes; 4, hardly ever; 5, never.

Similarly, Section E was on students' use of devices, apps, and platforms to obtain health information. Students were required to respond with Yes or No to their use or nonuse of selected devices, apps, and platforms. Section F focused on use of health information obtained by respondents using the Internet. Here too, students were required to respond with Yes or No to selected use of health information obtained. Under Section G, participants were required to rate the importance of identified factors affecting their decision to use apps, platforms, and websites as sources of health information. Specifically, participants were to indicate whether the selected factors were not important, fairly important, or very important. Section H, the last section, focused on how the health information obtained using the Internet had helped improve students' personal health.

4.3. Validity and Reliability of the Questionnaire. The researchers took measures to ensure validity of the developed questionnaires. Before the actual data collection, the questionnaire was reviewed by 2 academics including one statistician and one medical geographer. Also, 5 postgraduate students including 3 from Kwame Nkrumah University of Science and Technology and 2 from the University of Ghana reviewed the questionnaire for content validity. Modifications were made based on the feedback from the reviewers. With the aim of improving its reliability, the questionnaire was then pretested on 15 university students who were not part of the actual survey. Modifications were also made based on the results of the pretesting. Internal consistency reliability was ensured by calculating Cronbach's alpha coefficient of internal consistency. A value of .697 was obtained as Cronbach's alpha coefficient, indicating acceptable level of internal consistency in the questionnaire.

4.4. Data Collection. The questionnaires were administered by the researchers with the help of three trained graduate students. The questionnaires were sent to the assistants from the 3 selected universities via email to be printed for administration. The assistants were first taken through the questionnaire to ensure familiarity and ease of handling. Participation in the study was voluntary, and informed consent was obtained before the questionnaire administration began. To ensure consistency, the questionnaire was designed and printed in the English language, which is the official language of instruction in Ghanaian academic institutions.

4.5. Data Analysis. Data were analyzed using frequencies and percentages, as well as means and standard deviations. Descriptive statistics were calculated for the following: sociodemographics, access and general use of the Internet,

use of Internet for health purpose, usage of health information sought, and rating of the importance of criteria for evaluating health websites, apps, and platforms, as well as the importance of health information sought in improving students' health. Data analysis was done using the IBM SPSS Statistics version 20.

5. Results

5.1. Characteristics of the Sample. Table 1 presents the background characteristics of the study participants. Variables of interest are age, gender, level of study, and place of residence. Participating in the study were 650 students from three (3) Ghanaian universities. The participants in the study were aged between 18 and 37 years, with an average age of 27 years. For the age groups, the majority (35.5%) belonged to the 20–24 category, followed by those aged 25–29 years (23.8%).

The majority of the respondents were males ($n = 383$, 58.9%). By level of study, undergraduate students formed the majority ($n = 409$, 62.9%), followed by master's students ($n = 186$, 28.8%), with only a few doctoral students ($n = 55$, 8.5%). The students either lived on campus in the traditional halls of residence ($n = 234$, 36.0%), or in private hostels ($n = 30.3\%$), or stayed with their families at varying distances from the main campus (206, 31.7%).

5.2. Students' Access and Use of Internet. Table 2 presents results on students' access to Internet services. All of the 650 participants confirmed that they access and use the Internet, and a great majority ($n = 509$, 78.3%) reported Internet use every day. Also, most students had used the Internet for more than five years, with as many as 48.5% ($n = 315$) having used the Internet between 5 and 9 years. Another 28.6% ($n = 186$) indicated Internet use for a continuous period of not less than 10 years. Per duration of interne use a day, most students use the Internet for up to seven hours a day, and specifically 37.5% ($n = 244$) use Internet for a maximum of three hours a day, followed by usage of between 4 to 7 hours a day by 33.4% (217) of students. Few students ($n = 60$, 9.2%) use the Internet for more than 10 hours daily.

The students mostly accessed internets using mobile data bundles ($n = 268$, 41.2%) and campus WiFi ($n = 195$, 30.0%). Few students ($n = 33$, 5.1%) use Local Area Network (LAN). On the place of primary Internet access, students access Internet services mostly on campus (WiFi and labs) ($n = 294$, 45.2%) and halls and hostel ($n = 229$, 35.2%). Only a few accessed Internet from their homes ($n = 107$, 16.5%). The students' experience in using Internet was acceptable, as the majority of them rated their level of experience in using Internet as fair ($n = 364$, 56.0%), followed by those who rated themselves as very experienced ($n = 251$, 38.6%). Few students rated themselves as not experienced ($n = 22$, 3.4%).

The students were asked to indicate the main challenge that they face in accessing and using Internet. More than half ($n = 351$, 54.0%) indicated unreliable and slow connection as their main challenge. Other challenges reported on were high cost of Internet and devices, reported by 14.9% ($n = 97$), problems of viruses and malware (7.8%), and congestion at ICT centres where Internet is accessed (6.0%). Unreliable

TABLE 1: Background characteristics of respondents.

Variable	Category	Frequency ($n = 650$)	Percentage
	<20	139	21.4
	20–24	231	35.5
	25–29	155	23.8
Age (years)	≥30	115	17.7
	Missing	10	1.5
	Mean	**27.40**	
	SD	**3.47**	
Gender	Male	383	58.9
	Female	267	41.1
	Undergraduate	409	62.9
Level of study	Master's	186	28.6
	Doctoral	55	8.5
	Campus	234	36.0
	Hostel	197	30.3
Place of residence	Home	206	31.7
	Missing	13	2.0

power connection was surprisingly not an issue, reported by only 5.5% of the sampled students.

5.3. Students' Use of the Internet for Health Purpose. The students were asked about their extent of use of Internet for health purposes. They were first asked whether or not they used the Internet for health purposes or to seek health information. The results are presented in Table 3 which also presents results on the reasons for their use of Internet for health purposes. Out of the 650 students, the overwhelming majority 67.7% ($n = 440$) use Internet for health purposes or to seek health information.

The study also enquired about factors that students take into consideration in their selection of the means of accessing the Internet for health information and support. As shown in Table 4, currency of information was the most important factor, followed by ease of understanding of information. The least important factors were quality of links and comprehensiveness.

The students use the online health information to take several important decisions and actions concerning their health. As shown in Table 5, greater majority of the students reported that they mostly use the health information obtained as a basis for lifestyle change ($n = 315, 72.4\%$). There is a big lag between this response and the next important use of online health information, which is "discussing health issues with health professionals" ($n = 170, 39.5\%$). Other self-reported uses of online health information are "changing medication" ($n = 102, 23.7\%$), and making, cancelling, or changing appointments with doctor ($n = 63, 14.7\%$).

The survey further revealed the extent of self-reported improvement in students' health conditions by using information sought using the Internet. As shown in Table 6 majority ($n = 144, 40.1\%$) revealed that their health conditions have "improved a lot," followed by those whose health has "improved somehow" ($n = 112, 33.5\%$). Altogether,

these two responses show a positive impact of online health information on respondents' health as they make up 73.6% of responses.

Only a small 1.2% ($n = 4$) of students reported that online health information had not had any effect at all on their overall health situation.

6. Discussion

This study provides insight into the extent of Internet use for online health information and support among university students in Ghana. The study revealed that all the university students use the Internet. This finding is not surprising, looking at the rising popularity of the Internet among the youth and the ease of access by android, IOS, and Microsoft-powered smart phones and other hand-held devices. Earlier studies have found an extensive use of Internet among adolescents and young adults including university students [5, 20, 21, 23–26]. Most tertiary institutions in Ghana currently provide Internet connections for their students whether in their halls and hostels or on campus by means of campus-wide WiFi and computer laboratories. Respondents in this study primarily accessed the Internet on campus as well as in the halls and hostels, possibly because such places mostly offer reliable Internet services at low costs. They are also places where students undertake academic and research activities whether in their busy or leisure periods. This finding is consistent with previous studies [5, 11, 21, 24, 25, 27–29].

The survey revealed that more than half of all participants use the Internet to obtain health information and support (among other uses), specifically finding information about illnesses and interacting with health professionals via emails, Facebook pages, and other social media platforms such as Whatsapp, where contact details of selected health professionals at the university hospitals have been made available. This implies that there is a great potential of the Internet as

TABLE 2: Internet access and use by students.

Variable	Categories	Frequency (n = 650)	Percent
Use of Internet	Yes	645	100.0
	No	0	0.0
Years of Internet use	<1	8	1.2
	1–4	126	19.4
	5–9	315	48.5
	≥10	186	28.6
	Missing	16	2.3
Use of Internet everyday	Yes	509	78.3
	No	136	20.9
	Missing	5	.8
Hours of daily use Internet	1–3	244	37.5
	4–7	217	33.4
	8–10	86	13.2
	>10	60	9.2
	Missing	43	6.6
	Mean	**5.41**	
	SD	**3.28**	
Type of Internet	Mobile data	268	41.2
	Campus WiFi	195	30.0
	LAN	33	5.1
	All	149	22.2
	Missing	5	.8
Place of primary Internet access	Campus labs and WiFi	294	45.2
	Halls and hostels	229	35.2
	Home	107	16.5
	Missing	20	3.1
Level of experience	Very experienced	251	38.6
	Fairly experienced	364	56.0
	Not experienced	22	3.4
	Missing	13	2.0
Barriers to Internet use	Unreliable and slow connection	351	54.0
	High cost of internet and devices	97	14.9
	Congestion at ICT centres	39	6.0
	Unreliable power supply	36	5.5
	Viruses and malware	51	7.8
	No challenge	71	10.9
	Missing	5	.8

an important channel for health information and support, for not only university students, but also the general population. This is particularly so as the Internet offers suitable, a lot of, and cheap information as noted by Horgan and Sweeney [6]. Also, the Internet is seen as the acceptable and practicable tool for behavioural intervention for university students as noted by Zabinski et al. [30] and Escoffery et al. [31] and adults in general as noted by Tate et al. [32].

The survey also revealed that about 68% of the sampled university students in Ghana sought for health information or support online. This result compares with other studies globally, including a study on predictors of online health seeking behaviour among Egyptian adults which shows that

Internet was the main source for health information [33]. It also confirms the result of a survey in 7 European countries (Denmark, Norway, Germany, Poland, Greece, Portugal, and Latvia) in 2005 which revealed that, on average, about 63% of individuals aged 8–29 years were online health seekers [34]. Also, the result of a survey in Italy in 2010 showed that 65% and 60% of young Italian females and males (between 18–29 years) respectfully used the Internet for health-related purposes [35]. It also confirms a study in the United States on health information seeking behaviour among US adults using data from four cycles (2011–2014) of the Health Information National Trends Survey (HINTS) that found that a greater percentage of US adults use the

TABLE 3: Students' use of Internet for health purpose.

Response	n	%
Use of Internet for health purpose		
Yes	440	67.7
No	205	31.5
Missing	4	.8
Total	650	100.0
Reasons for using Internet for health purpose		
Vast amount of valuable information available	249	56.6
Anonymous, private, and confidential	340	77.3
Easy to find information	421	95.7
Cheap	170	38.6
Convenient	310	70.5
Easy to communicate with peers	280	63.6
Less embarrassing than talking to a professional	216	49.1

TABLE 4: Factors considered in seeking online health information.

Factor	Ratings			Total
	Not important	Fairly important	Very important	
	n (%)	n (%)	n (%)	
Accuracy of information	1 (1.4)	175 (40.9)	247 (57.7)	428
Currency of information	16 (3.7)	184 (43.0)	288 (67.3)	428
Comprehensiveness	11 (2.6)	215 (50.0)	204 (47.4)	430
Ease of understanding	10 (2.3)	156 (36.0)	267 (61.7)	433
Content readability	3 (.7)	178 (41.6)	247 (57.7)	428
Confidentiality	63 (14.5)	204 (47.1)	166 (38.3)	433
Interactivity	74 (17.1)	233 (53.8)	126 (29.1)	433
Quality of links	33 (7.6)	220 (50.8)	180 (41.6)	433
Use of multimedia	68 (20.6)	164 (49.7)	98 (29.7)	330
Appearances	36 (10.9)	174 (52.7)	120 (38.4)	330

Internet as the first place they go for health information [36]. A systematic literature review on the use of social media for retrieving health information by patients and healthcare consumers revealed that there is a high use of social media by patients and healthcare consumers in retrieving health-related information [37]. Several other studies in the United States of America [31, 32], Italy [35], and Israel [38] have also reported lower levels of Internet use for health purposes than those found in the present study. Reasons for the higher use of the Internet for health purposes by the university students could be the abundance of Internet access on campus including campus-wide WiFi and computer pools and the comfortability with which students find their use [4, 38]. There is little wonder then that more than half of the students reported being experienced with the Internet. The level of Internet use for health purpose in this study was however lower than level reported in Australia [39] where two-thirds of the participants use Internet for health purposes. Also, in the United States, the Pew Research Center's Internet & American Life Project in 2012 showed that 72% of people aged 18–29 years were online health seekers [40].

The wealth of health websites and online information available to the public has raised numerous concerns about how accurate the information on such websites and platforms is as well as the possibility of harm as a result of inaccurate information [4, 41]. Criteria for assessing which websites and platforms to use to gain access to health information varied from accuracy, currency of information, comprehensiveness, ease of understanding, readability, confidentiality, interactivity, and quality of links to use of multimedia and appearances. Barnes et al. [42] found that the important criteria among adult Internet users included authority of the sources, ease of use, attribution, disclosure of authors, accessibility, and availability. This study consequently confirms that the credibility of the websites, platforms, and information is critical for consumers of online health information. However, the students may face some difficulties with regard to quality and accuracy of health-related information obtained. It is therefore essential to help them search and use the most suitable and quality online health information. This can be achieved by targeting the main way of Internet use, which is identified to be the social networks. Social networks could be established as a place for health professionals to help the youth deal with online information as noted by Buame [20].

Finally, 72% of the students who use Internet for health purpose reported having had their lifestyle or health

TABLE 5: Decisions students make with online health information.

Use of online health information	Response				Total
	Yes		No		
	Freq.	%	Freq.	%	
Making, canceling, or changing appointment with doctor	63	14.7	367	85.3	430
Discussing health issues with health professional	170	39.5	260	60.5	430
Changing medication, without discussing with professional	102	23.7	328	76.3	430
Change of lifestyle	315	72.4	120	27.6	435

TABLE 6: Extent of improvement in students' health by online health information.

Extent of improvement	Frequency	Percentage
A lot	134	40.1
Somehow	112	33.5
Only a little	84	25.1
Not at all	4	1.2
Total	334	100.0
Missing	106	

behaviour change after their contact with online information. It is possible that the changes in question reflect improved healthy lifestyles (e.g., good eating habit, adequate exercise, reducing alcohol intake, and smoking).

7. Conclusions

This study reveals that Ghanaian university students are active users of the Internet, including use for health purpose (i.e., searching for health information and support). The results justify the increase in efforts over the past several years by the various universities in Ghana to provide cheap and accessible Internet for students for various purposes, most of which are development-oriented and life-enhancing.

This study concludes that the Internet is assuming a more and more important role in the lives of the youth especially students in higher education institutions and that its use is not only limited to purely academic and leisure purposes, but also used for life-supporting and sustaining purposes including searching for health information. There is therefore the need to promote e-health in the country as a viable platform for health interventions and healthcare. This would, among other benefits, provide quick, accessible, and affordable access to healthcare and health information. It would also ease the pressure and congestion that characterize physical healthcare services in the country, leading to overall improvement in healthcare delivery. For the youth and especially tertiary students, providing on-the-go access to healthcare via e-health fits into their lifestyle and is therefore very appropriate. In this vein, it is expected that, as per results of this study, the Ghana Health Service and its supervising Ministry of Health will take the giant steps of making healthcare truly accessible to all as enshrined in international and national protocols by promoting e-health through design of responsive websites, platforms, and applications for accessing healthcare.

It is envisaged that the integration of technology in healthcare, by promoting Internet-based access to healthcare especially with university students and other qualified groups in the population, will go a long way to address problems of access and quality in healthcare delivery in the country. However, it would be equally prudent to be aware of online safety issues for students and other users of Internet for health-based information. Piracy issues will also have to be addressed, together with providing information on privacy options.

There are limitations to the work. The study was conducted among university students and thus cannot lay claim to be representative of the behaviour of all young people in the country. The study also assumes that Internet-based health information is wholesome and appropriate to the needs of seekers, which might not necessarily be so. There is junk information out there, and the extent to which this might impact health outcomes must be investigated and safeguarded. In pursuit of this, there is the need for a thorough evaluation of the various websites, apps, and platforms that are health related, so that those that are not health-enhancing could be avoided.

Ethical Approval

This study was part of student's project which was conducted under the general internal review of the substantive supervisors. Hence, all respondents were made to sign informed consent prior to participation, and benefits, intent, procedure, and expected risks were all explained to them. The privacy and anonymity of all participants were protected, both during and after the research. Also, oral permission was sought from the head of every department from which a participant was selected.

References

[1] Computer Hope, "Information superhighway," 2010, http://www.computerhope.com/jargon/i/inforsupe.htm.

[2] G. A. Ajuwon, "Internet accessibility and use of online health information resources by doctors in training healthcare institutions in Nigeria," *Library Philosophy and Practice*, vol. 2015, no. 1, article 1258, 2015.

[3] C. Lagoe and D. Atkin, "Health anxiety in the digital age: An exploration of psychological determinants of online health information seeking," *Computers in Human Behavior*, vol. 52, article no. 3508, pp. 484–491, 2015.

[4] A. Mills and N. Todorova, "An integrated perspective on factors influencing online health-information seeking behaviours," in *Proceedings of the In Australasian Conference on Information Systems*, vol. 4, 2016.

[5] C. Escoffery, K. R. Miner, D. D. Adame, S. Butler, L. McCormick, and E. Mendell, "Internet use for health information among college students," *Journal of American College Health*, vol. 53, no. 4, pp. 183–188, 2005.

[6] Á. Horgan and J. Sweeney, "Young students' use of the internet for mental health information and support," *Journal of Psychiatric and Mental Health Nursing*, vol. 17, no. 2, pp. 117–123, 2010.

[7] S. Fox, L. Rainie, and J. Horrigan, *The Online Health Care Revolution: How the Web Helps Americans Take Better Care of Themselves*, Pew Internet & American Life Project, Washington, DC, USA, 2017.

[8] S. Fox, *The social life of health information, 2011*, Pew Internet & American Life Project, Washington, DC, USA, 2011.

[9] S. Gallagher, D. D. Tedstone, R. Moran, and Y. Kartalova-ODoherty, *Internet use and seeking health information online in Ireland: demographic characteristics and mental health characteristics of users and non-users*, Health Research Board, Dublin, Ireland, 2008.

[10] E. Renahy, I. Parizot, and P. Chauvin, "Health information seeking on the Internet: A double divide? Results from a representative survey in the Paris metropolitan area, France, 2005-2006," *BMC Public Health*, vol. 8, article 69, 2008.

[11] World Health Organisation, "Ghana Annual Report 2014," June 2015.

[12] E. E. Badu and E. D. Markwei, "Internet Awareness and Use in the University of Ghana," *Information Development*, vol. 21, no. 4, pp. 260–268, 2005.

[13] D. L. G. Borzekowski, J. N. Fobil, and K. O. Asante, "Online access by adolescents in accra: Ghanaian teens' use of the Internet for health information," *Developmental Psychology*, vol. 42, no. 3, pp. 450–458, 2006.

[14] United States Censu Bureau, "Internet Penetration Rate and Population Data from "Countries and Areas Ranked by Population: 2012," Population data, International Programs, U.S. Census Bureau, 2017.

[15] D. Laary, "Ghana: Mobile phone penetration soars to 128%—West Africa," 2015, http://www.theafricareport.com/West-Africa/ghana-mobile-phone-penetration-soars-to-128.html.

[16] H. K. Andreassen, M. M. Bujnowska-Fedak, C. E. Chronaki et al., "European citizens' use of E-health services: A study of seven countries," *BMC Public Health*, vol. 7, article 53, 2007.

[17] F. Beck, J.-B. Richard, V. Nguyen-Thanh, I. Montagni, I. Parizot, and E. Renahy, "Use of the internet as a health information resource among French young adults: Results from a nationally representative survey," *Journal of Medical Internet Research*, vol. 16, no. 5, article e128, 2014.

[18] Y. J. Lee, B. Boden-Albala, E. Larson, A. Wilcox, and S. Bakken, "Online health information seeking behaviors of hispanics in new york city: A community-based cross-sectional study," *Journal of Medical Internet Research*, vol. 16, no. 7, 2014.

[19] S. Santana, B. Lausen, M. Bujnowska-Fedak, C. E. Chronaki, H.-U. Prokosch, and R. Wynn, "Informed citizen and empowered citizen in health: Results from an European survey," *BMC Family Practice*, vol. 12, article 20, 2011.

[20] K. E. Buame, "Internet Using Habit among Junior High School Students of Nima," *International Journal of ICT and Management*, vol. 1, no. 3, pp. 133–138, 2013.

[21] R. Hinson and M. Amidu, "Internet adoption amongst final year students in Ghana's oldest business school," *Library Review*, vol. 55, no. 5, pp. 314–323, 2006.

[22] R. Wynn, E. Kwabia, and F. Osei-Bonsu, "Internet-based provider-patient communication in Ghana: recent findings," *International Journal of Integrated Care*, vol. 16, no. 5, article 47, 2016.

[23] S. M. Vambheim, S. C. Wangberg, J.-A. K. Johnsen, and R. Wynn, "Language use in an internet support group for smoking cessation: Development of sense of community," *Informatics for Health and Social Care*, vol. 38, no. 1, pp. 67–78, 2013.

[24] MO. Awoleye, WO. Siyanbola, and OF. Oladipupo, "Adoption assessment of Internet usage amongst undergraduates in Nigeria Universities-a case study approach," *Journal of Technology Management Innovation*, vol. 3, no. 1, pp. 84–89, 2008.

[25] T. Batane, "Internet Access and Use among Young People in Botswana," *International Journal of Information and Education Technology*, pp. 117–119, 2013.

[26] S. O. Oyeyemi, E. Gabarron, and R. Wynn, "Ebola, Twitter, and misinformation: A dangerous combination?" *BMJ (Online)*, vol. 349, Article ID g6178, 2014.

[27] M. P. Wang, K. Viswanath, T. H. Lam, X. Wang, and S. S. Chan, "Social Determinants of Health Information Seeking among Chinese Adults in Hong Kong," *PLoS ONE*, vol. 8, no. 8, Article ID e73049, 2013.

[28] J. A. Gilmour, S. D. Scott, and N. Huntington, "Nurses and Internet health information: A questionnaire survey," *Journal of Advanced Nursing*, vol. 61, no. 1, pp. 19–28, 2008.

[29] H. S. Shubha, "Relationship between internet use and health orientation: a study among university students," *Online Journal of Communication and Media Technologies*, 2015.

[30] M. F. Zabinski, D. E. Wilfley, M. A. Pung, A. J. Winzelberg, K. Eldredge, and C. Barr Taylor, "An interactive internet-based intervention for women at risk of eating disorders: A pilot study," *International Journal of Eating Disorders*, vol. 30, no. 2, pp. 129–137, 2001.

[31] C. Escoffery, C. DiIorio, K. A. Yeager et al., "Use of computers and the Internet for health information by patients with epilepsy," *Epilepsy and Behavior*, vol. 12, no. 1, pp. 109–114, 2008.

[32] D. F. Tate, R. R. Wing, and R. A. Winett, "Using internet technology to deliver a behavioral weight loss program," *The Journal of the American Medical Association*, vol. 285, no. 9, pp. 1172–1177, 2001.

[33] M. Ghweeba, A. Lindenmeyer, S. Shishi, M. Abbas, A. Waheed, and S. Amer, "What predicts online health information-seeking behavior among egyptian adults? a cross-sectional study," *Journal of Medical Internet Research*, vol. 19, no. 6, article e216, 2017.

[34] National Communications Authority, "Quarterly Statistical Bulletin on Communications in Ghana," vol. 1, no. 2, 2016.

[35] R. Siliquini, M. Ceruti, E. Lovato et al., "Surfing the internet for health information: An italian survey on use and population choices," *BMC Medical Informatics and Decision Making*, vol. 11, no. 1, article 21, 2011.

[36] W. Jacobs, A. O. Amuta, K. C. Jeon, and C. Alvares, "Health information seeking in the digital age: An analysis of health information seeking behavior among US adults," *Cogent Social Sciences*, vol. 3, no. 1, Article ID 1302785, 2017.

[37] A. Cordoş, S. Bolboacă, and C. Drugan, "Social Media Usage for Patients and Healthcare Consumers: A Literature Review," *Publications*, vol. 5, no. 2, p. 9, 2017.

[38] Y. Neumark, C. Lopez-Quintero, B. S. Feldman, A. J. Hirsch Allen, and R. Shtarkshall, "Online health information seeking among jewish and arab adolescents in Israel: Results from a national school survey," *Journal of Health Communication*, vol. 18, no. 9, pp. 1097–1115, 2013.

[39] C. Wong, C. Harrison, H. Britt, and J. Henderson, "Patient use of the internet for health information," *Australian Family Physician*, vol. 43, no. 12, pp. 875–877, 2014.

[40] S. Fox and M. Duggan, "Health online 2013," Pew Internet & American Life Project, Washington, DC, USA, 2017.

[41] Á. Horgan and J. Sweeney, "University students' online habits and their use of the internet for health information," *CIN - Computers Informatics Nursing*, vol. 30, no. 8, pp. 402–408, 2012.

[42] M. D. Barnes, C. Penrod, B. L. Neiger et al., "Measuring the relevance of evaluation criteria among health information seekers on the Internet," *Journal of Health Psychology*, vol. 8, no. 1, pp. 71–82, 2003.

18

Telemedical Coaching Improves Long-Term Weight Loss in Overweight Persons

Kerstin Kempf ⓘ,[1] Martin Röhling ⓘ,[1] Monika Stichert,[2,3] Gabriele Fischer,[3] Elke Boschem,[4] Jürgen Könner,[2] and Stephan Martin[1]

[1] West-German Centre of Diabetes and Health, Düsseldorf Catholic Hospital Group, Düsseldorf, Germany
[2] Occupational Health Services, Kassenärztliche Vereinigung Nordrhein, Düsseldorf, Germany
[3] Occupational Health Services Ärztekammer Nordrhein, Düsseldorf, Germany
[4] Occupational Health Services Eickhoff GmbH, Bochum, Germany

Correspondence should be addressed to Martin Röhling; martin.roehling@vkkd-kliniken.de

Academic Editor: Aura Ganz

Background. Lifestyle interventions have shown to be effective when continuous personal support was provided. However, there is lack of knowledge whether a telemedical-approach with personal coaching contributes to long-term weight losses in overweight employees. We, therefore, tested the hypothesis that telemedical-based lifestyle interventions accompanied with telemedical coaching lead to larger weight losses in overweight persons in an occupational health care setting. *Methods*. Overweight employees (n=180) with a body mass index (BMI) of >27 kg/m^2 were randomized into either a telemedical (TM) group (n=61), a telemedical coaching (TMC) group (n=58), or a control group (n=61). Both intervention groups were equipped with scales and pedometers automatically transferring the data into a personalized online portal, which could be monitored from participants and coaches. Participants of the TMC group received additionally one motivational care call per week by mental coaches to discuss the current data (current weight and steps) and achieving goals such as a healthy lifestyle or weight reduction. The control group remained in routine care. Clinical and anthropometric data were determined after the 12-week intervention. Additionally, weight change was followed up after 12 months. *Results*. Participants of TMC (-3.1 ± 4.8 kg, p<0.0001) and TM group (-1.9 ± 4.0 kg; p=0.0012) significantly reduced weight and sustained it during the 1-year follow-up, while the control group showed no change. Compared to the control group only weight loss in the TMC group was significantly different (p<0.001) after 12 months. TMC and TM group also reduced BMI, waist circumference, and LDL cholesterol. Moreover, TMC group improved additionally systolic and diastolic blood pressure, total cholesterol, HDL cholesterol, and HbA1c. *Conclusions*. Telemedical devices in combination with telemedical coaching lead to significant long-term weight reductions in overweight persons in an occupational health care setting. This study is registered with NCT01868763, ClinicalTrials.gov.

1. Introduction

Positive energy balance and reduced physical activity are common reasons for weight gain [1]. Overweight and obesity not only increase the risk for several cardiometabolic diseases such as type 2 diabetes or coronary heart disease [1], but are also associated with sick leave days and increased disease costs [2]. Weight reduction and a healthy diet and a physically active lifestyle are generally recommended for overweight people to prevent type 2 diabetes [3, 4]. An analysis of the German socioeconomic panel data estimated costs of 2.5-5.4 billion EUR caused by overweight- and obesity-related sick leave days [2]. Therefore, companies should have an essential interest in effective health care programs for weight control of their employees. Accordingly, there is a strong need for effective lifestyle-based approaches and programs [5], particularly with psychosocial support [6]. Several worksite behavioral lifestyle interventions have shown to be feasible and effective in improving risk factors (e.g., weight loss, HbA1c) for diabetes and cardiovascular disease [7, 8]. Beneficial effects of lifestyle programs in an occupational health care setting comprise improvements in (i) absenteeism, (ii) productivity, and (iii) health care costs for employers [9, 10]. Therefore, lifestyle interventions have been successfully implemented in multiple community settings [11–14]. However, occupational health care settings have not been extensively examined [8, 15, 16]. In this context, telemedical and technology-based interventions comprise numerous advantages over traditional clinical settings such as convenience, cost, and the ability to tailor plans and feedback to a participant's individual needs. Nonetheless, telemedical interventions are facing certain problems such as absence of face-to-face interaction [17, 18]. Nevertheless, studies have already shown that telemedical coaching or telemonitoring can contribute to large reductions of body weight of more than 5% [19, 20]. However, the scientific discussion concerns the added value of telemedical coaching on telemonitoring alone [21, 22]. Nonetheless, in a previously published study, it has been shown that an additional personal support during a lifestyle intervention is essential and more effective in reducing weight and achieving goals than without human encouragement [23]. Continuous external feedback not only offers patients an additional contact person for medical questions regarding healthy diet and physical activity but also supports patients to further focus on their goals and stay motivated [24]. Furthermore, telephonically delivered lifestyle coaching interventions have been shown to support weight reduction and improve quality of life in different cohorts, even in patients with serious mental illnesses [19, 25].

In previous uncontrolled trials we had already evaluated the efficacy of a telemedical mental motivation program [26, 27], telemedically supported blood glucose self-monitoring [28, 29], and telemedical coaching [30]. However, there is still a lack of knowledge whether a telemedical-approach with in-person contact and personal coaching contributes to long-term weight losses and improvements in other cardiometabolic parameters.

We, therefore, tested in the present randomized controlled study the hypothesis that (i) a telemedical intervention with or without telemedical coaching leads to long-term weight losses and other beneficial clinical outcomes and (ii) whether telemedical coaching shows an additional impact on the results in overweight participants in an occupational health care setting.

2. Materials & Methods

2.1. Study Population. In an occupational health care setting overweight employees of the companies *"Gebr. Eickhoff Maschinenfabrik"*, the *"Ärztekammer Nordrhein"*, and the *"Kassenärztliche Vereinigung Nordrhein"* were invited by their medical corporate department for participation in the study. Eligible volunteers (n=180; inclusion criteria: 18-75 years old, body mass index (BMI) ≥ 27 kg/m^2; exclusion criteria: acute diseases, severe illness with in-patient treatment during the last 3 months, weight reduction >2 kg/week during the last month, smoking secession during the last 3 months, drugs for active weight reduction, pregnancy, and breastfeeding) were randomized according to an electronically generated randomization list into three parallel groups. In detail,

each participant was assigned a serial study identifier (ID). For each ID there was a closed envelope with the group assignment. The first participant was enrolled on 16.07.2012 and the last participant finished the study in 05.02.2014. The study was conducted at the West-German Centre of Diabetes and Health (WDGZ) in Düsseldorf, Germany, in accordance with the ethical standards laid down in the 1964 Declaration of Helsinki and its later amendments. The research protocol was approved by the ethics committee of the Ärztekammer Nordrhein, Düsseldorf, and was registered at clinicaltrials.gov under the number NCT01868763. All participants gave written informed consent prior to their inclusion into the study.

2.2. Study Design. Participants in the telemedical (TM) and telemedical coaching (TMC) group were equipped with telemetric scales (smartLAB scale W; HMM Holding AG, Dossenheim, Germany) and pedometer (smartLAB walk P+; HMM Holding AG, Dossenheim, Germany) automatically transferring recorded data into a personalized online portal. These data could be monitored from both, participant and the coaching team of the WDGZ. Participants in the TM group could monitor their body weight and steps (daily, weekly or average) but got no further support during the 12 weeks of intervention. The TMC group got additionally weekly care calls from trained coaches. These care calls included information about overweight or obesity-related diseases like type 2 diabetes, healthy diet, physical activity, and coping strategies for lifestyle changes. Moreover, acquired data were discussed (i.e., steps and weight) and participants were further motivated to achieve their individual goals (i.e., weight goals and healthy lifestyle changes) using a mental motivation program [26, 27] (Supplementary material). The control group remained in routine care. After the intervention phase telemetric devices remained in possession of the participants of both groups, and the participants were instructed to carry on measuring their weight and steps after the 12-week intervention period.

At baseline and after 12 weeks of intervention participants visited their medical corporate department for determination of anthropometric and clinical data (i.e., age, sex, body weight, height, BMI, waist circumference, blood pressure, total cholesterol, high-density lipoprotein (HDL) cholesterol, low-density lipoprotein (LDL) cholesterol, triglycerides, and hemoglobin A1c (HbA1c)). The assessors were blinded for group allocation. Body weight was measured in light clothing to the closest 0.1 kg, height to the closest 0.5 cm, and waist circumferences at the minimum abdominal girth (midway between the rib cage and the iliac crest). Blood pressure was measured after a five-minute rest in a sitting position on both arms. Venous blood was collected by inserting an intravenous cannula into the forearm vein and laboratory parameters were analyzed at the local laboratory. One year after the end of the intervention weight data out of the online portal were used for the follow-up analysis. These weight data were continuously recorded during the follow-up period and automatically transferred to the online portal by the scales. Afterwards, the online portal was closed after the 12-month follow-up.

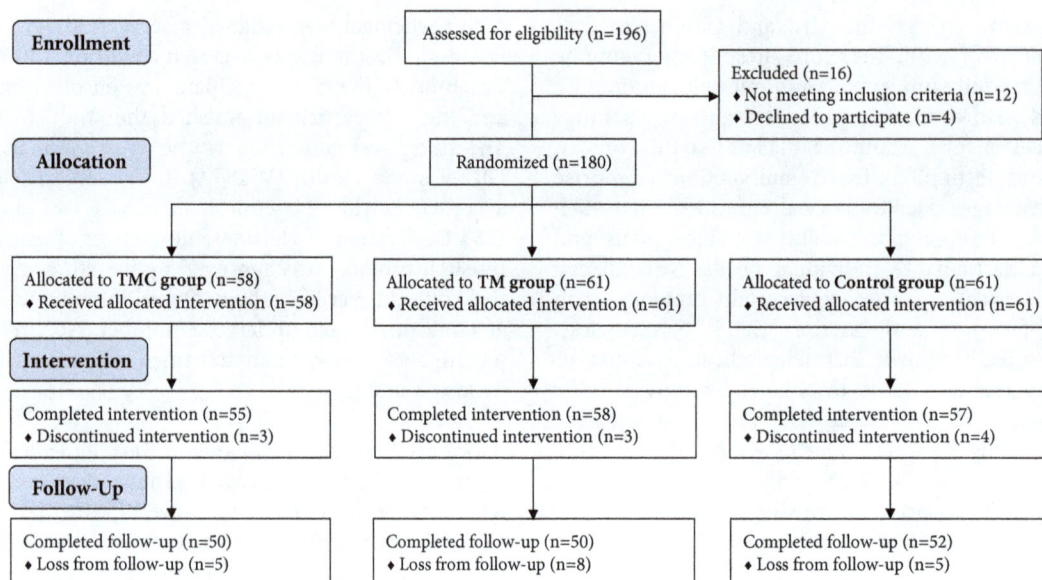

FIGURE 1: Flow diagram.

2.3. Statistical Analysis. Primary endpoint was the reduction of body weight after 12 weeks of intervention and its later course during the 12-month follow-up compared between all of the three groups. Secondary endpoints were the changes in BMI, waist circumference, systolic and diastolic blood pressure, total cholesterol, HDL cholesterol, LDL cholesterol, triglycerides, and HbA1c after 12 weeks of intervention. Sample size had been calculated assuming that telemedical coaching might affect body weight. Our data indicated that due to telemedical lifestyle intervention a reduction of 2.3 kg in body weight in the TMC group can be assumed, while for the control group a reduction of only 1.0 kg was estimated. To be able to measure such a difference with a power of 90% and a level of significance of 5%, at least 50 datasets per group were needed. Since a dropout rate of 20% was estimated, the plan was to recruit 60 subjects per group, i.e., a total of 180 persons. Intention-to-treat analyses were performed. Missing values were substituted by the "last-observation-carried-forward" principle. Means ± standard deviations or standard error of means are shown, as appropriate. Baseline differences had been analyzed by using the Chi square test or Kruskal-Wallis test for nonparametric data and the ANOVA test for parametric data. The Wilcoxon signed-rank test was used for the analysis of differences within all the groups. The Kruskal-Wallis statistics with Dunn's multiple comparisons test was conducted for the comparison of Δ-values. The Friedman test with Dunn's multiple comparisons test was used to test the within group differences between time points. The Bonferroni correction was applied to adjust for multiple testing. Level of significance was set at p=0.05. Statistical analyses were performed using GraphPad Prism 6.04 (GraphPad Software, San Diego, CA, USA) and SAS statistical package version 9.3 (SAS Institute, Cary, NC, USA).

3. Results

3.1. Study Population. Fifty-eight participants were randomized to the TMC group, 61 to the TM group, and 61 to the control group (Figure 1). Baseline data did not differ significantly between all groups (Table 1). Distribution of BMI categories was also not different at baseline between all of the groups (Table 2). Fifty-five (95%) participants of TMC, 58 (95%) of TM, and 57 (93%) of the control group completed the 12-week intervention phase. Follow-up data after 12 months were available from 50 (86%), 50 (82%), and 52 (85%) participants, respectively. Main reasons for dropout were "personal/private reasons" and loss of motivation.

3.2. Weight Loss and Improvement of Cardiometabolic Risk Factors during the 12-Week Intervention. Participants of the TMC (98.9 ± 18.7 kg to 95.8 ± 16.9 kg (-3.1 ± 4.8 kg; p<0.0001) and the TM group (97.9 ± 17.4 kg to 96.0 ± 16.7 kg (-1.9 ± 4.0 kg; p=0.0012)) significantly reduced weight (Table 1). However, the weight of the control group remained statistically unchanged throughout the 12-weeks intervention. Compared to the control group, weight loss was only significant in the TMC group (p<0.001) after 12 weeks. The distribution of categories for weight changes differed significantly between groups (p=0.043 for TMC versus TM and p=0.0002 for TMC versus control; Figure 2). While the majority of participants in the TMC group achieved a weight loss, the proportion of participants with unchanged weight or weight gain was highest in the control group. Accordingly, a significant reduction of BMI was observed in the TMC group (p<0.0001) and in the TM group (p=0.0014). In comparison to the control group BMI reduction was only significant in the TMC group (p<0.001; Table 1). A significant reduction of waist circumference (p=0.0002 for the TMC, p=0.0033 for the TM, and p=0.0109 for the control group) was observed

TABLE 1: Study population characteristics.

	TMC group (n=58)			TM group (n=61)			Control group (n=61)		
Sex (male /female) [%]	52 / 48			39 / 61			44 / 56		
Age [years]	44 ± 10			45 ± 10			47 ± 10		
	Baseline	End of intervention	Δ	Baseline	End of intervention	Δ	Baseline	End	Δ
Weight [kg]	98.9 ± 18.7	95.8 ± 16.9 * * * *	-3.1 ± 4.8 ##	97.9 ± 17.4	96.0 ± 16.7 **	-1.9 ± 4.0	101.7 ± 17.7	100.8 ± 17.8	-0.8 ± 3.1
Body Mass Index [kg/m²]	32.7 ± 4.6	31.7 ± 3.8 * * * * *	-1.0 ± 1.6 ##	32.9 ± 4.3	32.3 ± 4.1 **	-0.6 ± 1.3	34.0 ± 5.3	33.8 ± 5.4	-0.3 ± 1.0
Waist circumference [cm]	109 ± 12	106 ± 10 * * *	-3 ± 6	109 ± 13	108 ± 13 **	-2 ± 4	112 ± 13	111 ± 14 *	-2 ± 5
Systolic blood pressure [mmHg]	141 ± 24	138 ± 24 *	-4 ± 17	141 ± 23	139 ± 24	-3 ± 17	141 ± 17	140 ± 19	-1 ± 17
Diastolic blood pressure [mmHg]	90 ± 13	86 ± 12 *	-4 ± 11	88 ± 14	88 ± 13	0 ± 10	89 ± 12	88 ± 11	-1 ± 12
Triglycerides [mg/dl]¹	191 ± 120	169 ± 94	-22 ± 77	167 ± 83	169 ± 153	-5 ± 115	191 ± 119	181 ± 127	-10 ± 62
Total cholesterol [mg/dl]¹	218 ± 33	207 ± 33 *	-10 ± 28	210 ± 37	204 ± 36 *	-5 ± 15	225 ± 44	226 ± 46	1 ± 22
HDL cholesterol [mg/dl]¹	51 ± 15	53 ± 15 *	2 ± 7	51 ± 14	52 ± 13	1 ± 6	54 ± 18	55 ± 22	1 ± 11
LDL cholesterol [mg/dl]¹	135 ± 28	130 ± 29 **	-5 ± 22	131 ± 31	126 ± 32 **	-5 ± 14	140 ± 39	141 ± 41	1 ± 18
HbA1c [%]¹	5.6 ± 0.3	5.5 ± 0.3 *	-0.1 ± 0.2	5.6 ± 0.3	5.5 ± 0.3	0.0 ± 0.1	5.7 ± 0.5	5.7 ± 0.4	0.0 ± 0.3
HbA1c 5.7-6.4% [%]	28	21	7	39	33	6	43	43	0

Shown are means ± standard deviations. Baseline differences had been analyzed by using the Chi square test and the ANOVA test. The Wilcoxon signed rank test was conducted for analysis of differences within all of the groups (*, p<0.05; **, p<0.01; ***, p<0.001; * * * *, p<0.0001). Kruskal-Wallis test with Dunn's multiple comparisons test was used to compare changes after 12 weeks of intervention between the intervention groups and the control group (#, p<0.05; ##, p<0.01; ###, p<0.001; ####, p<0.0001 compared to the control group). Bold written numbers indicate differences that remain statistically significant after Bonferroni correction for multiple testing. ¹ missing values: n=6 in the telemedical coaching ('TMC) group; n=3 in the telemedical (TM) and in the control group. HDL, high-density lipoprotein; LDL, low-density lipoprotein; HbA1c, hemoglobin A1C.

TABLE 2: Distribution of BMI categories between groups at baseline.

	TMC group (n=58)	TM group (n=61)	Control group (n=61)
Overweight (BMI <30 kg/m^2) [n]	19 (32.8%)	17 (27.9%)	14 (23.0%)
Moderately obese (BMI 30-34,9 kg/m^2) [n]	20 (34.5%)	26 (42.6%)	25 (41.0%)
Severely obese (BMI 35-39,9 kg/m^2) [n]	16 (27.6%)	13 (21.3%)	13 (21.3%)
Very severely obese (BMI >40 kg/m^2) [n]	3 (5.2%)	5 (8.2%)	9 (14.8%)

TMC, telemedical coaching group; TM, telemedical group. Frequency of BMI categories was not different between all groups.

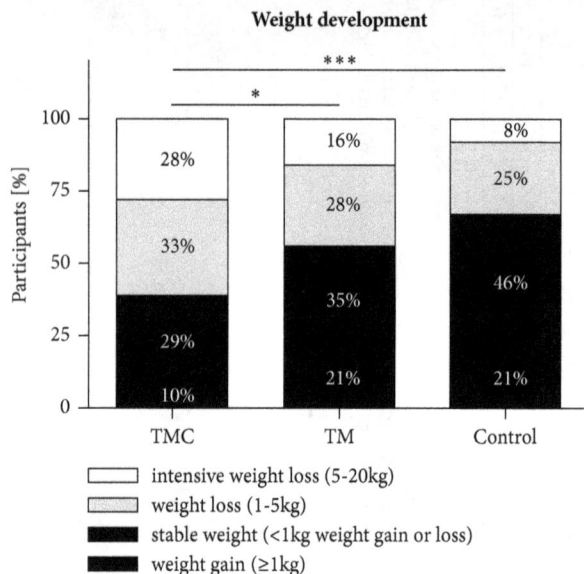

FIGURE 2: **Weight changes and differences after 12 weeks of intervention.** Participants of the telemedical coaching (TMC; n=58) group, the telemedical (TM; n=61) group, and the control group (n=61) were classified according to their weight change after 12 weeks of intervention into one of four categories: (1) ≥1 kg weight gain (black), (2) stable weight with <1 kg weight change (dark grey), (3) weight loss of 1-5 kg (light grey), or (4) weight loss of 5-20 kg (white). Shown are percentages. Differences in frequency distribution of weight change between the three groups were analyzed by using the Chi square test (∗, p<0.05; ∗ ∗ ∗, p<0.001).

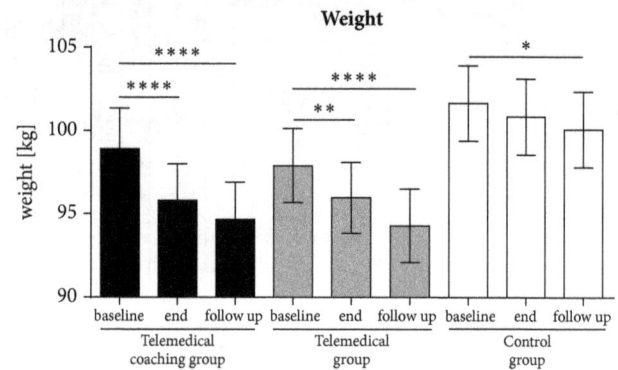

FIGURE 3: **Weight change and long-term effect.** Weight was determined at baseline, after 12 weeks of intervention and at the 52-week follow-up. Shown are means ± standard error of means. The Friedman test with Dunn's multiple comparisons test was used to test the within group differences between time points (∗, p<0.05; ∗∗, p<0.01; ∗ ∗ ∗, p<0.001; ∗ ∗ ∗∗; p<0.0001).

in all of the groups. However, the reduction in the control group did not remain statistically significant after correction for multiple testing. Moreover, cardiometabolic risk factors, i.e., systolic (p=0.039) and diastolic blood pressure (p=0.012), total cholesterol (p=0.014), HDL cholesterol (p=0.043), LDL cholesterol (p=0.006), and HbA1c (p=0.013) significantly improved in the TMC group, while only total cholesterol (p=0.013) and LDL cholesterol (p=0.006) improved in the TM group. Furthermore, proportion of persons with prediabetes (i.e., HbA1c: 5.7-6.4%) decreased by 7% in the TMC and by 6% in the TM group after 12 weeks of intervention.

3.3. Weight Change after 12 Months. Follow-up analysis of body weight demonstrated that participants of both intervention groups were further able to reduce weight after 12 months (Figure 3). In detail, participants of the TMC group further decreased their weight from 95.8 ± 16.9 kg to 94.7 ± 17.0 kg (-1.1 ± 2.4 kg; p<0.0001) in the period from week 12 to week

52. In sum, this represents a mean reduction of -4.2 ± 6.1 kg from baseline to week 52. The TM group decreased weight from 96.0 ± 16.7 kg to 94.3 ± 17.2 kg (-1.7 ± 4.8; p<0.0001) in the same study phase from week 12 to week 52. This represents a total reduction of 3.6 ± 6.1 kg from baseline to week 52. The control group showed also a slight decrease from 101.7 ± 17.7 kg to 100.1 ± 17.8 kg (-1.6 ± 3.5; p<0.05) after the 12-month follow-up.

4. Discussion

In the present randomized controlled three-armed study we could show that telemedical-based lifestyle interventions are applicable to motivate overweight individuals for lifestyle changes resulting in long-term weight reductions. In particular, the combination of telemedical devices and telemedical coaching led to greater reductions in body weight as well as improvements in cardiometabolic risk factors.

Other studies with different cohorts (e.g., persons with serious mental illness or obese patients with at least one cardiovascular risk factor) confirm our results and demonstrate that telemedical coaching or telemonitoring can contribute to relevant reductions of body weight of more than 5% [19, 20]. In particular, monitoring of physical activity (determined by accelerometers), body weight (daily recorded), and calorie intake (daily recorded) seems to be crucial for long-term (1-year period) weight management programs in obese patients, which is in line with our results [31]. Furthermore, the landmark study from Appel et al. investigated the effects of in-person support (face-to-face) in comparison to telemedical coaching (without face-to-face support) during a weight loss intervention program. Both lifestyle interventions achieved a meaningful weight reduction during a period of 24 months in obese patients. These important results underpin the potential of telemedical coaching and telemonitoring and indicate an effective solution for weight management support in the primary care and may be also for an occupational health care setting, even without face-to-face contact [20]. However, it has been shown that telephone calls alone, without telemedical coaching and monitoring, were not sufficient to sustainably influence behavior and reduce weight [21, 22] and demonstrated higher dropout rates as well [32]. In contrast, it has been shown due to a web-based weight management program that particularly the combination of automated web-based telemonitoring and basic nurse support (coaching) is an effective alternative for traditional weight management programs. The additional in-person support was essential for the weight reduction in comparison to the group without human encouragement. This relationship elucidates the necessity of external experts and coaching in telemedical interventions [23]. Moreover, Wi-Fi scales and other devices (e.g. smartphones or tablets with software applications) make it easier and more convenient for individuals to monitor their lifestyle, i.e. physical activity, diet, or weight measure. These behaviors are critical for short- and long-term weight control [33].

Besides the reduction of body weight, there were further relevant improvements in cardiovascular risk factors such as BMI, LDL cholesterol, and waist circumference in the present study. In line with other lifestyle intervention studies with electronic devices (web-, app- or SMS-based lifestyle interventions), external motivation, electronically transmitted reminders, or personalized coaching contribute to meaningful improvements in cardiovascular risk factors [20].

The present study was well tolerated. The overall dropout rate after 12 weeks of intervention and during the 12-month follow-up was 6% and 14%, and no adverse events were reported. This low dropout rate was also shown in patients with heart diseases during their cardiac rehabilitation (<10%) which was characterized by using telemedical devices (pedometers) accompanied by telephone coaching [34]. Possible explanations for these low dropout rates could be the flexible and easy contact with health experts as well as the more intense motivational coaching for lifestyle changes. Therefore, the number of telemedical lifestyle programs for the treatment of chronic diseases is increasing [35]. In light of this background, telemedical and telemonitoring channels (e.g., by call centers, internet-based programs, text messaging, or social networking sites) should improve their dissemination of intensive lifestyle programs to further improve the treatment of obesity. This development must be accompanied by far greater public health system efforts to prevent the development of obesity [33].

In a cohort of obese employees with a mean age of 47 years, 470-600 EUR additional costs per year for obesity-related sick leave days had been estimated [2]. Even with a conservative estimation, assuming constant costs, despite the

increasing age and increasing number of comorbidities as well as early retirement, spending of 9.400-12.000 EUR per person during the next 20 years will arise. Since qualified telemedical coaching programs are available for less than 50 EUR per month [24] companies should rethink their current health care strategies and consider other options. Therefore, an external telemedical health care provider might be a cost-saving and promising alternative [36, 37]. The total for each patient in the present study was around 400 EUR including costs for equipment, coaching calls, and maintenance costs for the access to the online portal during the 12-week intervention phase. As the results of this trial are promising regarding weight control (4% weight reduction within 1 year), future occupational health care initiatives could use this treatment approach. When comparing the costs of the TMC program with the expanses for sick leave days [2], obesity-related drug costs [38], and considering the huge burden for the global or national health care systems [39, 40], one could argue that this telemedical treatment approach could be an efficient alternative. Furthermore, the possibility of repeating the program as well as the not-existing side-effects underline the usefulness of this treatment approach.

There are strengths and limitations in our study that should be mentioned. Overweight employees had been invited by their medical corporate department for participation in this study. Therefore, there could be a chance for a selection bias if only motivated employees agreed to participate. However, randomization into one of the three parallel groups should have abolished any potential effect, particularly, because baseline characteristics of the three groups were not different. On the other hand, a high motivation might have led to the low dropout rate of only 6% observed in our trial. According to the study size with 180 participants, the results of the present study might not be generalizable or transferable to other nonoccupational cohorts. In contrast to that, the study of Luley et al. demonstrated higher dropout rates of 9-12% during a 1-year lifestyle telemonitoring program for weight loss in obese patients with metabolic syndrome [31]. This difference could be the result of a less intense mentoring program with only monthly calls or weekly letters. Another limitation of the present study is the lack of data regarding diet of the participants during the study. Future studies should collect these data and analyze and follow up changes of eating behavior during and after the initial intervention phase. Furthermore, missing values were imputed by the LOCF approach in the present study. This procedure is a conservative method to estimate treatment effects of an intervention. Therefore, our results might have been underestimated by this approach, which should be considered when interpreting the data.

In sum, telemedical-based interventions are effective for long-term weight reductions in overweight employees. Especially in combination with continuous telephone coaching telemedical-based interventions demonstrated large effects on weight reduction and cardiovascular risk factors. These results underline the potential usefulness of telemedical monitoring and coaching for an occupational health care setting and could be an effective approach for preventive health care programs.

Disclosure

Kerstin Kempf and Martin Röhling share the first authorship. HMM Holding AG had no influence on study design, data collection, data analysis, manuscript preparation, and/or publication decisions.

Authors' Contributions

Kerstin Kempf and Stephan Martin contributed to conception and design of the study. Monika Stichert, Gabriele Fischer, Elke Boschem, and Jürgen Könner helped in data collection. Kerstin Kempf and Martin Röhling contributed to analysis and interpretation of data and drafting of the manuscript. Kerstin Kempf, Martin Röhling, Monika Stichert, Gabriele Fischer, Elke Boschem, Jürgen Könner, and Stephan Martin approved the final version of the manuscript. Kerstin Kempf and Martin Röhling equally contributed to manuscript.

Acknowledgments

The authors thank their coaches B. Prete and I. Grafflage for their excellent work and the HMM Holding AG for providing scales and 3D-step counters.

References

[1] W. C. Knowler, S. E. Fowler, R. F. Hamman, C. A. Christophi, H. J. Hoffman, and A. T. Brenneman, "10-year follow-up of diabetes incidence and weight loss in the Diabetes Prevention Program Outcomes Study," *The Lancet*, vol. 374, no. 9702, pp. 1677–1686, 2009.

[2] T. Lehnert, N. Stuhldreher, P. Streltchenia, S. G. Riedel-Heller, and H.-H. König, "Sick leave days and costs associated with overweight and obesity in germany," *Journal of Occupational and Environmental Medicine*, vol. 56, no. 1, pp. 20–27, 2014.

[3] American Diabetes Association, "Executive summary: standards of medical care in diabetes—2014," *Diabetes Care*, vol. 37, supplement 1, pp. S5–S13, 2014.

[4] D. M. Nathan, E. Barrett-Connor, J. P. Crandall et al., "Long-term effects of lifestyle intervention or metformin on diabetes development and microvascular complications over 15-year follow-up: The Diabetes Prevention Program Outcomes Study," *The Lancet Diabetes & Endocrinology*, vol. 3, no. 11, pp. 866–875, 2015.

[5] CIPD. Absence Management. A survey of Policy and Practice. Annual Survey Report 2005.

[6] E. Demou, J. Brown, K. Sanati, M. Kennedy, K. Murray, and E. B. Macdonald, "A novel approach to early sickness absence management: The EASY (Early Access to Support for You) way," *Work*, vol. 53, no. 3, pp. 597–608, 2016.

[7] M. K. Kramer, D. M. Molenaar, V. C. Arena et al., "Improving employee health: Evaluation of a worksite lifestyle change program to decrease risk factors for diabetes and cardiovascular disease," *Journal of Occupational and Environmental Medicine*, vol. 57, no. 3, pp. 284–291, 2015.

[8] G. M. Dallam and C. P. Foust, "A Comparative Approach to Using the Diabetes Prevention Program to Reduce Diabetes Risk in a Worksite Setting," *Health Promotion and Practice*, vol. 14, no. 2, pp. 199–204, 2013.

[9] Centers for Disease Control and Prevention Atlanta (GA): CDC 2014, Workplace health promotion: benefits of health promotion programs. http://www.cdc.gov/workplacehealth-promotion/businesscase/benefits/index.html.

[10] American Heart Association Position Statement on Effective Worksite Wellness Programs. 2014, http://www.startwalking-now.org/documents/AHApositionstatementoneffectivework-sitewellnessprograms.pdf.

[11] M. K. K. Kramer, J. R. McWilliams, H.-Y. Chen, and L. M. Siminerio, "A Community-Based Diabetes Prevention Program," *The Diabetes Educator*, vol. 37, pp. 659–668, 2011.

[12] J. Ma, V. Yank, L. Xiao et al., "Translating the diabetes prevention program lifestyle intervention for weight loss into primary care: a randomized trial," *JAMA Intern Med*, vol. 28, no. 173, pp. 113–121, 2013.

[13] G. A. Piatt, M. C. Seidel, R. O. Powell, and J. C. Zgibor, "Comparative effectiveness of lifestyle intervention efforts in the community: Results of the rethinking eating and ACTivity (REACT) study," *Diabetes Care*, vol. 36, no. 2, pp. 202–209, 2013.

[14] L. Ruggiero, S. Oros, and Y. K. Choi, "Community-based translation of the diabetes prevention program's lifestyle intervention in an underserved Latino population," *The Diabetes Educator*, vol. 37, no. 4, pp. 564–572, 2011.

[15] K. Barham, S. West, P. Trief, C. Morrow, M. Wade, and R. S. Weinstock, "Diabetes prevention and control in the workplace: a pilot project for county employees," *Journal of Public Health Management and Practice*, vol. 17, no. 3, pp. 233–241, 2011.

[16] K. K. Giese and P. F. Cook, "Reducing obesity among employees of a manufacturing plant: Translating the diabetes prevention program to the workplace," *Workplace Health and Safety*, vol. 62, no. 4, pp. 136–141, 2014.

[17] A. Sineath, L. Lambert, C. Verga, M. Wagstaff, and B. C. Wingo, "Monitoring intervention fidelity of a lifestyle behavioral intervention delivered through telehealth," *mHealth*, vol. 3, article 35, 2017.

[18] V. L. Webb and T. A. Wadden, "Intensive Lifestyle Intervention for Obesity: Principles, Practices, and Results," *Gastroenterology*, vol. 152, no. 7, pp. 1752–1764, 2017.

[19] H. Temmingh, A. Claassen, S. Van Zyl et al., "The evaluation of a telephonic wellness coaching intervention for weight reduction and wellness improvement in a community-based cohort of persons with serious mental illness," *The Journal of Nervous and Mental Disease*, vol. 201, no. 11, pp. 977–986, 2013.

[20] L. J. Appel, J. M. Clark, H.-C. Yeh et al., "Comparative effectiveness of weight-loss interventions in clinical practice," *The New England Journal of Medicine*, vol. 365, no. 21, pp. 1959–1968, 2011.

[21] P. J. O'Connor, J. A. Schmittdiel, R. D. Pathak et al., "Randomized trial of telephone outreach to improve medication adherence and metabolic control in adults with diabetes," *Diabetes Care*, vol. 37, no. 12, pp. 3317–3324, 2014.

[22] K. L. Stuart, B. Wyld, K. Bastiaans et al., "A telephone-supported cardiovascular lifestyle programme (CLIP) for lipid reduction and weight loss in general practice patients: A randomised controlled pilot trial," *Public Health Nutrition*, vol. 17, no. 3, pp. 640–647, 2014.

[23] L. Yardley, L. J. Ware, E. R. Smith et al., "Randomised controlled feasibility trial of a web-based weight management intervention with nurse support for obese patients in primary care," *Interna-*

tional Journal of Behavioral Nutrition and Physical Activity, vol. 11, article 67, 2014.

[24] K. Kempf, B. Altpeter, J. Berger et al., "Efficacy of the telemedical lifestyle intervention program TeLiPro in advanced stages of type 2 diabetes: A randomized controlled trial," *Diabetes Care*, vol. 40, no. 7, pp. 863–871, 2017.

[25] S. Ayisi Addo and M. Steiner-Asiedu, "Telephone based weight loss intervention: Relevance for developing countries," *Critical Reviews in Food Science and Nutrition*, pp. 1–7, 2018.

[26] S. Martin, M. Dirk, H. Kolb, K. Kempf, A. Hebestreit, and G. Bittner, "Kognitive Verhaltenstherapie bei Typ 2 Diabetes: Ergebnisse einer Pilotstudie mit einem strukturierten Programm," *Diabetologie und Stoffwechsel*, vol. 4, pp. 370–373, 2009.

[27] K. Kempf, M. Dirk, H. Kolb, A. Hebestreit, G. Bittner, and S. Martin, "The da Vinci Medical-mental motivation program for supporting lifestyle changes in patients with type 2 diabetes," *Deutsche Medizinische Wochenschrift*, vol. 137, no. 8, pp. 362–367, 2012.

[28] K. Kempf, J. Kruse, and S. Martin, "ROSSO-in-praxi: A self-monitoring of blood glucose-structured 12-week lifestyle intervention significantly improves glucometabolic control of patients with type 2 diabetes mellitus," *Diabetes Technology & Therapeutics*, vol. 12, no. 7, pp. 547–553, 2010.

[29] K. Kempf, J. Kruse, and S. Martin, "ROSSO-in-praxi follow-up: Long-term effects of self-monitoring of blood glucose on weight, hemoglobin a1c, and quality of life in patients with type 2 diabetes mellitus," *Diabetes Technology & Therapeutics*, vol. 14, no. 1, pp. 59–64, 2012.

[30] M. Dienstl, K. Kempf, C. Schulz, J. Kruse, and S. Martin, "Einfluss von telemedizinischer Betreuung auf Stoffwechseleinstellung und Lebensqualität bei Patienten mit Typ-2-Diabetes mellitus," *Diabetologie und Stoffwechsel*, vol. 6, no. 03, pp. 164–169, 2011.

[31] C. Luley, A. Blaik, A. Götz et al., "Weight loss by telemonitoring of nutrition and physical activity in patients with metabolic syndrome for 1 year," *Journal of the American College of Nutrition*, vol. 33, no. 5, pp. 363–374, 2014.

[32] C. Holzapfel, M. Merl, L. Stecher, and H. Hauner, "One-year weight loss with a telephone-based lifestyle program," *Obesity Facts*, vol. 9, no. 4, pp. 230–240, 2016.

[33] T. A. Wadden, V. L. Webb, C. H. Moran, and B. A. Bailer, "Lifestyle modification for obesity: new developments in diet, physical activity, and behavior therapy," *Circulation*, vol. 125, no. 9, pp. 1157–1170, 2012.

[34] J. Sangster, S. Furber, M. Allman-Farinelli et al., "Effectiveness of a Pedometer-Based Telephone Coaching Program on Weight and Physical Activity for People Referred to a Cardiac Rehabilitation Program: A randomized controlled trial," *Journal of Cardiopulmonary Rehabilitation and Prevention*, vol. 35, no. 2, pp. 124–129, 2015.

[35] Y. Zhai, W. Zhu, Y. Cai, D. Sun, and J. Zhao, "Clinical- and cost-effectiveness of telemedicine in type 2 diabetes mellitus: a systematic review and meta-analysis," *Medicine*, vol. 93, no. 28, article e312, 2014.

[36] A. G. Tsai, T. A. Wadden, S. Volger et al., "Cost-effectiveness of a primary care intervention to treat obesity," *International Journal of Obesity*, vol. 37, supplement 1, pp. S31–S37, 2013.

[37] W. Hollingworth, J. Hawkins, D. A. Lawlor, M. Brown, T. Marsh, and R. R. Kipping, "Economic evaluation of lifestyle interventions to treat overweight or obesity in children," *International Journal of Obesity*, vol. 36, no. 4, pp. 559–566, 2012.

[38] D. E. Arterburn, M. L. Maciejewski, and J. Tsevat, "Impact of morbid obesity on medical expenditures in adults," *International Journal of Obesity*, vol. 29, no. 3, pp. 334–339, 2005.

[39] T. Andreyeva, R. Sturm, and J. S. Ringel, "Moderate and severe obesity have large differences in health care costs," *Obesity Research*, vol. 12, no. 12, pp. 1936–1943, 2004.

[40] M. Tremmel, U. Gerdtham, P. Nilsson, and S. Saha, "Economic Burden of Obesity: A Systematic Literature Review," *International Journal of Environmental Research and Public Health*, vol. 14, no. 4, p. 435, 2017.

19

An HTML5-Based Pure Website Solution for Rapidly Viewing and Processing Large-Scale 3D Medical Volume Reconstruction on Mobile Internet

Liang Qiao,[1,2] Xin Chen,[3] Ye Zhang,[1] Jingna Zhang,[1] Yi Wu,[4] Ying Li,[4] Xuemei Mo,[4] Wei Chen,[5] Bing Xie,[5] and Mingguo Qiu[1]

[1]Department of Medical Image, College of Biomedical Engineering, Third Military Medical University, Chongqing, China
[2]Department of Computer Science, College of Biomedical Engineering, Third Military Medical University, Chongqing, China
[3]College of Software and Computer, Chongqing Institute of Engineering, Chongqing, China
[4]Department of Digital Medicine, College of Biomedical Engineering, Third Military Medical University, Chongqing, China
[5]Department of Radiology, Southwest Hospital, Third Military Medical University, Chongqing, China

Correspondence should be addressed to Mingguo Qiu; bobqiao@163.com

Academic Editor: Manolis Tsiknakis

This study aimed to propose a pure web-based solution to serve users to access large-scale 3D medical volume anywhere with good user experience and complete details. A novel solution of the *Master-Slave* interaction mode was proposed, which absorbed advantages of remote volume rendering and surface rendering. On server side, we designed a message-responding mechanism to listen to interactive requests from clients (*Slave* model) and to guide *Master* volume rendering. On client side, we used HTML5 to normalize user-interactive behaviors on *Slave* model and enhance the accuracy of behavior request and user-friendly experience. The results showed that more than four independent tasks (each with a data size of 249.4 MB) could be simultaneously carried out with a 100-KBps client bandwidth (extreme test); the first loading time was <12 s, and the response time of each behavior request for final high quality image remained at approximately 1 s, while the peak value of bandwidth was <50-KBps. Meanwhile, the FPS value for each client was ≥40. This solution could serve the users by rapidly accessing the application via one URL hyperlink without special software and hardware requirement in a diversified network environment and could be easily integrated into other telemedical systems seamlessly.

1. Introduction

The 3D visualized reconstruction, which is built from sectional medical images (SMIs), such as CT, has an advantage of directly displaying the focus of a disease and is widely used in many fields, including diagnoses, case discussion, education, and patient consultation [1, 2]. In the era of mobile Internet (WIFI or 3G as fundamental carrier), with increasingly large amounts of SMI data of high quality, people desire to rapidly view and process this 3D visualized reconstruction of high quality in a diversified network environment via different client devices without installing special software [3]. In particular, many studies have reported that there were no significant differences of diagnostic accuracy regarding more and more diseases between mobile devices and the

traditional workstations that promoted the further development of medical imaging technology on mobile Internet [4–9]. Presently, the 3D visualized reconstruction techniques in medicine have fallen into the following two main categories: surface rendering and volume rendering [10], both with their own characteristics to adapt to the Internet application.

Surface rendering in medicine extracts the interested surface contour of the anatomical representation from SMIs into a 3D geometrical model, which is usually stored as a VRML, VTK, or X3D file [1, 11, 12]. Some Web3D technologies, such as WebGL, could directly support these models via most of the major web browsers [13] with a very good native user experience and that is a popular way to utilize Internet applications for medical 3D visualization. However, because the information integrity depends on presetting the interested area, the client user cannot arbitrarily view the internal anatomy structure or analyze the complex organization relationship. Therefore, surface rendering technology has been mainly used for special disease with specific requirements [11, 12, 14], and it could not adapt to the custom behavior of the client user in mobile Internet very well.

Volume rendering describes a wide range of techniques to generate images from 3D scalar data [15]. It is very convenient to view the internal anatomy structure and describe the complex organizational relationship through user adjustment of the parameters of color and opacity on each voxel [16]. However, volume rendering requires a complete computation of the original volumetric data for each user's behavior event, the cost of computation being much higher than that for surface rendering. Thus, volume rendering technology is often deployed on a dedicated image workstation and in a private network environment, where the scope of application is limited. Some low-level graphics APIs, such as OpenGL ES 2.0, have been integrated into WebGL for Internet application, which could be theoretically enabled to support GPU-based direct volume ray-casting implementations, or support some slice-based sampling techniques to get close to the imaging result of ray-casting-based implementations. Nevertheless, the imaging quality and efficiency is very limited, not just because of performance of common GPU, but also because of the limited performance of web pages [7–9]. Furthermore, there is still high requirement to network for original volumetric data transmission. Currently, there is a remote volume rendering scheme to solve the limit. This scheme deploys the volume rendering job on the server side to a real-time response to behavior instructions from the client and transmits the 2D projection image from volume rendering to the client display, where the client is only an interface for sending instructions and displaying results [9, 17–20]. For example, the user slides the mouse from point A to point B to express an operation of 3D rotation on the client side, and the server just calculates the final viewing angle from A to B and sends the final result to the user. Because there is no original data downloading and no rendering cost on the client side, the network load and computing pressure of the client could be significantly reduced. However, this interaction model of "the client sends one operation request, the server replies one result at a time" may cause a bad user experience. Specifically, it may lose the value of Frames Per Second (FPS), one of the most important parameters of the 3D interactive experience. Therefore, all of [9, 17–20] discretized the trajectory of one single operation request from the client into several request points to request continuous responses from the server. For example, if the path between mouse points A and B were converted into several separated remote volume rendering requests from the client, the sever would respond to each request and send continuous 2D projection images to the client. Thus, the value of FPS could be increased; however, it may lead to a huge pressure on the server load (response to a large amount of requests) and network load (continuous data stream). Additionally, [9, 17–19] ask the client to install customized software or plug-ins, which may lead to a lack of compatibility. Therefore, existing remote volume rendering methods do not adapt to the mobile Internet application characteristics of lightweight [21] very well, which ask for lower resources of network and computing, and avoid unnecessary installation.

In this study, we plan to combine the advantage of surface rendering technology based on WebGL with the advantage of remote volume rendering to design a solution for viewing and processing 3D medical volume reconstruction in a pure webpage environment. Finally, a visualization interaction platform would be built. This platform could be used anywhere, in a diversified network environment and diversified client devices, with a good user experience similar to the native application.

2. Computational Methods and Theory

The core concept includes the Slave model and Master volume. The Slave model is a contour model rendered by surface rendering technology, running on WebGL as a 3D interactive interface on the client side. The *Master* volume is a volumetric data rendering from original SMIs on the server side. The final required image of high quality is a projection drawing from the *Master* volume according to the behavior instructions from the *Slave* model. This solution could be named the *Master-Slave* dual-channel interaction mode and is expected to enhance the user experience similar to the native application in a pure web page, to reduce the pressure of the server load and network load, and to meet the requirement of lightweight volumetric data sharing in a mobile Internet application.

2.1. Design of the Master-Slave Dual-Channel Interaction Mode. The architecture of this solution constitutes the following two parts: the server side and client side. The server side renders the *Master* volume to generate the final required image of high quality, while the client side provides the *Slave* model's interactive navigation.

The detailed procedures are as follows (schematic diagram is shown in Figure 1):

On the server side, in zone ①, groups of SMIs could be uploaded to the server through the network interface of PACS or removable storage medium. Thereafter, the relevant *Slave* models could be automatically pregenerated by rough contour extraction. The listener in zone ② accepts the user's web behavior request (instructions) in real-time and guides zone ③ to load and render the relevant SMIs in memory, which is defined as the *Master* volume, generating a 2D projection image from the rendered result for client downloading.

On the client side, while the user wants to view and process a group of SMIs, the client could download the corresponding *Slave* model from the server and reconstruct it locally in zone ④; meanwhile, request the server to load and render relevant SMIs in memory. Thereafter, in zone ④, the user could view and process the local *Slave* model arbitrarily and submit the final behavior request (instructions) to the server to acquire the required projection image from the *Master* volume in zone ② ③ ⑤.

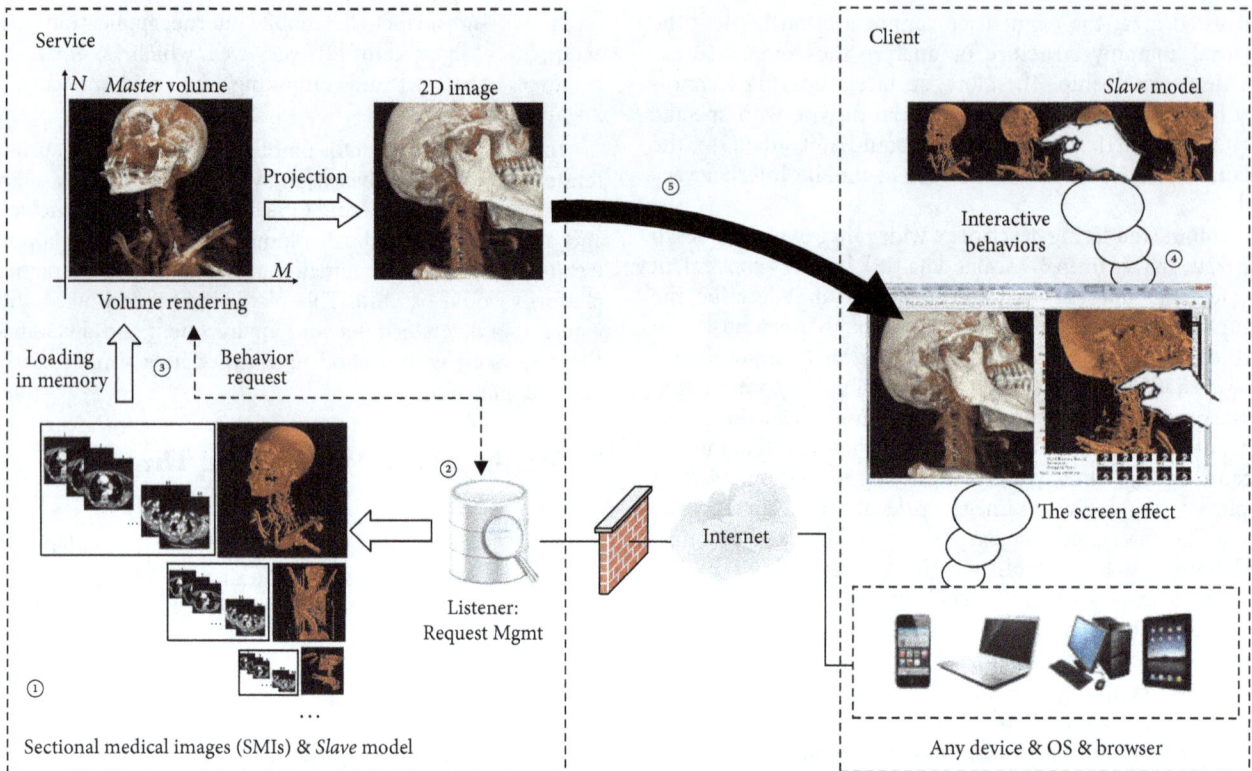

FIGURE 1: Architecture of the pure web-based solution via the *Master-Slave* dual-channel interaction mode.

Here, the client could be a pure web browser running on diversified devices, supporting the WebGL technique. That means there is no installation for the client.

2.2. Rendering of the Master Volume.

We adopted the ray-casting algorithm [22] to reconstruct the *Master* volume of SMIs. The algorithm is a direct volume rendering method that has been widely used for radiodiagnosis but requires a high computing performance of the device. First, we transformed the SMIs into volume voxels in 3D space (Figure 2(a)) and then simulated rays to cast each voxel with a customized color and opacity [23] into 2D space (Figure 2(b)). This method could be used to describe a complex organization relationship. Furthermore, it could display internal anatomy structure via removing (clipping) part of the voxels that simulate a user's behavior of dissection (Figure 2(c)).

Here, we directly used the VTK (Visualization Toolkit) library [24] to realize the ray-casting algorithm. For customized color and opacity, several frequently used schemes could be deployed on the server side in advance; a dropdown list was designed on the user interface to correspond to each scheme for remote volume rendering [25, 26]. For clipping, VTK provides a class of vtkPlane to build a virtual Clipping plane to guide the voxel removal [27]. It means the clipping job only needs the specific location of the virtual Clipping plane in the 3D coordinate system. The specific location could be described by the following two parameters in the computer graphics method: *normal vector* from the origin point to the plane and the *coordinate position of a point* on the Clipping plane, both from the client submission.

2.3. Generation and Interaction of the Slave Model.

The *Slave* model was pregenerated on the server side and was designed to be a navigational tool to interact with the Web page. While clients want to view and process the *Master* volume, the *Slave* model could be downloaded to the client and reconstructed on the client side.

2.3.1. Generation and Slimming of the Slave Model.

To interact with mobile Internet, the data size of the model should be as small as possible (much slimmer), while the clarity of the contour is acceptable. However, using the traditional compression-decompression algorithm may ask the client to install additional software. Hence, the steps in the generation of a smaller *Slave* model can be designed as follows (Figure 3). Here, we used a group of SMIs of the head and neck CT as an example, and the resolution of voxels is $512 \times 512 \times 495$, 249 MB (testing data (1) in Section 4).

Step 1 (resampling the original SMIs for first slimming). Load the corresponding SMIs into memory; shrink each sectional image to a standard size of $32 * 32$ via the resampling of the 2D space (Figures 3(a) and 3(b)).

Step 2 (building the 3D geometrical contour model). A marching cubes algorithm [28], one of the most common methods of surface rendering, was used to extract the interested surface contour of the anatomical representation from resampling SMIs into a 3D geometrical contour model. Here, according to the feature of the CT grayscale [29], we set a particular contour value at -800 or 200 that could separate the skin or skeleton of the body from the resampling

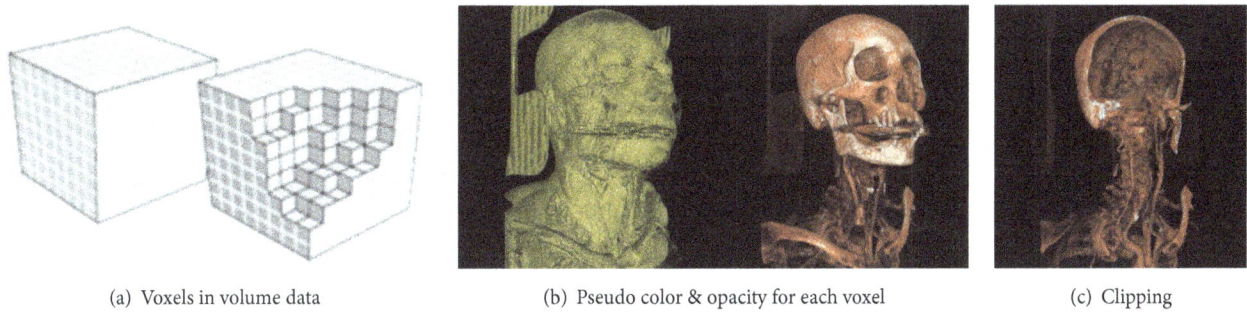

(a) Voxels in volume data   (b) Pseudo color & opacity for each voxel   (c) Clipping

FIGURE 2: Schematic diagram of the direct volume rendering method.

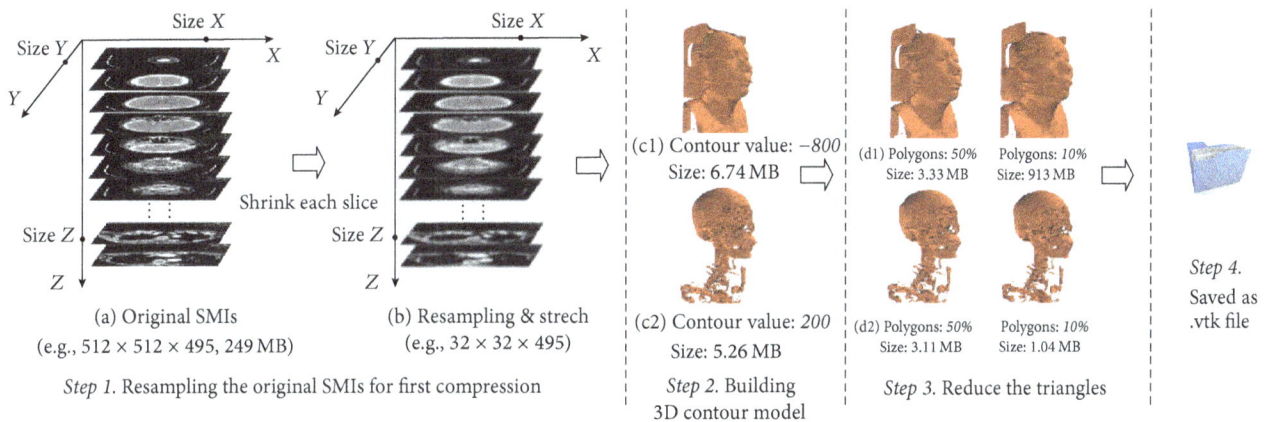

(a) Original SMIs
(e.g., 512 × 512 × 495, 249 MB)

(b) Resampling & strech
(e.g., 32 × 32 × 495)

(c1) Contour value: −800
Size: 6.74 MB

(c2) Contour value: 200
Size: 5.26 MB

(d1) Polygons: 50%
Size: 3.33 MB

Polygons: 10%
Size: 913 MB

(d2) Polygons: 50%
Size: 3.11 MB

Polygons: 10%
Size: 1.04 MB

Step 4.
Saved as
.vtk file

Step 1. Resampling the original SMIs for first compression

Step 2. Building
3D contour model

Step 3. Reduce the triangles

FIGURE 3: Schematic diagram of the generation and compression of the *Slave* model.

SMIs, respectively, to acquire a skin model or skeleton model (Figures 3(c1) and 3(c2)). In this case, the data size of the skin model and skeleton model could be reduced to 6.74 MB and 5.26 MB, respectively.

Step 3 (reducing the total number of polygons for second slimming). The 3D geometrical contour model from Step 2 is constitutive of polygons, and we could reduce the total number of polygons to further reduce the data size. In this case, the number was reduced to 50% and 10%, and the data sizes were reduced to approximately 3 MB and 1 MB, respectively (Figures 3(d1) and 3(d2)).

Step 4 (saved as *.vtk* model file). The slimmed model would be saved in a file of the *.vtk* format, which is a storage format of the geometrical model supported by WebGL, and then stored in the same directory with original SMIs.

The result of Figures 3(d1) and 3(d2) preliminarily showed that the *Slave* model whose data size is approximately 1 MB still could be fit for interactive navigation (more experiments detailed in Section 4.1). Moreover, an additional mutual interface of the client was designed as a remote parameter setting of the contour value and the total number of polygons, to permit users to customize the *Slave* model as desired.

2.3.2. Design and Quantization of the Interactive Behaviors in the Slave Model. For a friendly interactive experience on the client side, a simple style of interactive behaviors of the client and corresponding quantitative methods should be designed

to guide remote volume rendering, including the *viewing angle request* and *clipping request*.

For the Viewing Angle Request. The interaction of *viewing angle* includes rotation, flipping, zooming, and panning [30]. We defined the interactive 3D scene including only one *Slave* model and one camera and customized an interactive mode of the camera in VR technology to meet our requirement. Figure 4(a) shows the principle of the interaction of the *viewing angle* between the camera and *Slave* model. We limited the lens of the camera to always be taken on point $P1$ $(0, 0, 0)$, which was the origin of the world coordinate system. The interactive behaviors of the *viewing angle* were carried out by only changing the camera position except panning. For panning, it was carried out by changing the *Slave* model position; see examples in Figure 4(b).

According to the definition, while sending request instructions to the server for remote volume rendering, the instructions only include three quantization parameters from the client to accurately describe the interactive behavior of the *viewing angle request* to the *Slave* model. The three quantization parameters include the following: attribute *view up direction*, attribute *position* of camera, and attribute *position* of the center point of the *Slave* model.

Here, attribute *view up direction* of camera indicates the direction of the top of the camera. For example, $(0, -1, 0)$, a value of the *View Up direction*, indicates the camera is perpendicular to the XZ plane in the world coordinate system, and the top of the camera is in the opposite direction

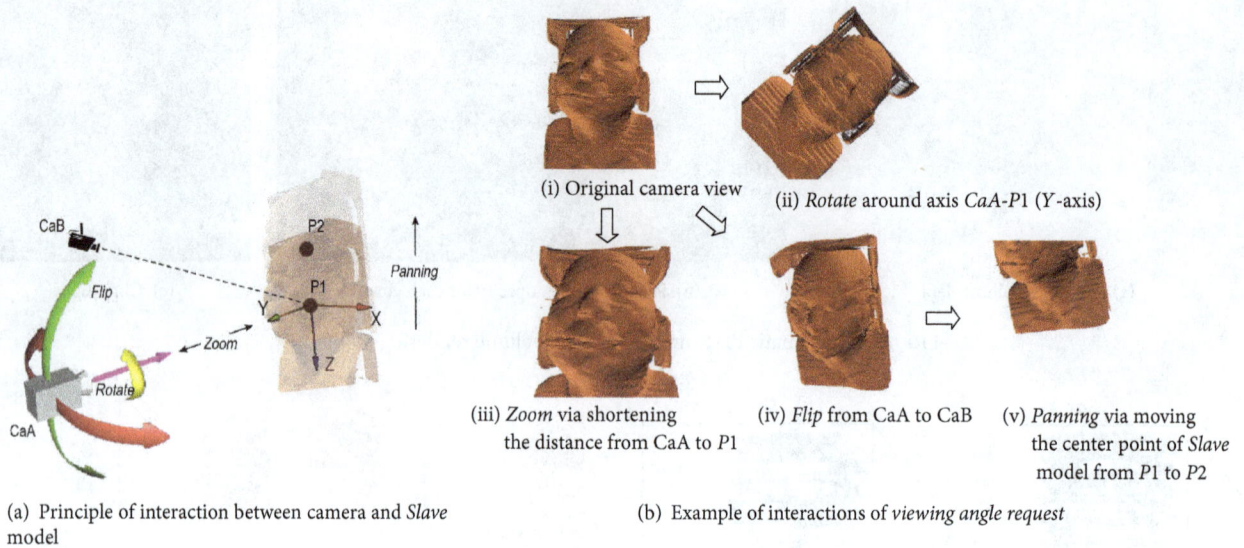

(i) Original camera view

(ii) *Rotate* around axis *CaA-P1* (*Y*-axis)

(iii) *Zoom* via shortening the distance from CaA to *P1*

(iv) *Flip* from CaA to CaB

(v) *Panning* via moving the center point of *Slave* model from *P1* to *P2*

(a) Principle of interaction between camera and *Slave* model

(b) Example of interactions of *viewing angle request*

FIGURE 4: Principle of the interaction of the *viewing angle* between the camera and *Slave* model and the corresponding example.

along the Z-axis (see the relationship between camera CaA and *Slave* model in Figure 4(a), and corresponding example (i) *original camera view* in Figure 4(b)).

In fact, WebGL has provided some interaction methods of the moving camera to view 3D objects via mouse- and gesture-based interactive behaviors, which were packaged into a library of TrackballControls.js for a web page script. We could directly utilize the js library to acquire the three quantization parameters. However, we need to rewrite the js library to restrict and customize the interactive mode of the camera that we have defined, to ensure the consistency of the interactive rule between the *Master* and *Slave* side.

For the Clipping Request. For arbitrarily clipping and viewing the internal anatomy structure of the *Master* volume, a green rectangle object, named the Clipping plane, was added in the above defined interactive 3D scene, to allow users to mimic the clipping behavior in the *Slave* model; see Figures 5(a) and 5(b). Here, a virtual control panel was designed separately to support the interactive behaviors of users using the Clipping plane (Figure 5(c)).

During the initialization phase, the Clipping plane covers the XY plane in the world coordinate system (Figure 5(a)). Its specific location could be accurately described by the following two quantization parameters in the computer graphics method: *normal vector* from the origin point to the Clipping plane, and the *coordinate position of a point* on the Clipping plane. Here, its default *normal vector* was $\{0, 0, 1\}$; one *point P* on the plane was on the position $(0, 0, 0)$.

For intuitive operation of the user experience, the interactive behaviors regarding the Clipping plane include rotation and panning, and both can be operated by a virtual control panel. However, for the accurate description of the request instructions for remote volume rendering, the two quantization parameters should be used.

Therefore, formula (1) was deduced to calculate the *normal vector* from the angles of rotation.

$$normal\ vector = \{\sin(\theta_y), -\sin(\theta_x)$$
$$\cdot \cos(\theta_y), \cos(\theta_x) \cdot \cos(\theta_y)\}. \tag{1}$$

Here θ_x, θ_y are the final rotation angles that rotate the Clipping plane clockwise around the X-axis and Y-axis, respectively.

For example, in Figure 5(b), a user rotated the Clipping plane 30 degrees clockwise around the Y-axis, and -15 degrees clockwise around the X-axis, and then panned the Clipping plane 95 pixels in the positive direction along the Z-axis. While submitting for remote volume rendering, $\theta_x = -15$, $\theta_y = 30$, the *normal vector* was $\{0.5, 0.2241, 0.8365\}$ according to formula (1). Meanwhile, according to the characteristic of monolithic translation, the one *point P* on the Clipping plane was moved to *position* $(0, 0, 95)$. That would be the two quantization parameters of request instructions for clipping.

2.4. Remote Interaction between the Server and Client. The interactive behaviors of the *Slave* model include *viewing angle request* and *clipping request*. Moreover, *color/opacity request* is operated by the dropdown list of the preset schemes (detailed in Section 2.2). All of these requests would be submitted to the server in the form of quantization parameters, which are named as request instructions.

However, in addition to responding to the client's instructions, the server has to find an efficient way to manage and allocate system resources, to enhance the robustness of the high frequency of interaction among multiple users, for example, to reduce the probability of deadlock, cumulative delay, and task-pipeline crossing.

In our system, we used relational database schema to manage the request instructions from the client and to

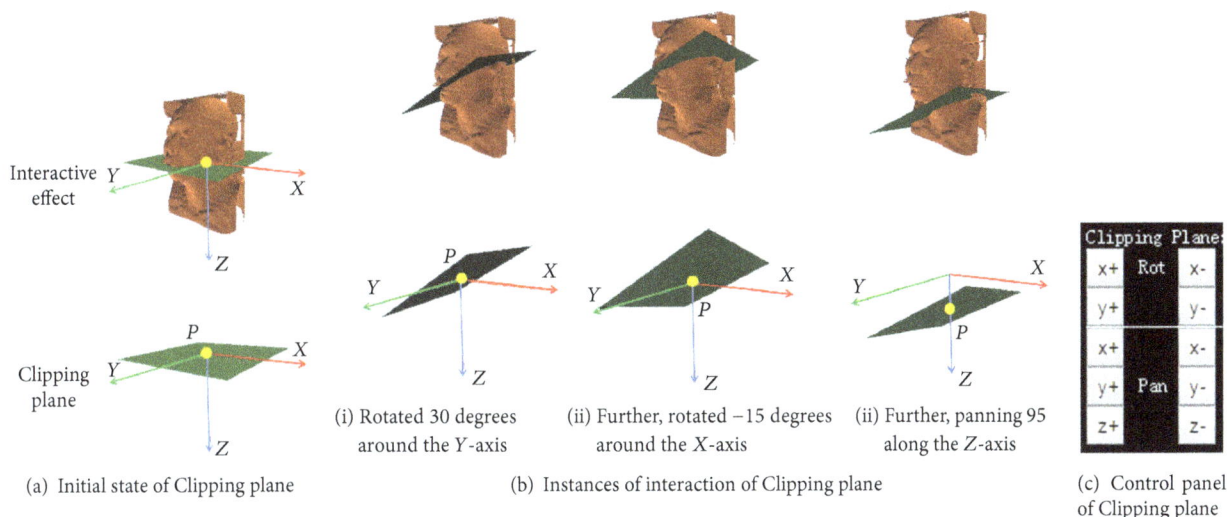

FIGURE 5: Design of the interaction of clipping to the *Slave* model and corresponding example.

allocate the system resources for guiding 3D rendering. The core tables and their data storage structure are designed in Table 1.

According to Table 1, if a user chooses a group of SMIs from a list, derived from the *base table*, the server would query the *pipeline table* whether the SMIs is serving the client. If No, the SMIs would be loaded in memory, and a task-pipeline between the user and SMIs would be built. Thereafter, the *state* of the *pipeline table* would be changed to "Yes." While being Yes, the client would be permitted to make the next interactive request. After that, for each request from the client, the server must query the *state* of the *behavior table* whether the pipeline is "pending" or "processing." If No, the server would accept the request with a record of a "pending" *state*. Additionally, the listener on the server would real-time arrange these pending requests to the server rendering in queue. While a request is being rendered, the corresponding *state* of *behavior table* would be changed as "processing" to prevent malignant submission. While the job is finished, the *state* would be changed to "finished," and a 2D projection image would be generated and saved in the specified HTTP sharing path.

The client adopted AJAX (Asynchronous JavaScript and XML) [31] to dynamically query the *state* of *behavior table* from the server at a fixed frequency of 300 ms. While rendering was finished, the client would download and update the 2D projection image via the HTML + js web page technique.

3. System Description

3.1. System Architecture. While Figure 1 depicts the *Master-Slave* dual-channel interaction mode, it also presents the overall architecture of the final platform. Here, we adopted the browser/server architecture, for which the communication with each other was via the HTTP protocol. The server side consists of the *Listener & Request Management Server* (in zone ②) and *Rendering Server* (in zone ③). The former accepts and manages the requests from the client

and guides the *Rendering Server* to an orderly response. The latter renders the SMIs and generates a 2D projection image for the client downloading via HTTP. At the same time, the client side was designed by the standard of HTML5 [32]. We used <img>, an HTML image tag, to display the 2D projection image in the form of pseudo 3D, and used AJAX + js technology to realize flicker-free page updates and client RIA (rich Internet application) over diversified web browsers without installation. Moreover, HTML5 includes the WebGL standard, and the *Slave* model could run on any HTML5-supporting web browsers without any web plug-ins or special software tools. Thus, the whole platform system could run under mature network technologies.

3.2. System Front-End. System front-end is an HTML5-based pure website that provides entrance to SMI access and 3D presentation. The users require a username and password to enter the system, or any experts could be invited to enter a specific task-pipeline with one URL hyperlink from a help seeker. In brief, using an HTML5-supporting web browser, including the major versions of Firefox, chrome, Opera, safari, IE 10+, the 3D volume can be viewed and processed as in Figure 6 and the Supplementary Materials available online at https://doi.org/10.1155/2017/4074137 (1. Demonstration of the operation procedure on laptop via website .mp4).

Here, the interactive behaviors of the user include the *viewing angle, clipping,* and *color/opacity* transformation. The first two items were operated on the *Slave* model, which was reconstructed on the client side. While the user wants to observe the final required image of high quality, the user just presses the submit button to submit the current behavior request instruction to the server and waits for the final 2D projection image to be updated.

Figure 6(a) presents the initial state of the *Slave* model (right) and 2D projection image (left). In Figure 6(b), mouse or hand gesture is used to operate the *Slave* model to

TABLE 1: Relational data storage structure of request behaviors from client and resource allocation on the server.

Table	Field	Note
Base table	DICOMs_ID	PRIMARY KEY, the unique identifier of a group of SMIs	To record the basic information of SMIs on the server side
	Storage path	The storage path of SMIs on the server side	
Pipeline table	pipeline_ID	PRIMARY KEY, the unique identifier of a pipeline for viewing a group of SMIs between the client and server	Based on *base table*, to record the connected relationship between the SMIs rendering in memory on the server and remote user on the client
	DICOMs_ID	FOREIGN KEY of *base table*, to declare which group of SMIs the client is viewing	
	Client	Client user	
	IP address	IP address of the committer	
	State	Whether the SMIs finished rendering in memory on the server? *Yes*, allow the client to next operation. *No*, prompt for waiting	
Behavior table	behavior_ID	PRIMARY KEY, the unique identifier of each behavior request event from the client	Based on *pipeline table*, to record operation requests from the client user and their process state
	pipeline_ID	FOREIGN KEY of *pipeline table*, to declare which pipeline on viewing and processing	
	Behavior type	Including *viewing angle, clipping, or color/opacity* transformation	
	Behavior-instruction	From the client, to transfer the parameters in terms of the corresponding behavior type, recorded in the form of quantization parameters	
	State	*Pending, processing, or finished*	

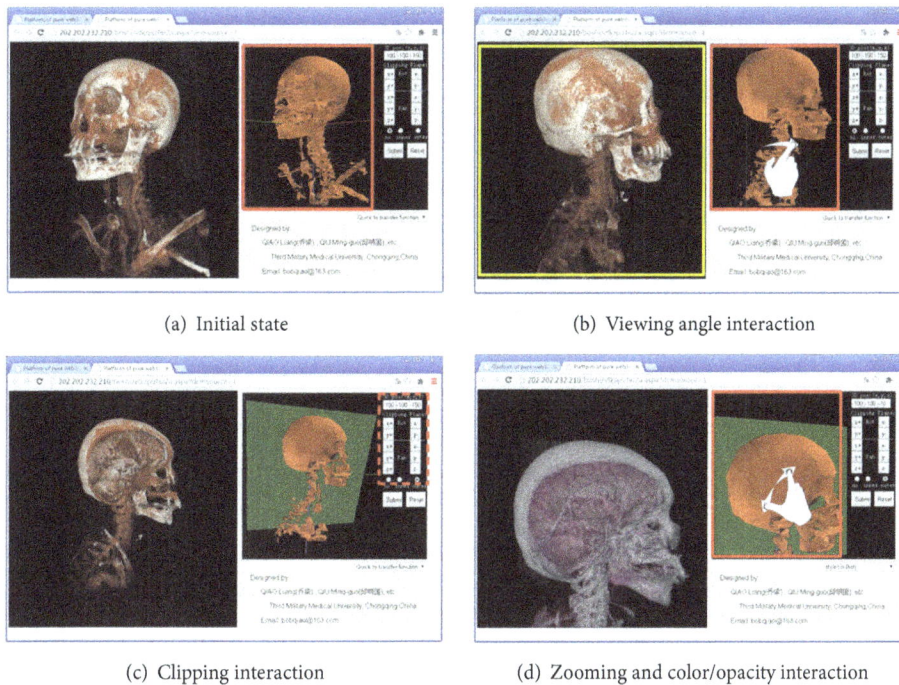

(a) Initial state

(b) Viewing angle interaction

(c) Clipping interaction

(d) Zooming and color/opacity interaction

FIGURE 6: Screenshot and operational demonstration.

transform the *viewing angle* from Figure 6(a) to Figure 6(b) (red solid box), and then the submit button is pressed to send the behavior request instruction to the server to require an updated projection image from the *Master* volume (yellow solid box). In Figure 6(c), using virtual control panel (red dashed box) to operate Clipping plane, after submitting, the new projection image was then updated (left). In Figure 6(d), the mouse wheel or hand gesture is used to zoom the *Slave* model, and then the color/opacity theme is submitted via the dropdown list (bottom right corner) to guide remote volume rendering.

4. Mode of Availability of the System

In this paper, we designed a *Master-Slave* dual-channel interaction mode to improve a problem of remote visualization interaction of the volume reconstruction of SMIs, which usually have a huge data size and calculation cost. Finally, a visualization interaction platform has been built. Particularly, there is no special software and hardware requirement for the clients, and no special network environment is needed.

To measure whether the effectiveness and performance to adapt to the mobile Internet application has characteristics of lightweight, three radiologists with more than 3 years of experience were invited to test the interactive experience, imaging quality, and compatibility over diversified Internet devices. Moreover, four junior students majoring in Biomedical Engineering were invited to test and quantize the network load and response time.

Testing Data. 3 groups of SMIs from the radiology department of Southwest Hospital of Chongqing include the following:

(1) head and neck CT with 495 slices, $512 * 512$, 249.4 MB, (2) trunk CT with 609 slices, $512 * 512$, 306.5 MB, and (3) thorax and mandible CT with 500 slices, $512 * 512$, 251.6 MB. *Server.* An IBM X3650M4 workstation (CPU: $4 \times$ E5-2603, RAM: 16 GB, OS: Windows Server 2008) was connected to the Internet via 10 Mbps. The 2D projection image was set as the resolution of $512 * 512$ with high quality JPEG compression (level-8).

Client. 4 Internet devices were located at the 3G or WIFI mobile Internet with the server. In Figure 7(a), there is a Founder E520 personal computer running on winXP with Firefox 46 web browser via 3G usb card. In Figure 7(b), there is an Acer E15 laptop running on win7 with chrome 43 web browser at WIFI. In Figure 7(c), there is a HuaWei Honor 6 smart phone running on EMUI 3.0, which is developed from Android 4.4.2 with the Opera 37 web browser at 3G net. In Figure 7(d), there is an iPad mini running on IOS6 with safari at WIFI. All of them could be representative in the mobile Internet. Additionally, each was limited to a 100-KBps wireless bandwidth by 360 security firewall for extreme test [33].

4.1. Interactive Experience, Imaging Quality, and Compatibility. To ensure the consistency of the context, the testing data (1) were considered as the main object of reference. Here, the demonstration and effect of the testing data (1) are shown in Figure 6.

Figure 6 shows that this *Slave* model of the testing data (1), which was compressed to 1.04 MB, could be fit to the demands of interactive navigation to accurately guide remote volume rendering, and shows that the projection image could be displayed to keep the original quality.

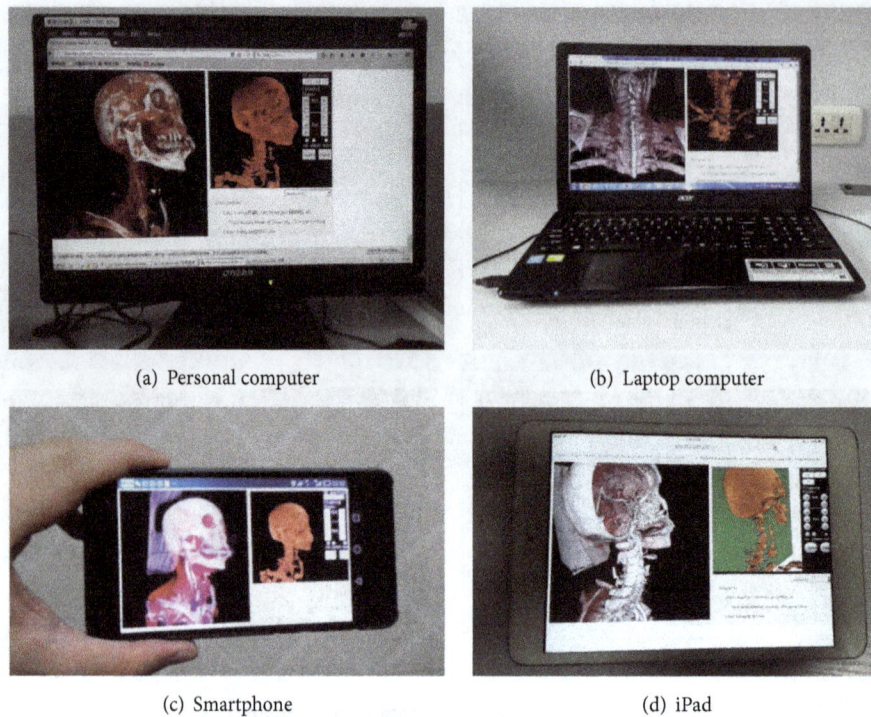

(a) Personal computer

(b) Laptop computer

(c) Smartphone

(d) iPad

FIGURE 7: The system is accessed via four different devices and web browsers under extreme bandwidth.

For further validation, three radiologists were invited to test the platform with the similar behaviors in Figure 6. This job was repeated to operate three groups of different testing data through different web browsers and Internet devices that were all aforementioned. Additionally, a five-point scale was designed to respond to the radiologists' requests (Table 2).

Table 2 presents a very positive evaluation from the statistical result of the imaging quality and interactive experience, and all three radiologists expressed that is an interesting way, whether as a gesture-based or mouse-based interaction. No installations were required from the client, and good compatibility was obtained (same result is shown in Table 3). However, one radiologist thought the default *Slave* model of the testing data (1), with a skeleton model of 1.04 MB (Figure 3(d2)), was a little rough. He suggested to use the skeleton model of 5.26 MB or skin model of 913 KB (Figures 3(c1) and 3(c2)) instead of the 1.04 model, both of which are the alternatives from the mutual interface for the client, as detailed in Section 2.3.1. Additionally, all three radiologists claimed that the response time for final high quality image is always about 1 second that is consistent with the test result in Section 4.2. However, they did accept the performance, because they could directly operate the *Slave* model smoothly without any delay on client side; thus a short wait for final high quality image had little influence. Moreover, one of the radiologists specifically expressed the native application of 3D rendering on desktop PC also needs 1 or 2 seconds' delay for final image; this performance of the solution running on smart phone is similar to the native application on PC and is very good.

4.2. Response Time and Network Load between the Client and Server. The response time can be defined as the time interval between the user sending a behavior request to the system and web browser loading the response results completely. The network load can be defined as the amount of data transmission of each interactive behavior. Four junior students majoring in Biomedical Engineering were invited to simultaneously test the platform for one hour. During the test, all of the students, respectively, viewed and processed the testing data (1) through the platform and performed similar behaviors to those detailed in Figure 6. This test was repeated by each student with different web browsers and Internet devices, all of which were aforementioned. Here, we trained the students to record the real-time network traffic by the 360 security firewall and the time interval by the script log. The results are showed in Table 3.

In Table 3, for each device, the amount of data transmission and response time of the *first loading* are much higher than the *behavior request* and *idle status* because the *first loading* asks the client to download the necessary *Slave* model. The response time of the *first loading* is <12 s at 100-KBps client bandwidth, which is similar to the total time spent on *Slave* model downloading. In fact, the response time of *first loading* also includes the cost time of SMI loading and rendering on the server side, but the server monitor presents the cost time as <7 s because SMI loading and *Slave* model downloading are simultaneous, and this cost could be neglected.

After the first loading, the network load of the *behavior request* for final image is spent on request instructions submission, final projection image downloading, and the server processing status querying at a fixed frequency of 300 ms,

TABLE 2: Statistic results of the five-point scale concerning the interactive experience and imaging quality.

Focus	Subject		Very agree	Agree	Uncertainty	Disagree	Very disagree
Interactive experience: Mouse-based △ Gesture-based ▲	The operation of viewing and processing is accurate	△	3				
		▲	3				
	Simple and easy to use without training	△	2	1			
		▲	3				
	A good user experience similar to native application	△	2	1			
		▲	2	1			
Imaging quality	*Slave* model could meet demands of navigation		2	1			
	2D image from *Master* volume could provide high quality reconstruction result via utilizing the display capability of Internet terminals		3				
Others	Latency time for final high quality images		3				

TABLE 3: Average response time and amount of data transmission from the different behaviors and devices at 100-KBps.

Devices	First loading (average value)		Behavior request for final image (average value)		Idle status of bandwidth occupation (KBps)	Frames Per Second (FPS)
	Amount of data trans (KB)	Response time (seconds)	Amount of data trans (KB)	Response time (seconds)		
PC (3G net)	1085.44	11.23	47.10	1.12	0.23	48–60
Laptop (WIFI)	1064.96	10.51	46.08	0.89	0.31	48–60
iPad mini (WIFI)	1079.41	10.93	44.03	0.95	0.35	50–60
Smartphone (3G net)	1075.02	10.72	39.94	1.02	0.28	30–40

where the projection image downloading is the main part. The results present a complete amount of data transmission of each behavior request is close to 50 KB, but the corresponding response time for final image is approximately 1 s in 100 KBps. That is because, besides the network load, the rest of time is spent on server processing and time interval of querying (300 ms). The short delay could be acceptable for practical applications, as detailed in Section 4.1.

While in the *idle status*, including the user's interactive behavior (operation) on the *Slave* model, the bandwidth occupation is almost negligible. Moreover, there are no significant differences among diversified devices and networks at 100-KBps client bandwidth.

Additionally, the FPS of *Slave* model rendering on the client side is measured via stats.min.js, which is a library packaged from WebGL. When the client rendering is completed, FPS could remain at the upper limit.

5. Discussion and Comparison

Due to the nonprivate network environment and diversified purposes, application software on one device must compete for limited resources of the network and computing. Thus lightweight, which requires lower resources of the network and computing and avoids unnecessary installation, could be an important characteristic of mobile Internet application. Additionally, to avoid compatibility problems caused by different operating systems and client hardware characteristics,

using HTML5 and related web technologies running on major web browsers may be a choice to adapt to cross-platform deployment and the characteristics of lightweight [21].

Therefore, this article described research on a method for the *Master-Slave* dual-channel interaction mode, which is based on the HTML5 standard (also a wider web compatibility standard of WebGL), to permit users viewing and processing million-megabyte-class SMIs via different client devices (without hardware or operating system constraints), over a pure web page (without installing special software) and in a diversified network environment.

Compared with the traditional PACS mode of "image compression, transmission, local reconstruction," because our method does not transfer original SMIs to the client, it neither needs to wait for a long time to download nor requests special demands of the software environment on the client device. Moreover, compared with the state of the art of local volume rendering based on WebGL and HTML5 technology [7–9], our methods have no special demands of client hardware for computation that may reduce battery consumption [9] and enhance the compatibility of the client devices; our methods may be more fit for mobile Internet application. Additionally, the client does not access the original SMIs, which could be much safer.

Compared with popular solutions based on absolute surface rendering technology [11, 12, 14], our method has locally used this technique to only support light *Slave* model for interactive navigation; therefore, the demands of the network bandwidth and device rendering capability are almost negligible in our method. Moreover, the final required image of high quality is a projection drawing from volume rendering technology, indicating that our method could be convenient for users to view the internal anatomy structure and complex organization relationship; however, surface rendering technology could not support these characteristics of volume.

Compared with solutions based on absolute remote volume rendering methods, our method adopted the *Master-Slave* dual-channel interaction mode to strengthen the user experience, which is an entirely different approach from the mode of "continuous request, continuous response" of studies of [9]. Although studies of [17–19] proposed several methods to improve the mode to reduce the network load, including video-compressed transmission [17], tile-based transmission [18], and variable resolution transmission [19], the pressure of server load and real-time data stream increased. We used the same SMI data (testing data (1)), the same quality of final required image, and the same server configuration and volume rendering algorithm in Section 4 to test the methods in [17–19]. For quantitative test, we formulated an interactive trajectory with fixed 30 request points, theoretically, assuming 30 rendering requests triggered per 1 second; there should be 30 fps render effects. On this basis, [17] adopted 512 ∗ 512 mpeg-4 compression for transmission, [18] adopted 8 ∗ 8 blocks to segment each 512 ∗ 512 frame and transfer the blocks which are different from previous frame in the process of interaction, and [19] adopted 64 ∗ 64 resolution transmission in the process of interaction, but 512 ∗ 512 for end frame. The test was repeated for 5 times under the condition of one single client monopolizing the bandwidth and server under ideal WIFI environment. The results showed that the total amount of data transmission for each interaction test of [17–19] was 298.0 KB, 603.6 KB, and 371.3 KB, respectively, the average response time of first frame was 1.10 seconds, 0.59 seconds, and 0.52 seconds, and the average cumulative response time of end frame (30th frame which is the final required image) was 21.31 seconds, 17.61 seconds, and 16.01 seconds. The response time contains the factors of server continuous rendering response, server continuous frame-encoding, and so forth (more than 70% server CPU utilization during interaction), but the network factors could be tentatively neglected under the ideal single-user WIFI environment. Assuming that we can improve the server's processing ability to completely eliminate the server response delay (perfect 30 fps interaction effect), the theoretical value of the bandwidth could be 298.0 KBps, 603.6 KBps, and 371.3 KBps, respectively. In summary, the FPS value, one of the most important parameters of the 3D interactive experience, of the studies of [17–19] was correlated reciprocally with the number of simultaneous tasks on the server side (server task-pipelines), server processing ability, and network bandwidth, and an obvious delay of interaction was clearly presented. By contrast, all of the Internet devices chosen to test our method could provide an FPS value at 30–60, and the FPS value was not correlated with server tasks, server processing ability, and network bandwidth, but with

the device GPU (Graphics Processing Unit). Undoubtedly, almost all GPUs of Internet devices in the market could meet the demands of our light *Slave* model rendering. Moreover, the peak value of the bandwidth under the behavior request for final image was less than 50 KBps and less than 1 KBps at idle (including the operation of *Slave* model); thus, both were far below those tests of methods of [17–19]. Thus, our method could be more suitable for a complex mobile Internet environment. Moreover, the complex compression transmission methods of [17–19] were built on customized software of plug-ins for the client, which is hard to apply to pure web pages and falls short of wide compatibility. By contrast, that is our method's advantage.

For the server load, because the *Master* volume in our method only responds to the final behavior request (instructions) instead of the continuous request of the studies of [9, 17–19], the test showed that server CPU utilization was less than 20% at idle (including the operation of *Slave* model), and less than 30% for responding to behavior request; thus, it was far below of those tests of methods of [17–19] with nearly a full load during all the operation time under the same conditions of SMI data, quality of final required image, server configuration, and volume rendering algorithm. Theoretically, our platform can respond to more independent tasks (pipelines) at the same time. Table 2 shows that while the server was running four independent tasks simultaneously, the response time of our method remained at approximately 1 s in the 100-KBps client bandwidth, much better than [17–19], which was with more than 16 seconds' delay of end frame in the single task status. In fact because user viewing and processing of the 3D medical volume occurred via interaction on the *Slave* model, the delay experience was much fewer than that in [17–19], as detailed in Section 4.1. That indicates our method could have some more advantages, including much less network load and server load, to serve much more independent tasks and users.

In addition, [17–19] did not propose an effective interactive method to clip the 3D volume, what our method has accomplished.

6. Conclusion

This paper proposed a *Master-Slave* dual-channel interaction mode, which absorbed the advantages of the surface rendering of WebGL and remote volume rendering, to build a visualization interaction platform to rapidly view and process 3D medical volume reconstruction in a pure webpage environment. This platform could be used in a diversified network environment (100-KBps bandwidth for extreme) and diversified client devices (no special hardware and operating system constraints), without any special installation but with a good user experience similar to native application. These features could serve authorized users to conveniently access SMIs and present 3D visualization anywhere and could be a technological basis of online communication among doctors and patients [34]. Or, at least, it could help clinicians to arbitrarily acquire 3D image according to their clinical needs instead of the static pictures that radiologists drafted. For example, clinicians could conveniently observe the complicated relationship of skull base bone and blood vessel via this platform (Figure 6(d)); in the past, this piece of information was provided by a few static images generated from radiologist's understanding.

Additionally, this solution is designed to be followed as an HTML5 standard interface, indicating any authorized user could rapidly access the application via one URL hyperlink, and the platform could be easily integrated into other telemedical systems seamlessly as a third-party application, for example the Supplementary Materials (2. Demonstration of the operation procedure on laptop linked by email.mp4, and 3. Demonstration of the operation procedure on iPad via website.mp4). These features may play an assistant role to improve work patterns and extend the range of application of traditional medical image systems. For example, it can be applied to regional health, telemedicine, and medical imaging education at a low cost because there is no special cost of deploy and upgrade of software, network, and hardware on the client side. And more importantly, a teacher can vividly show the students the image characteristics of the disease anywhere; a clinician can intuitively introduce disease to the patients anywhere and ask experts' help anywhere. That may promote the development of mobile medical technology to a certain degree.

Acknowledgments

This work was supported by the National Natural Science Foundation of China (no. 81171866), the National Key Basic Research Program of China (no. 2014CB541602), and the Social Livelihood Science and Technology Innovation Special Project of CSTC (no. cstc2015shmszx120002).

References

[1] Q. Zhang, M. Alexander, and L. Ryner, "Synchronized 2D/3D optical mapping for interactive exploration and real-time visualization of multi-function neurological images," *Computerized Medical Imaging and Graphics*, vol. 37, no. 7-8, pp. 552–567, 2013.

[2] S. Zimeras and L. G. Gortzis, "Interactive tele-radiological segmentation systems for treatment and diagnosis," *International Journal of Telemedicine and Applications*, vol. 2012, Article ID 713739, p. 15, 2012.

[3] S. E. Mahmoudi, A. Akhondi-Asl, R. Rahmani et al., "Web-based interactive 2D/3D medical image processing and visualization software," *Computer Methods and Programs in Biomedicine*, vol. 98, no. 2, pp. 172–182, 2010.

[4] L. Faggioni, E. Neri, I. Bargellini et al., "IPad-based primary 2D reading of CT angiography examinations of patients with suspected acute gastrointestinal bleeding: preliminary experience 1L," *British Journal of Radiology*, vol. 88, no. 1047, Article ID 20140477, 2015.

[5] J. B. Park, H. J. Choi, J. H. Lee, and B. S. Kang, "An assessment of the iPad 2 as a CT teleradiology tool using brain CT with subtle intracranial hemorrhage under conventional illumination," *Journal of Digital Imaging*, vol. 26, no. 4, pp. 683–690, 2013.

[6] P. T. Johnson, S. L. Zimmerman, D. Heath et al., "The iPad as a mobile device for CT display and interpretation: diagnostic accuracy for identification of pulmonary embolism," *Emergency Radiology*, vol. 19, no. 4, pp. 323–327, 2012.

[7] J. M. Noguera and J. R. Jiménez, "Visualization of very large 3D volumes on mobile devices and WebGL," in *Proceedings of the 20th International Conference in Central Europe on Computer Graphics, Visualization and Computer Vision, WSCG 2012*, pp. 105–112, June 2012.

[8] J. Congote, A. Segura, L. Kabongo et al., "Interactive visualization of volumetric data with WebGL in real-time," in *Proceedings of the 16th International Conference on 3D Web Technology, (Web3D '11)*, pp. 137–145, June 2011.

[9] A. Schiewe, M. Anstoots, and J. Krüger, "State of the art in mobile volume rendering on iOS devices," in *Proceedings of the Eurographics Conference on Visualization (EuroVis '15)*, 2015.

[10] A. Evans, M. Romeo, A. Bahrehmand et al., "3D graphics on the web: a survey," *Computers & Graphics*, vol. 41, no. 1, pp. 43–61, 2014.

[11] M. Callieri, R. M. Andrei, M. D. Benedetto et al., "Visualization methods for molecular studies on the web platform," in *Proceedings of the 15th international conference on web 3D technology (Web3D '10)*, pp. 117–126, July 2010.

[12] J. Jiménez, A. M. López, J. Cruz et al., "A Web platform for the interactive visualization and analysis of the 3D fractal dimension of MRI data," *Journal of Biomedical Informatics*, vol. 51, pp. 176–190, 2014.

[13] WebGL, https://www.khronos.org/webgl/.

[14] C. R. Butson, G. Tamm, S. Jain, T. Fogal, and J. Krüger, "Evaluation of interactive visualization on mobile computing platforms for selection of deep brain stimulation parameters," *IEEE Transactions on Visualization and Computer Graphics*, vol. 19, no. 1, pp. 108–117, 2013.

[15] M. Levoy, "Display of surfaces from volume data," *IEEE Computer Graphics and Applications*, vol. 8, no. 3, pp. 29–37, 1988.

[16] E. Kotter, T. Baumann, D. Jäger, and M. Langer, "Technologies for image distribution in hospitals," *European Radiology*, vol. 16, no. 6, pp. 1270–1279, 2006.

[17] S. Park, W. Kim, and I. Ihm, "Mobile collaborative medical display system," *Computer Methods and Programs in Biomedicine*, vol. 89, no. 3, pp. 248–260, 2008.

[18] J. R. Mitchell, P. Sharma, J. Modi et al., "A smartphone client-server teleradiology system for primary diagnosis of acute stroke," *Journal of Medical Internet Research*, vol. 13, no. 2, p. e31, 2011.

[19] T. Hachaj, "Real time exploration and management of large medical volumetric datasets on small mobile devices—evaluation of remote volume rendering approach," *International Journal of Information Management*, vol. 34, no. 3, pp. 336–343, 2014.

[20] P. Quax, J. Liesenborgs, A. Barzan et al., "Remote rendering solutions using web technologies," *Multimedia Tools and Applications*, vol. 75, no. 8, pp. 4383–4410, 2016.

[21] D. Preuveneers, Y. Berbers, and W. Joosen, "The future of mobile E-health application development: exploring HTML5 for context-aware diabetes monitoring," *Procedia Computer Science*, vol. 21, pp. 351–359, 2013.

[22] J. M. Noguera, J. J. Jiménez, and M. C. Osuna-Pérez, "Development and evaluation of a 3D mobile application for learning manual therapy in the physiotherapy laboratory," *Computers and Education*, vol. 69, pp. 96–108, 2013.

[23] Y. S. Kang, "Volume rendering overview," in *GPU Programming and Cg Language Primer*, chapter 14, pp. 154-155, 1st edition, 2009.

[24] Visualization Toolkit (VTK), http://www.vtk.org/.

[25] vtkPiecewiseFunction Class Reference of VTK, http://www.vtk.org/doc/nightly/html/classvtkPiecewiseFunction.html.

[26] vtkColorTransferFunction Class Reference of VTK, http://www.vtk.org/doc/nightly/html/annotated.html.

[27] vtkPlane Class Reference of VTK, http://www.vtk.org/doc/nightly/html/classvtkPlane.html.

[28] L. Ma, D.-X. Zhao, and Z.-Z. Yang, "A software tool for visualization of molecular face (VMF) by improving marching cubes algorithm," *Computational and Theoretical Chemistry*, vol. 1028, pp. 34–45, 2014.

[29] G. F. Wang, J. Liu, and W. Liu, "DIB display and window transformation technology for DICOM medical images," *Chinese Journal of Medical Device*, vol. 18, no. 8, pp. 1–5, 2005.

[30] L. Qiao, X. Chen, L. X. Yang et al., "Development of medical image three-dimensional-visualization platform based on home network and pure web conditions," *Beijing Biomedical Engineering*, vol. 34, no. 3, pp. 229-233,286, 2015.

[31] M. Ying and J. Miller, "Refactoring legacy AJAX applications to improve the efficiency of the data exchange component," *Journal of Systems and Software*, vol. 86, no. 1, pp. 72–88, 2013.

[32] HTML5, http://www.w3.org/TR/2012/CR-html5-20121217/.

[33] QIHU 360 SOFTWARE CO. LIMITED, 360 Internet Security, http://www.360safe.com/Internet-security.html.

[34] L. Qiao, Y. Li, X. Chen et al., "Medical high-resolution image sharing and electronic whiteboard system: a pure-web-based system for accessing and discussing lossless original images in telemedicine," *Computer Methods and Programs in Biomedicine*, vol. 121, no. 2, pp. 77–91, 2015.

20

An Iterative, Mixed Usability Approach Applied to the Telekit System from the Danish TeleCare North Trial

Pernille Heyckendorff Lilholt, Clara Schaarup, and Ole Kristian Hejlesen

Department of Health Science and Technology, Aalborg University, Aalborg, Denmark

Correspondence should be addressed to Pernille Heyckendorff Lilholt; phl@hst.aau.dk

Academic Editor: Sotiris A. Pavlopoulos

Objective. The aim of the present study is to evaluate the usability of the telehealth system, coined Telekit, by using an iterative, mixed usability approach. *Materials and Methods.* Ten double experts participated in two heuristic evaluations (HE1, HE2), and 11 COPD patients attended two think-aloud tests. The double experts identified usability violations and classified them into Jakob Nielsen's heuristics. These violations were then translated into measurable values on a scale of 0 to 4 indicating degree of severity. In the think-aloud tests, COPD participants were invited to verbalise their thoughts. *Results.* The double experts identified 86 usability violations in HE1 and 101 usability violations in HE2. The majority of the violations were rated in the 0–2 range. The findings from the think-aloud tests resulted in 12 themes and associated examples regarding the usability of the Telekit system. The use of the iterative, mixed usability approach produced both quantitative and qualitative results. *Conclusion.* The iterative, mixed usability approach yields a strong result owing to the high number of problems identified in the tests because the double experts and the COPD participants focus on different aspects of Telekit's usability. This trial is registered with Clinicaltrials.gov, NCT01984840, November 14, 2013.

1. Introduction

Information technology has developed exponentially in recent years, influencing substantially the field of telehealth. Thus, the outcomes of trials of telehealth systems have demonstrated that telehealth can provide economic gains, superior continuity of care, and more self-sufficient patients [1–3]. The Danish cluster-randomised, controlled, large-scale trial, TeleCare North, is an example hereof. Tele-Care North was implemented in 2014-2015, recruiting a total of 1,225 patients from the North Denmark Region. The purpose of this trial was to assess the effectiveness and cost-effectiveness of a telehealth system (named Telekit) designed for patients with chronic obstructive pulmonary disease (COPD) compared with usual practice. In Denmark, *usual practice* includes care, monitoring, and treatment of patients, and these tasks are performed by general practitioners and municipality healthcare workers such as community nurses. The purpose of the Telekit system is to allow COPD patients to gain more insight into their own disease and to

support their skills and resources in relation to the management of their disease, thereby giving them greater control over their lives and hopefully enhancing their quality of life. The outcomes of the TeleCare North trial include changes in quality of life, mortality, physiological indicators, and the incremental cost-effectiveness ratio measured from baseline to follow-up at 12 months [4].

Self-management initiatives such as the TeleCare North trial are increasingly being integrated into healthcare as self-management initiatives are implemented to reduce admission rates, improve quality of life, and prevent worsening of the patient's condition. Despite the growing popularity of self-management initiatives, people encountering problems using systems commonly stop using the technologies or withdraw early from studies [5]. Identifying patient factors explaining this behaviour, extant literature suggests that many existing systems are directed towards clinical users and focus less on pertinent patient factors like technology needs, capabilities, and psychological and environmental barriers, and so forth. Even when patient factors are taken into account, they are often prioritized only when the user interface is prepared and less when the system is being conceived and designed [6].

Developing and implementing a system do not require attention only to the technical requirements. The processes also depend on user involvement and participation in the form of, for example, user satisfaction, usability, and a recognized need for the technology in daily life. The users' interaction with the telehealth technologies is therefore particularly important because their level of interaction shows whether they want to make use of the telehealth technologies or prefer opting out. Many patients using telehealth are elderly patients who suffer from chronic disease, have limited skills, and are socioeconomically disadvantaged. These limitations need to be considered throughout the design process of telehealth technologies [7, 8]. Patient safety is another important aspect because telehealth technologies involve transmitting information and communicating with patients. The healthcare professionals need to be sure that data are transmitted securely and that only relevant healthcare professionals have access to the transmitted data. To provide patient outcomes and clinical outcomes that are satisfactory, telehealth technologies need to show good usability [9].

Usability is defined as follows by the International Organisation for Standardisation (ISO 9241-11):

> The extent to which a product can be used by specified users to achieve specified goals with effectiveness, efficiency and satisfaction in a specified context of use [10].

Several different usability testing methods are available for collecting user perspectives with a view to improving the usability of telehealth technologies [11]. Usability testing measures the ease of use of a technology quantitatively or qualitatively. The literature on the topic indicates that several different methods should be used when testing usability as each method has strengths and limitations and provides different perspectives on usability [12–16]. The literature on this topic highlights the importance of using mixed usability methods iteratively. Iteration refers to the process by which development activities are repeated or looped during system development and how each loop is revised. Iteration, therefore, means going through multiple design versions of a system by conducting usability evaluations and revising the system based on the usability findings made [14, 15]. Usability expert Jakob Nielsen argues in favour of iterative usability testing; specifically, he recommends two iterations (one iteration is a redesign of two design versions) or more, because the first redesign will have many remaining problems [17].

Using an iterative, mixed usability approach, the purpose of this article was to evaluate the usability of the Telekit system from the Danish TeleCare North trial with a view to improving its quality and functionality. The usability methods were two heuristic evaluations (HE1, HE2) and two think-aloud tests (TA1, TA2). The usability evaluations were divided into a pretest and a posttest: (1) the pretest included usability evaluations (HE1, TA1) and was performed on two consecutive versions of the Telekit system in two previous studies [18, 19]. HE1 was performed early in Telekit's design process to assess potential usability problems that could complicate the implementation of the system. The problems found in HE1 have triggered several substantial changes and a number of updated versions of the Telekit system [17, 18]. After the heuristic evaluation (HE1), a think-aloud test (TA1) was performed to determine the users' experiences with the revised version of the Telekit system [20]. (2) The posttest included usability evaluations (HE2, TA2) performed after completion of the TeleCare North trial. Specifically, a second heuristic evaluation (HE2) and a second think-aloud test (TA2) were performed on the latest, updated version of the Telekit system.

Various evaluation methods and strategies have already been developed, and several studies have used different iterative usability testing methods in combination [20, 21]. The goal of this study was to evaluate the usability of the Telekit system through iterative, mixed usability testing. Quantitative results and qualitative findings were generated and these were compared in order to assess the usability of the Telekit system.

2. Materials and Methods

2.1. Study Population. The study population consisted of two different groups of participants. One group ($n = 10$) attended the heuristic evaluations (HE1, HE2) and another ($n = 11$) attended the think-aloud tests (TA1, TA2). All participants received verbal or written information about the study procedure and consented to participate in the study.

2.1.1. Study Population—Heuristic Evaluations (HE1, HE2). Five usability experts were invited to participate in each heuristic evaluation. Some experts (experts number (1) and number (3)) took part in both evaluations. All experts were biomedical engineers and were serving as Ph.D. fellows or associate/assistant professors with the Department of Health Science and Technology, Aalborg University, Denmark. They all had specific expertise in the health domain and in usability and the user interface being evaluated, which made it reasonable to denote them as double experts.

2.1.2. Study Population—Think-Aloud Test (TA1). Six participants (three men, three women) with COPD attended TA1 [20]. They were randomly selected among 17 pilot patients from the Danish TeleCare North trial [4]. Their average age was 69 years (min 65, max 73), and they represented different stages of COPD (one mild, one moderate, and four severe). The participants in the severe stage needed oxygen therapy. Their technology experiences varied; some were novices, some were knowledgeable, and some were daily users. The participants had 6 months of experience with the Telekit system before taking the TA1.

2.1.3. Study Population—Think-Aloud Test (TA2). Five participants (one man, four women) with COPD were recruited from the Danish TeleCare North trial [4]. We contacted the district nurses from the trial who then randomly selected potential users. Their average age was 65 years (min 50, max 72); and the participants had previously worked as childminder ($n = 1$), grocer ($n = 2$), housewife ($n = 1$), and a sandwich preparer ($n = 1$). Two participants had moderate COPD (lung capacity in the 50–80% range) and three had severe COPD (lung capacity 30–55%). Those in the severe stage of the disease were wheelchair users and required oxygen therapy.

Inclusion criteria were outlined before recruitment to the think-aloud test was initiated:

(i) Participants should have recently received the Telekit system (<3 months) because they had to maintain their curiosity and should not have developed habits in the use of the Telekit system.

(ii) Participants should have received the first of two training sessions before initiating the think-aloud test. This was important because they needed basic knowledge about the use of the Telekit system; otherwise, they would not be able to use the system during the test.

(iii) Participants should be fairly well functioning in order to be able to complete the think-aloud test. Thus, only patients who were able to express their experiences with the Telekit system could be included.

2.2. The Telekit System. The Telekit system was developed by Silverbullet A/S [22, 23] and was designed to support patients diagnosed with COPD, diabetes, and heart failure in the management of their disease, and also to reduce the healthcare costs associated with these diseases. Telekit operates on an open source platform, OpenTele, which is also used in two other Danish regions, besides the North Denmark Region. The OpenTele platform is a license-free platform that collects the patient's health data and health professionals' interaction with data and transports data to central databases [22].

The COPD patients receive instructions for the use of Telekit by community nurses either at home or at a healthcare center. Instructions are given as two training sessions. The Telekit system consists of a small portable carrying case containing a tablet (Samsung Galaxy TAB 2, 10.1, Samsung Electronics, Seoul, South Korea) [24]; a blood pressure monitor (Model UA-767, plus BT-C, Nonin Medical, Minnesota, USA) [25]; a fingertip pulse oximeter (Nonin, Onyx II 9560, A&D Medical, Tokyo, Japan) [26]; and the Precision Health Scale (UC-321 PBT-C, A&D Medical, Tokyo, Japan) [25]. The Telekit is an asynchronous solution that collects health data from patients at home via an application. The patients use an integrated application, which is available from the tablet. After login to the application, the patients are able to answer disease-related questions, such as: *Do you cough more than usual?* In addition to answering questions, the patients measure their blood pressure, oxygen saturation, heart rate, and weight 1-2 times a week as agreed with their doctor. The blood pressure monitor, fingertip pulse oximeter, and the health scale automatically transfer the measurements via Bluetooth to the application on the tablet. Thereafter, the data are sent to a web portal used by healthcare providers for their interaction with the patients. Using the web portal, healthcare providers receive and analyse the patients' health data on fixed days. The healthcare providers check if the patients' measurements are higher than expected and they also view

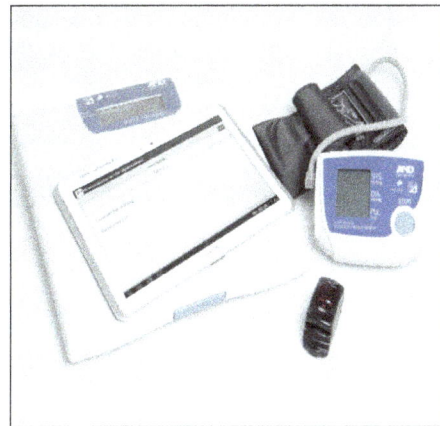

FIGURE 1: The Telekit system from the Danish TeleCare North trial. The COPD patients use Telekit to measure their vital signs.

the patients' answers to disease-related questions. In the light of this information, the healthcare providers can respond quickly and get the patients started on proper treatments [4]. Figure 1 shows the equipment that makes up the Telekit system.

2.3. Study Design and Data Collection. In this study, we evaluated the usability of the Telekit system from the Danish TeleCare North trial using an iterative, mixed usability approach. A pretest was conducted during the initial phase of the TeleCare North trial, and a posttest was performed after trial completion. In the pretest, a heuristic evaluation (HE1) and a think-aloud test (TA1) were performed on two consecutive versions (version: 1.5.0, version: 1.11.3) of the Telekit system [20, 21]. In the posttest, the same usability evaluations methods were used to test the latest version (version 1.29.0) of the Telekit system, yielding a second heuristic evaluation (HE2) and a second think-aloud test (TA2). The quantitative results and qualitative findings related to the pre- and posttest were then compared to each other.

2.3.1. Heuristic Evaluation. Heuristic evaluation is an inspection method in which a small set of experts inspect and evaluate a user interface of a system using a list of accepted usability principles (called heuristics). Each expert independently discovers system usability problems by identifying unmet heuristics, that is, heuristic violations, and assesses the severity of each violation. The evaluation produces a list of potential usability problems that may then serve as input for improving the system in a next round of iterations [14, 27].

In this study, the heuristic evaluations (HE1 and HE2) from the pre- and posttest were applied in laboratory settings in which two researchers participated (a moderator and an observer). The moderator's role was to interact with the experts and guide them with respect to operation of the Telekit system if problems occurred or if certain parts of the user interface needed to be explained. The observer's role was to note the experts' comments and to complete a checklist of the heuristic violations in collaboration with the experts.

In each heuristic evaluation, the five experts were asked to perform different representative tasks using the Telekit system. The tasks for both heuristic evaluations included (1) *login*; (2) *read and watch films about the Telekit system*; (3) *read and watch instructions about the Telekit system*; (4) *perform measurements* (blood pressure, heart rate, oxygen saturation, weight, etc.); (5) *find images presenting their measurements*; (6) *write a message to healthcare providers*, and (7) *logout*. Besides these tasks, they were also encouraged to inspect other aspects of the system.

Each expert identified problems in the Telekit system, classified these in accordance with Jakob Nielsen's ten heuristics (Table 1), and scored the severity of each problem (Table 2) [28]. The experts completed a checklist consisting of usability violations and violation severity scores and provided potential solutions. The severity rating scores were based on Rolf Molich's 5-point severity rating scale: 0: *improvements*; 1: *minor problem*; 2: *severe problem*; 3: *critical problem*; and 4: *malfunction* [29]. The total duration of each heuristic evaluation was 90 minutes including introduction, tasks, and debriefing.

2.3.2. Think-Aloud Tests. The goal of performing a think-aloud test is to record potential users' experiences and thoughts about a system. This can be done by giving the users tasks that they have to complete by using the system. The test encourages users to verbalise their thoughts and to express what they are thinking, doing, and feeling when they go through the user interface. The test makes it possible for the observer and moderator to see and understand the cognitive processes that users engage in during task completion [30].

To achieve as real a test setting as possible, the moderator and the observer chose to perform think-aloud tests (TA1, TA2) in the participants' homes. Furthermore, the patient's home provided a safe place and familiar surroundings for the test. The participants were asked to perform the same seven tasks as the experts performed in the heuristic evaluations. It was explained to the participants that the goal of the evaluations was to evaluate the system and not to test their ability to perform tasks. By providing this information, the moderator and the observer hoped that the participants would feel free to comment and criticise the Telekit system. The researchers were present during all the tests. The moderator's role was to interact with the participants, guide them through the tasks, and encourage them to think aloud during the tests. The moderator did not intervene or disrupt the thinking process; only if the participants actively asked for help were they guided to move forward with the system. The observer's role was to record the tests, collect field notes about verbalised and nonverbalised expressions, and furthermore take notes of observations made. In addition, the observer framed a summary of the participants' demographic characteristics (described in Sections 2.1.2 and 2.1.3). The duration of each think-aloud test was approximately 45 minutes including introduction, tasks, and debriefing.

2.4. Data Analysis. The data analysis was divided into three parts in order to compare the pre-and posttest of the Telekit system: (1) a pre- and posttest comparison of HE1 versus HE2,

(2) a pre- and posttest comparison of TA1 versus TA2, and (3) a posttest comparison of HE2 versus TA2.

The observer's notes from each heuristic evaluation and think-aloud test were computed and transferred to Microsoft Excel 2010. Data from the heuristic evaluation were departed into heuristics, problems, locations, solutions, and severity ratings. To uncover usability issues during the think-aloud tests, the participant comments and moderator observations were counted and categorised into overall usability themes regarding the contents of the identified usability findings. These themes were developed on the basis of discussions and reflections among the observer, the moderator, and the participants. In order to compare data from the mixed usability evaluation methods (HE2 and TA2), usability topics were created from the tasks that the participants and the experts were asked to perform in both usability evaluation methods. The moderator and the observer grouped together the number of identified usability problems during HE2 with the number of usability comments and the number of usability observations encountered in TA2 thereby forming these usability topics.

Spreadsheets were made for both of the heuristic evaluations, regarding distribution of usability problems by heuristic, distribution of the number of usability violations classified into heuristics per expert, and distribution of usability violations into severity degrees among experts. Spreadsheets were also made for both think-aloud tests and used to record the number and contents of usability findings identified by the participants and identified from observer notes. The spreadsheets made it possible to categorise the usability findings into themes and topics and to compare the pretest and the posttest.

3. Results

In this section, the results from pre-and posttest of the Telekit system will be presented in three parts: (1) HE1 versus HE2, (2) TA1 versus TA2, and (3) HE2 versus TA2.

3.1. Comparison of the Two Heuristic Evaluations (HE1 versus HE2). In total, the experts identified 152 problems of which 86 (57%) were unique to HE1. In HE2, the experts identified 223 problems of which 101 (45%) were unique. The number of unique usability problems was slightly higher in HE2 than in HE1.

Figure 2 presents the distribution of unique usability problems identified for each heuristic in HE1 and HE2, respectively. With the exception of heuristic number (9) (*help users recognize, diagnose, and recover from errors*), all heuristics were used in HE2. The heuristic which had the lowest number of usability problems in HE1 was number (10) (*help and documentation*) with only two (2%) usability problems.

Heuristic number (2) (*match between system and the real world*) with 27 (31%) problems and heuristic number (8) (*aesthetic and minimalist design*) with 11 (13%) problems were associated with the highest number of usability problems in HE1. In comparison with HE2, heuristic number (1) (*visibility of system status*) with 23 (23%) problems and heuristic number (4) (*consistency and standards*) with 22

TABLE 1: Jakob Nielsen's ten heuristics, including a description of each heuristics.

Jakob Nielsen's ten heuristics	Description of heuristics
(1) Visibility of system status	The system should always keep users informed about what is going on, through appropriate feedback within reasonable time.
(2) Match between system and the real world	The system should speak the users' language, with words, phrases, and concepts familiar to the user, rather than system-oriented terms. Follow real-world conventions, making information appear in a natural and logical order.
(3) User control and freedom	Users often choose system functions by mistake and will need a clearly marked "emergency exit" to leave the unwanted state without having to go through an extended dialogue. Support undo and redo.
(4) Consistency and standards	Users should not have to wonder whether different words, situations, or actions mean the same thing. Follow platform conventions.
(5) Error prevention	Even better than good error messages is a careful design which prevents a problem from occurring in the first place. Either eliminate error-prone conditions or check for them and present users with a confirmation option before they commit to the action.
(6) Recognition rather than recall	Minimize the user's memory load by making objects, actions, and options visible. The user should not have to remember information from one part of the dialogue to another. Instructions for use of the system should be visible or easily retrievable whenever appropriate.
(7) Flexibility and efficiency of use	Accelerators—unseen by the novice user—may often speed up the interaction for the expert user such that the system can cater to both inexperienced and experienced users. Allow users to tailor frequent actions.
(8) Aesthetic and minimalistic design	Dialogues should not contain information which is irrelevant or rarely needed. Every extra unit of information in a dialogue competes with the relevant units of information and diminishes their relative visibility.
(9) Help users recognize, diagnose, and recover from errors	Error messages should be expressed in plain language (no codes), precisely indicate the problem, and constructively suggest a solution.
(10) Help and documentation	Even though it is better if the system can be used without documentation, it may be necessary to provide help and documentation. Any such information should be easy to search, be focused on the user's task, list concrete steps to be carried out, and not be too large.

TABLE 2: Rolf Molich's severity rating scale.

Five-point severity rating scale	Description of severity ratings
(0) Improvement	Which does not substantially disturb the user's experience
(1) Minor problem	The user will be somewhat delayed (few minutes)
(2) Severe problem	The user will be much delayed (several minutes)
(3) Critical problem	The user cannot carry out the task
(4) Malfunction problem	The system does not work properly

Table 3 presents the number of usability violations classified into heuristics per expert for the two heuristic evaluations (HE1, HE2). Heuristic number (2) (*match between system and the real world*), heuristic number (4) (*consistency and standards*), and heuristic number (8) (*aesthetic and minimalist design*) were the most referred heuristics during both evaluations. The number of usability violations related to heuristic number (2) (*match between system and the real world*) decreased from 49 in HE1 to 29 in HE2. In contrast, heuristic number (4) (*consistency and standards*) and heuristic number (8) (*aesthetic and minimalist design*) increased from 20 usability violations to 43 and from 20 to 30 in HE2, respectively.

By comparing heuristic number (1) (*visibility of system status*) in HE1 and HE2, an increase from five usability violations in HE1 to 26 usability violations was identified. Heuristic number (7) (*flexibility and efficiency of use*) was associated with eight usability violations in HE1 and 22

(22%) problems were associated with the highest number of usability problems.

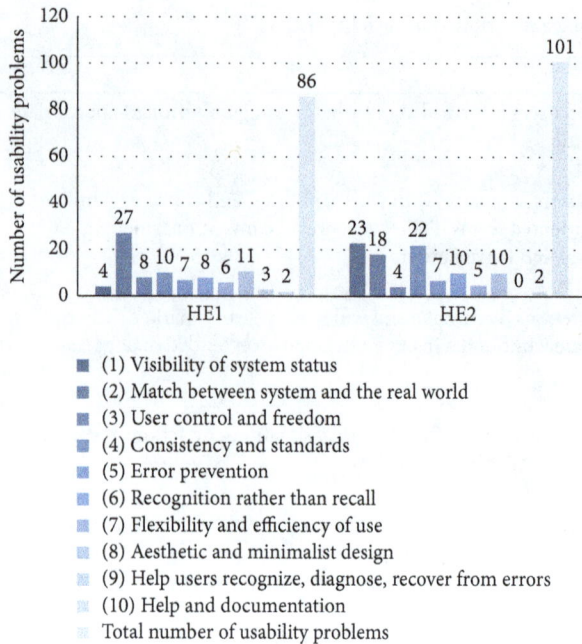

FIGURE 2: Distribution of usability problems by heuristic for both heuristic evaluations (HE1 and HE2).

■ (1) Visibility of system status
■ (2) Match between system and the real world
■ (3) User control and freedom
■ (4) Consistency and standards
■ (5) Error prevention
■ (6) Recognition rather than recall
■ (7) Flexibility and efficiency of use
▨ (8) Aesthetic and minimalist design
▨ (9) Help users recognize, diagnose, recover from errors
▨ (10) Help and documentation
□ Total number of usability problems

usability violations in HE2. Furthermore, in HE2, the number of usability violations relating to heuristic number (10) (*help and documentation*) was three times higher than in HE1.

Table 4 shows the distribution of severity degrees among experts for HE1 and HE2. The severity scores 0, 1, and 2 were the most frequently used in both heuristic evaluations. The severity scores 3 and 4 were used considerably more frequently in HE2 than in HE1, increasing from 4 to 23 the severity score *critical problem* and increasing from 4 to 25 the severity score *malfunction*.

3.2. Comparison of the Two Think-Aloud Tests (TA1 versus TA2).

Table 5 is divided into five columns representing the presence of themes (yes/no) in TA1/TA2 and a description of examples of usability findings commented on by the participants during TA1/TA2. The think-aloud tests produced 12 themes: (1) *habits*; (2) *lack of curiosity*; (3) *information level*; (4) *the Telekit system—know how*; (5) *comfortable with the Telekit system*; (6) *usability problems*; (7) *learnability*; (8) *system feedback*; (9) *content of the Telekit system*; (10) *measurements*; (11) *the Telekit design*; and (12) *relevance of the Telekit system*. The columns "Yes" and "No" in the table show which themes were present in TA1 and TA2, respectively. For instance, the theme *information level* was represented in TA2 but not in TA1 and therefore only the TA2 column contains an example/description of the usability finding. Table 5 shows only a selection of the usability problems and therefore the themes can contain several more usability problems than already presented in the table.

Through the participants' verbal and nonverbal language, it became clear that the theme *habits* was relevant for their interaction with the Telekit system. The observer noticed, for example, that during certain tasks the participants avoided using unknown functionalities of the system, and the participants also expressed this stating, "*Why do I have to use that function if the system works fine without it?*" The theme, *lack of curiosity*, was related to the participants' lack of need to build new habits given their existing use of the system. One example of this was a participant who was not interested in using the message functionality because the participant was not used to writing emails. The third theme, *information level*, was relevant because the participants lacked overall knowledge about the Telekit system and their COPD disease. The fourth theme, *the Telekit system—know how*, was related to their experiences with the Telekit system. Some of the participants were surprised to discover certain functionalities, for example, the zoom function or the scroll function.

The fifth theme, *comfortable with the Telekit system*, became relevant because several of the participants expressed that their relatives or doctors had made it clear to them that they could not do anything wrong when interacting with the system and that they could always ask for help if problems occurred. The sixth theme, *usability problems*, was created because several usability problems were identified by the participants during TA1 and TA2. As mentioned in Materials and Methods, before the present study, the participants had received training sessions containing instructions to using the Telekit system. The seventh theme, *Learnability*, was relevant because the majority of the participants reported that they had learned more about how to use the system and had started using some of the functionalities in their daily lives, for example, the functionality allowing them to measure their blood pressure.

The eighth theme, *system feedback*, was based on the technical feedback that participants became acquainted with during the tests. The ninth theme, *contents of the Telekit system*, included formulations, questions, descriptions, and functionalities that were visible in the system. One of the major tasks that participants needed to perform in the Telekit system was to measure their vital signs with different devices. Their ability to do so resulted in the tenth theme, *Measurements*. The eleventh theme, *The Telekit design*, was created by inspiration from Nielsen's heuristic number (8) named *aesthetic and minimalist design*. The theme included design aspects and visual suggestions to improve the system. The last theme, *relevance of the Telekit system*, arose because participants inadvertently verbalised their reflections stating how the Telekit system had suddenly become a very important part of their daily life as it helped them manage their COPD.

3.3. Comparison of the Heuristic Evaluation and the Think-Aloud Test (HE2 versus TA2).

In this section, we compare the usability findings identified during the posttest of the Telekit system. We compared the number of usability problems identified in HE2 with the number of usability comments and observations identified by participants and researcher in TA2. Table 6 below presents the number of problems per expert (E1-E5) classified as follows: (1) *misc.*; (2) *read and watch films*; (3) *read and watch instructions*; (4) *log in*; (5) *perform measurements*; (6) *write a message*; (7) *view images*, and (8) *log out*. The topics were created on the

TABLE 3: Distribution of the number of usability violations classified into heuristics per expert.

Heuristics	Expert 1		Expert 2		Expert 3		Expert 4		Expert 5		Total	
	HE1	HE2	HE1	HE2	HE1	HE2	HE1	HE2	HE1	HE2	HE1	HE2
(1) Visibility of system status	0	8	0	7	1	4	3	3	1	4	5	26
(2) Match between system and the real world	5	4	8	7	7	4	14	11	15	3	49	29
(3) User control and freedom	1	0	0	3	1	4	3	5	6	2	11	14
(4) Consistency and standards	7	11	3	5	2	18	6	2	2	7	20	43
(5) Error prevention	2	6	3	0	5	8	6	4	2	4	18	22
(6) Recognition rather than recall	2	7	3	9	1	10	2	0	5	1	13	27
(7) Flexibility and efficiency of use	3	5	2	3	0	6	1	4	2	4	8	22
(8) Aesthetic and minimalist design	5	3	3	4	5	19	4	0	3	4	20	30
(9) Help users recognize, diagnose, and recover from errors	2	0	1	0	0	0	0	0	2	0	5	0
(10) Help and documentation	1	1	0	0	0	5	1	3	1	1	3	10

TABLE 4: Distribution of usability violations on Rolf Molich's severity rating scale [29].

Severity degree	Expert 1		Expert 2		Expert 3		Expert 4		Expert 5		Total	
	HE1	HE2	HE1	HE2	HE1	HE2	HE1	HE2	HE1	HE2	HE1	HE2
(1) Improvement	12	16	11	5	10	17	14	2	14	3	61	43
(2) Minor problem	8	19	12	21	12	30	19	11	15	13	66	94
(3) Severe problem	3	6	0	9	0	7	7	8	7	8	17	38
(4) Critical problem	2	3	0	3	0	10	0	5	2	2	4	23
(5) Malfunction	3	1	0	0	0	14	0	6	1	4	4	25

TABLE 5: Usability findings from the think-aloud tests were classified into 12 themes. The table illustrates the themes and the presence of themes (yes/no) and provides examples of the usability findings from TA1 and TA2.

Themes	TA1	TA2	Examples from TA1	Examples from TA2
Habits	Yes	Yes	The users received the Telekit system half a year before and were offered education	The users read the questionnaire very superficially—they know what is going to happen in the subsequent step
Lack of curiosity	Yes	Yes	The users did not attempt to remember password and username	The users are not interested in using the message function for writing or sending messages; the users' curiosity is not aroused
Information level	No	Yes		Users did not use the message menu because they do not know its function
The Telekitsystem—know how	No	Yes		The users know the different icons
Comfortable with the Telekit system	Yes	Yes	The users were satisfied with the functionalities of the Telekit system. The users had no problems with navigation in the Telekit system	The users are not afraid of pressing the wrong key because they know that they always have a way out; the users are comfortable using Telekit
Usability problems	Yes	Yes	The users had difficulties obtaining a reaction from the touchscreen because of cold finger or long nails. The users had difficulties remembering username and password which prevented them from logging in	The users did not know how to pause the film. It was not easy to find the log-out button
Learnability	No	Yes		The users had no problems with the scroll function
System feedback	Yes	Yes	When the users pressed multiple times on the touchscreen, the Telekit system did not react to commands	The Telekit system's speed was too slow, could be faster
Content of the Telekit system	Yes	Yes	For the experienced users, a more flexible system with les text material would work better	It was nice to be asked about COPD symptoms. There was doubt about the meaning of the icons
Measurements	Yes	Yes	When users pressed the touchscreen multiple times, this resulted in incorrect answers and measurements. Users made mistakes in the sequences of actions so that the measurements were taken too early or too late because of the location and naming of keys	The users place the blood pressure cuff incorrectly. The users start the weight with their feet easily
The Telekit design	Yes	Yes	Some users had difficulties identifying keys on the Telekit keyboard. The users had no problems with the scroll function	There was lack of validation when the users change password. The typography was appropriate
Relevance of the Telekit system	No	Yes		The users had brought the Telekit system to their doctor

TABLE 6: The eight usability topics, participants' comments per usability, researcher observations, and expert-reported usability violations.

Usability topics within the Telekit system	Researcher observation in TA2						Participant comments in TA2						Expert-reported usability in HE2					
	P1	P2	P3	P4	P5	Total	P1	P2	P3	P4	P5	Total	E1	E2	E3	E4	E5	Total
Misc.	4	1	2	0	1	8	3	6	0	2	2	13	9	7	15	4	7	42
Read and watch films	4	0	0	0	0	4	3	2	0	2	2	9	5	4	11	4	5	29
Read and watch instructions	1	0	0	0	0	1	2	1	2	0	1	6	7	3	7	3	2	22
Log in	1	1	0	1	0	3	2	1	1	0	0	4	4	3	7	1	1	16
Perform measurement	6	3	1	0	2	12	5	5	7	6	2	25	15	16	26	15	5	77
Write a message	4	0	1	0	0	5	1	4	4	3	2	14	4	2	7	3	4	20
View images	3	0	1	1	1	6	2	0	0	0	1	3	1	3	5	2	6	17
Log out	1	0	0	0	0	1	0	0	1	1	0	2	0	0	0	0	0	0
Total	24	5	5	2	4	40	18	19	15	14	10	76	45	38	78	32	30	223

basis of the tasks the experts and participants were asked to perform during the mixed usability evaluation. Table 6 also illustrates the participants' (P1–P5) number of usability comments by topic and the researcher observations made during TA2. In HE2, the experts identified more usability violations than anywhere else (n = 77) in topic 5, *perform measurements*, and the second-largest number of violations was observed for topic 1, *misc.* (n = 42). In TA2, the participants and the researcher also had more comments for topic 5, *Perform measurements*, than for any other topic as a total of 25 comments and 12 observations were recorded.

In general, the number of problems identified in HE2 was higher than the number of problems identified in TA2. Overall, there were more expert-identified problems (n = 223) than participant comments (n = 76) and researcher observations (n = 40). Contrary to HE2, in TA2, the participants and the researcher identified the highest number of problems regarding usability topic 8, *log out*. These issues were not reported in HE2 (Table 6).

4. Discussion

Recent years have seen a boom in the development of telehealth technologies in the hope that they would save costs for society and provide benefits for patient. Evaluating usability is an important step in the development of telehealth technologies and it is a prerequisite to successful implementation [31–33]. Multiple usability evaluation methods may be used in the testing and evaluation of usability ranging from inspection methods such as heuristic evaluations to user tests such as think-aloud tests.

In the literature, the importance of working iteratively when developing and evaluating systems is often emphasised [19]. Furthermore, experiences and documentation of performed tests describe that using different methods and techniques to assess the usability of a system illuminates different and very important perspectives from the perspectives of both the user and the expert. The various usability methods complement each other, but some methods are preferable to others, depending on how far the system is in the development process. Thus, it is recommendable to combine the methods and to use iterative design processes in which systems are tested repeatedly through circular processes [14].

Some studies have already combined different usability evaluation methods and worked in iterative loops in the design and evaluation of systems [34–36]. Nevertheless, it has not been possible to find studies or other telehealth technologies that use the exact same setup as the present study. However, we did find examples of similar research of other technological systems [37]. For instance, one study has compared two prototypes of a digital emergency medical services system through heuristic evaluations and subsequently examined the validity of the heuristic evaluations in an ethnographic study [38]. Using a mix of usability methods iteratively is important because it allows us to adjust the design of the system. However, when working with usability, it should be remembered that it will always be possible to further improve a system and a "perfect" system will therefore be difficult to attain.

The present study aimed to evaluate the usability of the Telekit system from the Danish TeleCare North trial and to improve its quality and functionalities. Telekit was evaluated by the use of an iterative, mixed usability approach. Specifically, the evaluation included a pre- and posttest of the Telekit system, which uncovered knowledge about the prevalence, severity, and contents of the usability problems. Data were compared descriptively as follows: (1) comparison of HE1 versus HE2; (2) comparison of TA1 versus TA2, and (3) comparison of HE2 versus TA2.

4.1. Comparison of HE1 versus HE2. After HE1, Silverbullet received a list of well-documented recommendations to improve Telekit's interface in order to make it more user-friendly. How Silverbullet managed the recommendations was out of the researchers' hands. It is unsure whether the company followed the list to the letter, which is reflected by the usability issues identified through the posttest, HE2 (n = 101), and the pretest (n = 86). The company's prioritization of usability issues led to the need of further rounds of heuristic evaluations due to the experts' identification of the similar issues supplemented with new issues.

Another explanation could be that the experts had become more aware of any issues in the evaluation process after performing an evaluation of Telekit in the pretest phase. A third explanation may be that three new experts were performing the HE2 assessment instead of the five experts from HE1. From a comparison validity point-of-view, it would have been preferable to use the same experts for the pretest and the posttest. However, the new experts were selected based on the same criteria as the pretest experts in order to achieve the best possible match. These criteria encompassed that the experts should be double experts and have the same education, the same knowledge about the health domain, and the same expertise in the field of usability. However, the use of experts with different levels of familiarity with the assessed system has both pros and cons. The experts who were familiar with the system beforehand may have been affected by their previous experiences with the system. For example, they may have discovered so many errors during the pretest that they had formed a negative, initial opinion which may be difficult to ignore during the second evaluation of the Telekit system. The behaviour of expert number (3) indicates an already negative attitude towards the system, contrary to the negative attitude the expert could have increased the skills in identifying usability issues. Similarly, it may be advantageous to use new experts because they would see and assess the Telekit system with fresh eyes.

4.2. Comparison of TA1 versus TA2. The think-aloud tests produced twelve themes and examples of usability findings within these themes. The themes were characterised by both positive and negative findings and results. The majority of the themes appeared in the posttest, which can be explained by the improvements made in the Telekit system in the time between TA1 and TA2. A conflicting explanation may be that changes of the Telekit system after TA1 reduced the usability of Telekit rather than improving it, thus causing more themes to be observed in the posttest.

The think-aloud test was suitable for gaining insight into the COPD participants' thoughts and revealed usability problems encountered during their interaction with the Telekit system. One of the strengths of the think-aloud test is that it allows the collection of data on the users' cognitive processes and how they interact with the system. The test identified both positive and negative aspects of the Telekit system as experienced by the participants. The researchers intended to include the same participants in both tests but finally decided against this because the participants needed to maintain their curiosity and could have generated habits concerning the use of the system during the first test. It was also considered to include time as a result of the think-aloud test. However, it proved too complex to use the time as a measurement element because some parts of the conversations were small talk used to establish an atmosphere in which the participants felt that they were allowed to freely express their opinion. Small talk also helped create a relationship of trust between the participants and the researchers. These talks were deemed necessary since our evaluation of the Telekit system depended on a good relationship.

4.3. Comparison of HE2 versus TA2. During the posttest, we chose to perform a comparison across the two different evaluation methods. The Telekit system has undergone many improvements [21], and therefore we compared the results from the second heuristic evaluation (HE2) with the results of the second think-aloud test (TA2). It was desirable to compare the results collected from HE1 and HE2 with the results from TA1 and TA2, but we decided not to do so for the reasons stated above. In addition, data from TA1 and TA2 were not sufficiently comparable to allow for a detailed analysis of these results in comparison with HE1 and HE2 and because the number of participants varied between the pre- and posttest (5 and 6, resp.).

When comparing the results from HE2 and TA2, we found that more usability problems were identified through heuristic evaluation than through think-aloud tests. This may reflect the different scope and potential of the two usability evaluation methods. In contrast to the many problems found using the heuristic evaluation, the positive aspects of the system were not identified by experts but by the COPD participants through the think-aloud test. The COPD participants agreed on some aspects of system usability, but it was clear that they had a different perspective on usability. The experts focused on the system's functionality and interface in general, such as system feedback, navigation, and error prevention. In contrast, the participants focused more on integrating the system into their daily routines, and the themes from the think-aloud test were therefore less technical and more focused on whether the system was meaningful and relevant to them as human beings.

4.4. Methodological Considerations. Our results were analysed descriptively, which is an advantage in this type of study because this approach provides an overview of the contents and the scope of the problems. Another reason for performing descriptive analyses was that a large body of material was available for using descriptive analyses, which

made it more visually comprehensible. A disadvantage of the descriptive analysis was that statements in relation to the classification of usability problems were not fully exploited by this descriptive type of analysis. However, it was possible to minimise this issue by including two different types of tests representing different perspectives and views on various usability aspects.

The ten heuristics developed by the usability expert Jacob Nielsen and the 5-level severity rating scale given by Rolf Molich were used in both heuristic evaluation sessions [29, 39]. The use of same tool in both sessions enhances the probability of increasing the reliability of the two performed sessions. Many heuristics could have been employed, but by evaluating the Telekit system with the same ten heuristics in the two heuristic evaluation sessions, HE1 and HE2, we gained the possibility of comparing the results of the pretest and the posttest.

The present study has a number of limitations. First, it would have been preferable to use the same experts for both heuristic evaluations which would have made it possible to compare the experts' results individually.

Another limitation is that the pretest included two non-identical versions of the Telekit system, whereas the versions from the posttest were identical. This occurred because the results from the heuristic evaluation (HE1) led to changes in the Telekit system before the think-aloud test (TA1) had been established. The results from the heuristic evaluation (HE2) were not integrated into the Telekit system before the think-aloud test (TA2) was performed. The advantage of adopting this approach in the pretest phase was that HE1 cleaned the system's interface for potential usability problems which might otherwise have led to lack of interest among users. A disadvantage was that system development took longer time because corrections were made by Silverbullet [23] before new versions of the Telekit system were updated.

Based on the present study, we recommend taking a mixed usability approach and applying it iteratively in the development of medical healthcare systems and telehealth technologies. As an iterative, mixed usability approach was only implemented in a single system, the Telekit system from the Danish TeleCare North trial, we cannot generalise the quantitative results and qualitative findings collected in the present study to other telehealth technologies as the results will likely depend on the type of system, among others.

We adopted a holistic view to evaluate the usability of the Telekit system and followed the system's lifecycle which allowed us to analyse and to elicit the participants' needs and to identify required functionalities. This approach included building a full understanding of both COPD participants' and the experts' perspectives. Developing and evaluating new telehealth systems is an ongoing process. Predicting the duration of this process is no exact science, and when the process ends depends on the users who evaluate the systems and the setting in which the system is going to be implemented.

In the future, it would be interesting to compare the heuristic evaluations and think-aloud tests with a different type of usability evaluation method, such as eye-tracking. Eye-tracking provides objective results in terms of heat maps and subjective findings in the form of comments and statements regarding the heat maps [40]. The objective results and subjective heat maps seem to be a very relevant supplement to the present study because additional usability results may surface that were not identified by the other methods.

5. Conclusion

A mixed usability approach performed iteratively on the Telekit system was conducted. Quantitative results and qualitative findings indicated that, to achieve an effective and thorough usability evaluation, it is necessary to combine various methods and to apply these repeatedly. Based on the study results, the Telekit system seems promising as a tool supporting COPD patients in the management of their disease. The heuristic evaluation from the pretest triggered substantial changes in the Telekit system, and several new versions of the system have since been implemented. Thereafter, a think-aloud test was established where participants verbally expressed their experiences with the system. Approximately one year after the system was fully implemented and operational, a posttest was performed. In our comparison of pre- and posttest problems, we assumed that the posttest would identify fewer problems. This assumption was disconfirmed and this illustrates the importance of working iteratively. Furthermore, it is also appropriate to use a mix of usability evaluation methods as each usability method will illuminate different perspectives of usability. The Telekit system still needs functionality and design improvements. However, the system is fully implemented and the COPD patients from the Danish TeleCare North trial have already reported that they experience increased freedom, control, and security and greater awareness of their COPD symptoms when using the system [41]. Hence, we conclude that the Telekit system requires further usability evaluation and recommend mixed methods to be applied in this process. This study was valuable to enhance and customize the Telekit system based on the users' needs by performing extended evaluations and user tests.

Competing Interests

The authors declare that there are no competing interests regarding the publication of this paper.

Acknowledgments

The authors thank the healthcare professionals (district nurses and head nurses) who are affiliated to the TeleCare North trial for their cooperation and help in finding potential participants for their study. In this context, they also thank the participants who invited them into their homes and agreed to participate in the think-aloud tests. Furthermore, they extend their gratitude to the usability experts from the Department of Health Science and Technology, Aalborg University, for their constructive participation in the heuristic evaluations. Finally, they would like to thank Associate Professor Morten Pilegaard and Cand.ling.merc., Certified Translator Peter Steffensen for proofreading the manuscript. This study was funded by the North Denmark Region; 11 municipalities in the North Denmark Region; the Obel Family Foundation; the Danish Agency for Digitalization Policy and Strategy, and the European Social Fund.

References

[1] M. Cartwright, S. P. Hirani, L. Rixon et al., "Effect of telehealth on quality of life and psychological outcomes over 12 months (Whole Systems Demonstrator telehealth questionnaire study): nested study of patient reported outcomes in a pragmatic, cluster randomised controlled trial," BMJ, vol. 346, no. 7897, article f653, 2013.

[2] R. Wootton, "Twenty years of telemedicine in chronic disease management-an evidence synthesis," Journal of Telemedicine and Telecare, vol. 18, no. 4, pp. 211–220, 2012.

[3] S. McLean, U. Nurmatov, J. L. Liu, C. Pagliari, J. Car, and A. Sheikh, "Telehealthcare for chronic obstructive pulmonary disease," Cochrane Database of Systematic Reviews, no. 7, Article ID CD007718, 2011.

[4] F. W. Udsen, P. H. Lilholt, O. Hejlesen, and L. H. Ehlers, "Effectiveness and cost-effectiveness of telehealthcare for chronic obstructive pulmonary disease: study protocol for a cluster randomized controlled trial," Trials, vol. 15, no. 1, article 178, 2014.

[5] J. Cruz, D. Brooks, and A. Marques, "Home telemonitoring in COPD: a systematic review of methodologies and patients' adherence," International Journal of Medical Informatics, vol. 83, no. 4, pp. 249–263, 2014.

[6] J. Singh, C. Lutteroth, and B. C. Wünsche, "Taxonomy of usability requirements for home telehealth systems," in Proceedings of the 11th International Conference of the NZ Chapter of the ACM Special Interest Group on Human-Computer Interaction (CHINZ '10), pp. 29–32, July 2010.

[7] K. Horton, "The use of telecare for people with chronic obstructive pulmonary disease: implications for management," Journal of Nursing Management, vol. 16, no. 2, pp. 173–180, 2008.

[8] Y. J. Chun and P. E. Patterson, "A usability gap between older adults and younger adults on interface design of an Internet-based telemedicine system," Work, vol. 41, no. 1, pp. 349–352, 2012.

[9] T. Botsis and G. Hartvigsen, "Current status and future perspectives in telecare for elderly people suffering from chronic diseases," Journal of Telemedicine and Telecare, vol. 14, no. 4, pp. 195–203, 2008.

[10] N. Bevan, "International Standards for HCI," in Encyclopedia of Human Computer Interaction, pp. 1–15, 2006.

[11] M. Maguire, "Methods to support human-centred design," International Journal of Human Computer Studies, vol. 55, no. 4, pp. 587–634, 2001.

[12] A. Kushniruk, "Evaluation in the design of health information systems: application of approaches emerging from usability engineering," Computers in Biology and Medicine, vol. 32, no. 3, pp. 141–149, 2002.

[13] J. Horsky, K. McColgan, J. E. Pang et al., "Complementary methods of system usability evaluation: surveys and observations during software design and development cycles," Journal of Biomedical Informatics, vol. 43, no. 5, pp. 782–790, 2010.

[14] M. W. M. Jaspers, "A comparison of usability methods for testing interactive health technologies: methodological aspects and empirical evidence," International Journal of Medical Informatics, vol. 78, no. 5, pp. 340–353, 2009.

[15] R. R. Hall, "Prototyping for usability of new technology," *International Journal of Human Computer Studies*, vol. 55, no. 4, pp. 485–501, 2001.

[16] D. Castilla, A. Garcia-Palacios, J. Bretón-López et al., "Process of design and usability evaluation of a telepsychology web and virtual reality system for the elderly: butler," *International Journal of Human Computer Studies*, vol. 71, no. 3, pp. 350–362, 2013.

[17] J. Nielsen, "Parallel & Iterative Design+Competitive Testing = High Usability," 2011, https://www.nngroup.com/articles/parallel-and-iterative-design/.

[18] J. Nielsen, "Iterative Design of User Interfaces," 1993, http://www.nngroup.com/articles/iterative-design/.

[19] H. R. Hartson, T. S. Andre, and R. C. Williges, "Criteria for evaluating usability evaluation methods," *International Journal of Human-Computer Interaction*, vol. 13, no. 4, pp. 373–410, 2001.

[20] P. H. Lilholt, S. Heiden, and O. K. Hejlesen, "User satisfaction and experience with a telehealth system for the danish telecare north trial: A Think-Aloud Study," *Studies in Health Technology and Informatics*, vol. 205, pp. 900–904, 2014.

[21] P. H. Lilholt, M. H. Jensen, and O. K. Hejlesen, "Heuristic evaluation of a telehealth system from the Danish TeleCare North Trial," *International Journal of Medical Informatics*, vol. 84, no. 5, pp. 319–326, 2016.

[22] Silverbullet, *OpenTele | Architecture*, Opentele.Silverbullet.dk, 2013, http://opentele.silverbullet.dk/architecture/.

[23] Silverbullet, 2016, http://opentele.silverbullet.dk.

[24] Samsung, 2016, http://samsung.com.

[25] A. Medical, "Andonline," 2016, http://andonline.com.

[26] Nonin. Nonin, 2016, http://nonin.com.

[27] J. Nielsen, "How to conduct a heuristic evaluation," vol. 10, 2001, http://www.nngroup.com/articles/how-to-conduct-a-heuristic-evaluation/.

[28] J. Nielsen, *10 Heuristics for User Interface Design*, vol. 2013, 1995, http://www.nngroup.com/articles/ten-usability-heuristics/.

[29] R. Molich, *Usable Web Design*, Nyt Teknisk, Copenhagen, Denmark, 2007.

[30] M. Van Someren, Y. F. Barnard, and J. A. C. Sandberg, *The Think Aloud Method—A Pratical Guide to Modelling Cognitive Processes*, Academic Press, Amsterdam, The Netherlands, 1994.

[31] J. Polisena, K. Tran, K. Cimon et al., "Home telehealth for chronic obstructive pulmonary disease: a systematic review and meta-analysis," *Journal of Telemedicine and Telecare*, vol. 16, no. 3, pp. 120–127, 2010.

[32] S. Kitsiou, G. Paré, and M. Jaana, "Systematic reviews and meta-analyses of home telemonitoring interventions for patients with chronic diseases: a critical assessment of their methodological quality," *Journal of Medical Internet Research*, vol. 15, no. 7, article e150, 2013.

[33] S. McLean, U. Nurmatov, J. L. Y. Liu, C. Pagliari, J. Car, and A. Sheikh, "Telehealthcare for chronic obstructive pulmonary disease: cochrane review and meta-analysis," *British Journal of General Practice*, vol. 62, no. 604, pp. e739–e749, 2012.

[34] R. L. Yussof, T. N. Paris, H. Abas, and H. B. Zaman, "Mixed usability evaluation during the development cycle of 'MEL-SindD'," *Procedia—Social and Behavioral Sciences*, vol. 105, pp. 162–170, 2013.

[35] M. R. Boland, A. Rusanov, Y. So et al., "From expert-derived user needs to user-perceived ease of use and usefulness: a two-phase mixed-methods evaluation framework," *Journal of Biomedical Informatics*, vol. 52, pp. 141–150, 2014.

[36] H. C. Ossebaard, E. R. Seydel, and L. van Gemert-Pijnen, "Online usability and patients with long-term conditions: a mixed-methods approach," *International Journal of Medical Informatics*, vol. 81, no. 6, pp. 374–387, 2012.

[37] S. G. S. Shah and I. Robinson, "User involvement in healthcare technology development and assessment: structured literature review," *International Journal of Health Care Quality Assurance Incorporating Leadership in Health Services*, vol. 19, no. 6-7, pp. 500–515, 2006.

[38] Z. Tang, T. R. Johnson, R. D. Tindall, and J. Zhang, "Applying heuristic evaluation to improve the usability of a telemedicine system," *Telemedicine Journal and e-Health*, vol. 12, no. 1, pp. 24–34, 2006.

[39] J. Nielsen, *10 Heuristics for User Interface Design*, 1995, http://www.nngroup.com/articles/ten-usability-heuristics/.

[40] C. Schaarup, G. Hartvigsen, L. B. Larsen, Z.-H. Tan, E. Arsand, and O. K. Hejlesen, "Assessing the potential use of eye-tracking triangulation for evaluating the usability of an online diabetes exercise system," *Studies in Health Technology and Informatics*, vol. 216, pp. 84–88, 2015.

[41] P. H. Lilholt, L. K. Hæsum, and O. K. Hejlesen, "Exploring user experience of a telehealth system for the Danish TeleCare North Trial," *Studies in Health Technology and Informatics*, vol. 210, pp. 301–305, 2015.

21

Effect of Reinforcement of Oral Health Education Message through Short Messaging Service in Mobile Phones

Harish C. Jadhav,[1] Arun S. Dodamani,[1] G. N. Karibasappa,[1] Rahul G. Naik,[2] Mahesh R. Khairnar,[3] Manjiri A. Deshmukh,[4] and Prashanth Vishwakarma[1]

[1]*Department of Public Health Dentistry, JMF's ACPM Dental College, Dhule, Maharashtra 424001, India*
[2]*Department of Public Health Dentistry, Dr. Hedgewar Smruti Rugna Seva Mandal's Dental College, Hingoli, Maharashtra 431513, India*
[3]*Department of Public Health Dentistry, Bharati Vidyapeeth Dental College and Hospital, Sangli, Maharashtra 416416, India*
[4]*Department of Public Health Dentistry, Swargiya Dadasaheb Kalmegh Smruti Dental College, Nagpur, Maharashtra 441110, India*

Correspondence should be addressed to Harish C. Jadhav; drharishjadhav2003@gmail.com

Academic Editor: Carlos De Las Cuevas

Objective. This paper aims to assess the effectiveness of reinforcement of oral health education message through short messaging service (SMS) in mobile phones. *Material and Methods.* 400 subjects from two colleges (200 from each college) belonging to 18–20 years age group possessing mobile phones were randomly selected and baseline examination of oral hygiene and gingival status was carried out using Oral Hygiene Index (OHI) and Gingival Index (GI). Oral health education was provided to all the subjects. Oral health education message was reinforced through short messaging service (SMS) in mobile phones for the subjects belonging to the intervention group. There was no such reinforcement for the control group. Follow-up examinations were done at the end of 1st, 2nd, 3rd, and 6th month. After the 3rd month, subjects of the intervention group did not receive oral health education message through short messaging service (SMS) and were followed up after next three months. Compiled data was analyzed using SPSS version 16 statistical software. *Result.* Mean OHI and GI scores in intervention group were significantly ($p < 0.01$) less than those of control group after the 2nd, 3rd, and 6th month. *Conclusion.* Reinforcement of oral health education message through short messaging service (SMS) is effective media to improve oral health.

1. Introduction

Many current-day health problems in individual and community are associated with lifestyle changes. Adopting unhealthy lifestyle is responsible for chronic diseases such as obesity, heart diseases, and cancer [1]. Oral diseases are no exception to this. Oral diseases are predominantly man-made attributing to his/her lifestyle [1, 2].

Human society is undergoing continuous transformation through the harnessing of information and knowledge from the various technologies that in turn have affected our value systems, power structures, everyday routines, and environment [3]. The development in technology has influenced the individual and the society. One among them is the influence of mobile on all sections of society [4]. Mobile phone usage has increased globally; over half of the world's 6.5 billion people now use mobile phone services [5]. Total wireless subscription in India stands at 952.34 million (in urban 553.45 million whereas in rural 398.89 million) at the end of January 2015 [6]. Mobile based innovations are quickly emerging as the new frontiers in transforming health due to fast-growing penetration of mobile phones into remote areas [5]. Mobile short messaging service (SMS) has high penetration and developed into a powerful, real-time communication medium [7].

The innovations and increase in usage of mobile phones have prompted for rapid communication as well as utilization for accessing personal and reliable health information [8]. Health information regarding prevention and treatment of diseases can be given to people through an affordable and cost-effective medium like short messaging service. Health education is a process of transmission of knowledge. The goal of planned health education program is not only to bring about new behavior but also to reinforce and maintain healthy behavior that will promote and improve individual, group, or community health [9]. One to one approach in oral health education is promising in improving oral hygiene, but it is time-consuming and impractical from community perspective. Available health education models have their own limitations to adopt healthy lifestyles such as slow feedback mechanism, expensive apparatus and training required limited access in rural areas, and an inability of customization for the target population [10]. Substitution of personal instruction by other means of communication has been investigated, such as the use of self-educational manuals and audio-visual aids.

People can be motivated through periodic prompts that can encourage healthy behaviors in them [11]. Reinforcement is one of the most important principles of health education which helps to adopt healthy behavior and lifestyles [12]. Text messaging is able to elicit healthier behaviors, such as adherence to treatment guidelines, smoking cessation, dietary advice, and exercise regimes that can prevent the development of certain behavior-related diseases [12, 13]. Sparse data is available regarding the use of mobile to deliver dental health across the globe and in India. Moreover, there is limited literature evidence regarding the effect of reinforcement of oral health education message through mobile phones on oral health. Hence, an attempt has been made to assess the effectiveness of reinforcement of oral health education message through short messaging service (SMS) using mobile phones among 18–20-year-old BSW (Bachelors in Social Work) students of North Maharashtra University, Jalgaon, Maharashtra, India.

2. Material and Methods

The present study was a quasi-experimental controlled trial conducted on 400 subjects from two different social work colleges (P. J. Nehru College of Social Work, Amalner, Jalgaon, and Dr. Babasaheb Ambedkar College of Social Work, Morane (Nakane), Tal. Dist. Dhule) in North Maharashtra region. These two colleges were randomly selected from 5 social work colleges situated in North Maharashtra region using lottery method. Both colleges were well apart from each other (almost 45 kms) so that students of both colleges could not interact with each other and they were unaware about randomization and mode of intervention in the research. Permission to conduct the research was obtained from higher authorities of both colleges. Ethical clearance was obtained from Institutional Review Board of ACPM dental college, Dhule, and informed written consent was obtained from all the participants prior to the study.

2.1. Inclusion Criteria. Subjects in the age group of 18–20 years possessing personal mobile phones with SMS facility

and agreement to comply with the study visits were included in the study.

2.2. Exclusion Criteria. Subjects who did not have personal mobile phones and medically compromised subjects were excluded.

2.3. Study Design. Based on the data obtained from pilot study, keeping α at 5% ($p < 0.05$), power at 80%, considering Cohen's medium effect size 0.5, sample size for each group was determined to be 200. Since we had two groups (intervention and control), final sample size was determined to be 400.

Aim and objectives of the research were explicitly explained to both institutional higher authorities and permission to conduct the research was obtained from them. Thereafter details of the research were explained to all the students of both institutions and 200 subjects from each college satisfying the eligibility criteria were randomly selected. Baseline data using a specially prepared and pretested proforma was obtained from the 200 study subjects from each college which included demographic details. Intraoral examination was done to assess oral health using Oral Hygiene Index (given by John C. Green and Jack R. Vermillion in 1960) and Gingival Index (developed by Loe H. and Silness J. in 1963).

After the collection of baseline data, oral health education was provided to all the subjects of both colleges using common risk factor approach (oral hygiene practices, diet, habits such as smoking and alcohol use, stress, and trauma). As these causes are common to a number of other chronic diseases, adopting a collaborative approach is more rational than one that is disease specific [2]. Hence, common risk factor approach was employed in current study. Oral health education was given through PowerPoint presentation (20-minute presentation by investigator himself); demonstration of proper brushing technique on brushing model using "Modified Bass Technique" and information on use of interdental aids were also given. The benefit of using such audio-visual aids is that sound and sight can be combined together to create a better presentation in terms of better understanding on the part of the subjects. Subjects were then allowed to ask their doubts and comprehensive explanation was given to clarify their doubts.

Later intervention group and control group (college) were selected randomly by using lottery method by a person who was not known to the examiner. The examiner was blinded to the grouping. Oral health message included the information regarding proper oral hygiene practices, effects of harmful habits, and importance of proper intake of diet. The message was reinforced through short messaging service (SMS) from mobile phones for the subjects belonging to the intervention group. No other oral health information was provided to the intervention group during the study period. The messages were sent by the person who was unknown to the examiner and examiner was kept blind to the group receiving the message. Health related messages both in English and in local language (Marathi) were sent. Each of the two messages in both languages was sent to the intervention group twice a week for the period of 3 months. After the 3rd month, messages were ceased to be sent. No such oral health message or any such kind of health education was given to the participants belonging to the control group after randomization.

2.4. Following Oral Health Education Message Was Drafted through SMS to Be Sent to the Intervention Group. The message was as follows: "Hi, brush your teeth twice daily with toothbrush and toothpaste to avoid dental diseases. Avoid snacking in between the meals and rinse your mouth properly after every meal. Stay away from tobacco as it is the main cause of cancer, gum diseases, lung diseases and heart diseases."

2.5. Testing of the SMS. After the initial framing of the oral health education message, it was sent randomly to 30 subjects to assess their opinion regarding the comprehension, relevance, and practicality of following the message. The required and relevant changes were made in the SMS. Again the procedure was repeated and the oral health education message was finalized.

2.6. Examination and Calibration. All the oral examinations as well as oral health education presentations were performed by a single trained and calibrated examiner. Hence, only intraexaminer reliability was determined. To determine intraexaminer reliability, the oral examination of 25 randomly selected subjects was repeated on different dates. The results so obtained were subjected to Kappa Statistics. The Kappa coefficient value for intraexaminer reliability was 0.87 which is interpreted as very good.

The examination was performed under natural light in the classroom. A set of instruments, namely, mouth mirror, explorer numbers 5 and 23, and periodontal probe, were used for each individual patient separately. Intraoral examination was done using Oral Hygiene Index and Gingival Index to collect the clinical data after the 1st, 2nd, and 3rd months from both groups. After the 3rd month, SMS to reinforce health education were ceased to be sent to the intervention group. From the 3rd month to the 6th month, no other oral health education was imparted to study participants. Then intraoral examination of both groups was done using Oral Hygiene Index and Gingival Index after six months of baseline data collection.

2.7. Statistical Analysis. Compiled data was analyzed using Statistical Package for Social Science (SPSS) version 16 statistical software. The intervention and control groups were compared according to age and gender using nonparametric Pearson's chi square test. Continuous data was presented as mean and standard deviation. Mean OHI and mean GI at different intervals were compared in between all subjects of intervention and control group by unpaired *t*-test. Overall changes in mean OHI and mean GI scores within intervention and control groups were compared using ANOVA test followed by post hoc analysis.

TABLE 1: Gender-wise distribution between the intervention and control group.

| Gender | Group | | Total |
	Intervention	Control	
Male	137	149	286
Female	63	51	114
Total	200	200	400
p value		*p* > 0.05	

TABLE 2: Comparison of mean OHI score at different intervals between intervention and control group.

Mean OHI score	Intervention	Control	*p* value
At baseline	3.79 ± 1.54	3.63 ± 1.39	0.283 (NS)
After 1 month	3.14 ± 1.32	3.21 ± 1.31	0.580 (NS)
After 2 months	2.64 ± 1.14	3.38 ± 1.35	<0.01
After 3 months	2.32 ± 1.07	3.56 ± 1.37	<0.01
After 6 months	2.88 ± 1.11	3.99 ± 1.46	<0.01

NS, not significant.

TABLE 3: Comparison of mean GI score at different intervals between intervention and control group.

Mean GI score	Intervention	Control	*p* value
At baseline	0.31 ± 0.32	0.29 ± 0.29	0.394 (NS)
After 1 month	0.23 ± 0.26	0.24 ± 0.27	0.849 (NS)
After 2 months	0.15 ± 0.17	0.25 ± 0.28	<0.01
After 3 months	0.10 ± 0.13	0.28 ± 0.29	<0.01
After 6 months	0.16 ± 0.16	0.35 ± 0.32	<0.01

NS, not significant.

3. Results

3.1. Demographics of the Participants. Table 1 shows gender-wise distribution of study participants between the two groups. Chi square test showed no significant difference (*p* > 0.05) in the gender-wise distribution between intervention and control groups indicating a good match (Table 1).

3.2. Oral Hygiene Condition of Participants. Comparison of mean OHI score at different intervals between intervention and control groups showed no significant difference in mean OHI score at baseline (*p* = 0.283) and after 1st month (*p* = 0.580) in between intervention and control groups. However, mean OHI score in intervention group was significantly less than that of control group after the 2nd, 3rd, and 6th month (*p* < 0.01) (Table 2).

3.3. Gingival Condition of Participants. When mean GI scores between intervention and control group were compared at different intervals, it was found that there was statistically no significant difference in mean GI score at baseline (*p* = 0.394) and after 1st month (*p* = 0.849) in between intervention and control groups. But mean GI score in intervention group was less than that of control group after the 2nd, 3rd, and 6th month (*p* < 0.01) (Table 3).

TABLE 4: Within group comparison of mean OHI scores at each interval.

Groups	Interval	Mean	Standard deviation	F value	p value
Intervention	At baseline	3.79	1.540	109.211	<0.001
	After 1 month	3.141	1.3248		
	After 2 months	2.636	1.1441		
	After 3 months	2.319	1.0768		
	After 6 months	2.88	1.113		
Control	At baseline	3.63	1.393	108.454	<0.001
	After 1 month	3.213	1.3129		
	After 2 months	3.382	1.3529		
	After 3 months	3.561	1.3861		
	After 6 months	3.99	1.464		

TABLE 5: Pairwise comparison of mean OHI scores within intervention and control group using post hoc test.

Groups	(I)	(J)	Mean difference (I − J)	p value
Intervention	At baseline	After 1 month	0.651	<0.001
	At baseline	After 2 months	1.155	<0.001
	At baseline	After 3 months	1.472	<0.001
	At baseline	After 6 months	0.910	<0.001
	After 1 month	After 2 months	0.504	<0.001
	After 1 month	After 3 months	0.821	<0.001
	After 1 month	After 6 months	0.259	<0.001
	After 2 months	After 3 months	0.317	<0.001
	After 2 months	After 6 months	−0.245	<0.001
	After 3 months	After 6 months	−0.563	<0.001
Control	At baseline	After 1 month	0.420	<0.001
	At baseline	After 2 months	0.251	<0.001
	At baseline	After 3 months	0.072	0.172 (NS)
	At baseline	After 6 months	−0.357	<0.001
	After 1 month	After 2 months	−0.169	<0.001
	After 1 month	After 3 months	−0.348	<0.001
	After 1 month	After 6 months	−0.777	<0.001
	After 2 months	After 3 months	−0.180	<0.001
	After 2 months	After 6 months	−0.609	<0.001
	After 3 months	After 6 months	−0.429	<0.001

NS, not significant.

3.4. Post Hock Comparison. The mean OHI scores (Table 4) and the mean GI scores (Table 6) of the subjects in intervention and control groups were highly significantly different ($p < 0.001$) across baseline and after 1 month, 2 months, 3 months, and 6 months.

The result of the post hoc test (with least significant difference) shows difference of mean OHI scores between each of the two time intervals to be highly significant ($p < 0.001$) in both intervention and control groups except between baseline and 3 months scores in control group ($p = 0172$) (Table 5). Similarly, difference of mean GI scores between each of the two time intervals was highly significant ($p < 0.001$) in both intervention and control groups except between 2 months and 6 months ($p = 0.06$) in the intervention group and between baseline and 3 months ($p = 0.271$) which was not statistically significant (Table 7).

4. Discussion

From the results, it can be seen that, in intervention group, baseline mean OHI and GI scores linearly decreased up to the 3rd month and gradually increased thereafter till the 6th month, but it was less than baseline mean OHI score and GI score. In control group, mean OHI and GI scores showed reduction after one month but thereafter linearly increased up to the 6th month. After the 6th month, mean OHI and GI scores were more than those of baseline scores.

In the present study, there was an improvement in oral health from baseline to the 1st month in both intervention and control groups which was not statistically significant ($p = 0.58$). It may be due to the fact that oral health education provided before the start of the study might have the positive effect on the oral health behavior up till one month. Hence,

TABLE 6: Within group comparison of mean GI scores at each interval using ANOVA test.

Groups	Factor 1	Mean	Standard deviation	F value	p value
Intervention	At baseline	0.313	0.32	71.673	<0.001
	After 1 month	0.231	0.26		
	After 2 months	0.153	0.17		
	After 3 months	0.097	0.13		
	After 6 months	0.165	0.16		
Control	At baseline	0.287	0.29	71.787	<0.001
	After 1 month	0.236	0.27		
	After 2 months	0.254	0.28		
	After 3 months	0.278	0.29		
	After 6 months	0.352	0.32		

TABLE 7: Pairwise comparison of mean GI scores within intervention and control group using post hoc test.

Groups	(I)	(J)	Mean difference (I − J)	p value
Intervention	At baseline	After 1 month	0.082	<0.001
	At baseline	After 2 months	0.160	<0.001
	At baseline	After 3 months	0.216	<0.001
	At baseline	After 6 months	0.148	<0.001
	After 1 month	After 2 months	0.078	<0.001
	After 1 month	After 3 months	0.134	<0.001
	After 1 month	After 6 months	0.066	<0.001
	After 2 months	After 3 months	0.056	<0.001
	After 2 months	After 6 months	−0.012	0.064 (NS)
	After 3 months	After 6 months	−0.068	<0.001
Control	At baseline	After 1 month	0.052	<0.001
	At baseline	After 2 months	0.033	<0.001
	At baseline	After 3 months	0.009	0.271 (NS)
	At baseline	After 6 months	−0.064	<0.001
	After 1 month	After 2 months	−0.019	<0.001
	After 1 month	After 3 months	−0.042	<0.001
	After 1 month	After 6 months	−0.116	<0.001
	After 2 months	After 3 months	−0.024	<0.001
	After 2 months	After 6 months	−0.097	<0.001
	After 3 months	After 6 months	−0.074	<0.001

NS, not significant.

there was an improvement in mean OHI and GI scores of all the participants.

After baseline data collection, oral health message was reinforced through short messaging service (SMS) from mobile phones for only the subjects belonging to the intervention group, which might have kept them aware of the importance of oral health and motivated them to maintain proper oral health. Study participants in intervention group might have been more aware, concerned about their health, and more positive towards health, thus taking proper measures like proper brushing and flossing to maintain good oral health. It indicates that reinforcement at regular intervals through SMS helps to adopt healthier practices and improve oral health. These findings are in agreement with study conducted by Sharma et al. which shows that text messaging was more effective than pamphlets in improving knowledge, attitude, and practices of mothers [14]. Mean OHI and mean GI scores in intervention group were less than those of control group after the 2nd, 3rd, and 6th month. These results are in concordance with the studies conducted by Eppright et al. in orthodontic patients [15].

Limited literature is available on effect of reinforcement on oral health through SMS, but SMS reminders are effective in smoking cessation, treatment guidelines, behavior change, and so forth. The results are similar to the studies conducted by Shetty et al. showing significant improvements in the health outcomes of diabetic patients [16]. Similar results obtained in the study conducted by Koshy et al. on attendance reminders for ophthalmic patients showed that attendance rates were increased in patients who received SMS reminder compared to patients who did not receive SMS reminder [17]. Similarly Huang et al. indicated that SMS intervention enabled patients to consume their medication on time [18].

Apart from SMS intervention, other studies have been conducted using different health interventions showing positive effect on health [19, 20]. Approaches for oral health education other than personal approach have also been used which have resulted in improvement in oral health following intervention. One such study was conducted by Harnacke et al. who employed computer based training to teach either Fones technique or Modified Bass Technique. Computer presentation resulted in improvement of oral hygiene skills and gingivitis using Fones technique when compared to control groups [21]. However, no such difference was seen in participants following Modified Bass Technique. Similar results were obtained in a population based survey conducted by Gholami et al. using mass media campaign through TV channels. The study demonstrated a significant impact of the mass media campaign on Iranian adults' knowledge regarding periodontal health and disease [22]. Zotti et al. evaluated the influence of a mobile application-based approach for domestic oral hygiene maintenance in improving oral hygiene compliance and oral health in a group of orthodontic patients. The study showed positive results in improving oral hygiene compliance of adolescent patients and in improving their oral health [23].

The present study showed that maintenance of improved oral health over longer time periods requires prolonged, repeated instructions, as explained in a study conducted by Ivanovic and Lekic [24]. Apart from the reinforcement of health education through SMS to intervention group, regular visits of the investigator to collect the data, visit to dentist to seek care might have contributed to better oral health.

However, in control group, there was no improvement in oral health; probably lack of reinforcement might have resulted in poor oral health. Investigator's visit to both colleges for collecting data at every month during study period might have motivated maintaining good health behavior casting only for few days. Impact of dental examination alone might have been responsible for improvement of oral health but for limited time period. Later on the Hawthorne effect might have reduced reflecting the deterioration of oral health [25].

After cessation of intervention from the 3rd month to the 6th month in intervention group, there was an increase in mean OHI and GI scores similar to control group. Lack of oral health education through SMS within this period and lack of investigator's visits to participants might have resulted in relapse of OHI and GI scores towards baseline. Also subjects underwent their academic examinations within this period. Hence, they might have been suffering from stress due to which their oral health might have deteriorated [26]. These results are confirmatory with studies conducted by Schou showing the immediate effects on the dental health status, but these effects disappeared or decreased from the 3rd month to the 6th month after dental health education program [27].

The findings of the present study show that oral health is improved after provision of health education; reinforcing health education helped motivate maintaining good oral health. Still the study had an inherent limitation in terms of the design of the study, that is, quasi-experimental design which lacks a true randomization. Beholding the internal validity limitations of the study, generalization of the results seems to be questionable. Hence, we propose future research with the most valid study design among various population groups to assess the efficacy of this intervention.

5. Conclusion

SMS through mobile phone emerging as a new tool helps elicit healthier behaviors and reinforcement of oral health education message through short messaging service (SMS) using mobile phones can be effective media to improve oral health. As a Public Health Dentist, we should motivate the policy-makers to recommend telecom sector companies as a social responsibility to send free of cost oral health educational SMS at community level for taking the society to pinnacles of glory.

Acknowledgments

The authors would like to thank the participants for their cooperation and are very grateful to Dr. Prashant Patil, Assistant Professor, Department of Physiology, Shri Bhausaheb Hire Government Medical College, Dhule, Maharashtra, India, for helping them with statistical analysis.

References

[1] B. Purohit and A. Singh, "Lifestyle and oral health," *Advances in Life Science and Technology*, vol. 3, pp. 34–44, 2012.

[2] A. Sheiham and R. G. Watt, "The Common Risk Factor Approach: a rational basis for promoting oral health," *Community Dentistry and Oral Epidemiology*, vol. 28, no. 6, pp. 399–406, 2000.

[3] R. Linturi, "The role of technology in shaping human society," *Foresight*, vol. 2, no. 2, pp. 183–188, 2000.

[4] A. Addo, "The adoption of mobile phone: how has it changed us socially?" *Issues in Business Management and Economics*, vol. 1, no. 3, pp. 47–60, 2013.

[5] D. S. Thomas, "Affordable Mobile technology towards Preventive Health care: Rural India," *IOSR Journal of Dental and Medical Sciences*, vol. 3, no. 3, pp. 32–36, 2012.

[6] Telecom Regulatory Authority of India, *Highlights of Telecom Subscription Data as on 31st January, 2015 New Delhi, India*, 2015.

[7] C. M. Danis, J. B. Ellis, W. A. Kellog et al., "Mobile phones for health education in the developing world: SMS as a user interface," in *Proceedings of the 1st ACM Symposium on Computing for Development (ACM DEV '10)*, Article No. 13, London, UK, December 2010.

[8] K. Patrick, W. G. Griswold, F. Raab, and S. S. Intille, "Health and the mobile phone," *American Journal of Preventive Medicine*, vol. 35, no. 2, pp. 177–181, 2008.

[9] K. Park, *Textbook of Preventive and Social Medicine*, Banarasidas Bhanot, 20th edition, 2005.

[10] UWI The Caribbean Institute of Media and Communication, *Developing Communication Strategy Advantages and Disadvantages of Different Types of Media*, UWI The Caribbean Institute of Media and Communication, 2011.

[11] J. P. Fry and R. A. Neff, "Periodic prompts and reminders in health promotion and health behavior interventions: systematic review," *Journal of Medical Internet Research*, vol. 11, no. 2, article e16, 2009.

[12] A. Rodgers, T. Corbett, D. Bramley et al., "Do u smoke after txt? Results of a randomised trial of smoking cessation using mobile phone text messaging," *Tobacco Control*, vol. 14, no. 4, pp. 255–261, 2005.

[13] K. P. Kornman, V. A. Shrewsbury, A. C. Chou et al., "Electronic therapeutic contact for adolescent weight management: the Loozit study," *Telemedicine Journal and e-Health*, vol. 16, no. 6, pp. 678–685, 2010.

[14] R. Sharma, M. Hebbal, A. V. Ankola, and V. Murugabupathy, "Mobile-phone text messaging (SMS) for providing oral health education to mothers of preschool children in Belgaum city," *Journal of Telemedicine and Telecare*, vol. 17, no. 8, pp. 432–436, 2011.

[15] M. Eppright, B. Shroff, A. M. Best, E. Barcoma, and S. J. Lindauer, "Influence of active reminders on oral hygiene compliance in orthodontic patients," *The Angle Orthodontist*, vol. 84, no. 2, pp. 208–213, 2014.

[16] A. S. Shetty, S. Chamukuttan, A. Nanditha, R. K. C. Raj, and A. Ramachandran, "Reinforcement of adherence to prescription recommendations in Asian Indian diabetes patients using short message service (SMS)—a pilot study," *Journal of the Association of Physicians of India*, vol. 59, no. 11, pp. 711–714, 2011.

[17] E. Koshy, J. Car, and A. Majeed, "Effectiveness of mobile-phone short message service (SMS) reminders for ophthalmology outpatient appointments: observational study," *BMC Ophthalmology*, vol. 8, article 9, 2008.

[18] H.-L. Huang, Y.-C. J. Li, Y.-C. Chou et al., "Effects of and satisfaction with short message service reminders for patient medication adherence: a randomized controlled study," *BMC Medical Informatics and Decision Making*, vol. 13, article 127, 2013.

[19] A. J. Reynolds, J. A. Temple, S.-R. Ou et al., "Effects of a school-based, early childhood intervention on adult health and well-being," *Archives of Pediatrics and Adolescent Medicine*, vol. 161, no. 8, pp. 730–739, 2007.

[20] R. Yazdani, M. M. Vehkalahti, M. Nouri, and H. Murtomaa, "School-based education to improve oral cleanliness and gingival health in adolescents in Tehran, Iran," *International Journal of Paediatric Dentistry*, vol. 19, no. 4, pp. 274–281, 2009.

[21] D. Harnacke, S. Mitter, M. Lehner, J. Munzert, and R. Deinzer, "Improving oral hygiene skills by computer-based training: a randomized controlled comparison of the modified bass and the fones techniques," *PLoS ONE*, vol. 7, no. 5, Article ID e37072, 2012.

[22] M. Gholami, A. Pakdaman, A. Montazeri, A. Jafari, and J. I. Virtanen, "Assessment of periodontal knowledge following a mass media oral health promotion campaign: a population-based study," *BMC Oral Health*, vol. 14, no. 1, article 31, 2014.

[23] F. Zotti, D. Dalessandri, S. Salgarello et al., "Usefulness of an app in improving oral hygiene compliance in adolescent orthodontic patients," *Angle Orthodont*, vol. 86, no. 1, pp. 101–107, 2016.

[24] M. Ivanovic and P. Lekic, "Transient effect of a short-term educational programme without prophylaxis on control of plaque and gingival inflammation in school children," *Journal of Clinical Periodontology*, vol. 23, no. 8, pp. 750–757, 1996.

[25] S. J. Coombs and I. D. Smith, "The Hawthorne effect: is it a help or a hindrance in social research?" *Change: Transformations in Educations*, vol. 6, no. 1, pp. 97–111, 2003.

[26] R. Deinzer, N. Granrath, M. Spahl, S. Linz, B. Waschul, and A. Herforth, "Stress, oral health behaviour and clinical outcome," *British Journal of Health Psychology*, vol. 10, no. 2, pp. 269–283, 2005.

[27] L. Schou, "Active-involvement principle in dental health education," *Community Dentistry and Oral Epidemiology*, vol. 13, no. 3, pp. 128–132, 1985.

22

Noninferiority and Equivalence Evaluation of Clinical Performance among Computed Radiography, Film, and Digitized Film for Telemammography Services

Antonio J. Salazar,[1] Javier A. Romero,[2,3] Oscar A. Bernal,[3,4] Angela P. Moreno,[2] Sofía C. Velasco,[2,4] and Xavier A. Díaz[1]

[1]Electrophysiology and Telemedicine Laboratory, University of Los Andes, Carrera 1 Este No. 19A-40, Bogotá 11001, Colombia
[2]Department of Diagnostic Imaging, Fundación Santa Fe de Bogotá University Hospital, Calle 119 No. 7-75, Bogotá 11001, Colombia
[3]School of Medicine, University of Los Andes, Carrera 1 Este No. 19A-40, Bogotá 11001, Colombia
[4]School of Government, University of Los Andes, Carrera 1 Este No. 19A-40, Bogotá 11001, Colombia

Correspondence should be addressed to Antonio J. Salazar; ant-sala@uniandes.edu.co

Academic Editor: Manolis Tsiknakis

Objective. The aim of this study was to evaluate and compare the clinical performance of different alternatives to implement low-cost screening telemammography. We compared computed radiography, film printed images, and digitized films produced with a specialized film digitizer and a digital camera. *Material and Methods.* The ethics committee of our institution approved this study. We assessed the equivalence of the clinical performance of observers for cancer detection. The factorial design included 70 screening patients, four technological alternatives, and cases interpreted by seven radiologists, for a total of 1,960 observations. The variables evaluated were the positive predictive value (PPV), accuracy, sensitivity, specificity, and the area under the receiver operating characteristic curves (AUC). *Result.* The mean values for the observed variables were as follows: accuracy ranged from 0.77 to 0.82, the PPV ranged from 0.67 to 0.68, sensitivity ranged from 0.64 to 0.74, specificity ranged from 0.87 to 0.90, and the AUC ranged from 0.87 to 0.90. At a difference of 0.1 to claim equivalence, all alternatives were equivalent for all variables. *Conclusion.* Our findings suggest that telemammography screening programs may be provided to underserved populations at a low cost, using a film digitizer or a digital camera.

1. Introduction

Screening mammography programs, especially programs that use modern digital techniques such as computed radiography (CR) or full-field digital mammography (FFDM), have reduced the mortality rate associated with breast cancer [1, 2]. However, screening programs alone are inconclusive as they yield many false positives, and the definitive diagnosis of breast cancer is verified by biopsy and a histopathological examination of palpable lesions [3]. Therefore, the positive predictive value (PPV) of specific mammographic findings has been evaluated in several studies [4–6] and recently by

Venkatesan et al. [7]. Nevertheless, the evaluation of sensitivity is also very important in the evaluation of mortality associated with false negatives.

Telemedicine may help to provide widespread screening mammography services in underserved areas, and approaches such as CR or FFDM are useful in the implementation of telemammography. However, these technologies are still unaffordable in vulnerable areas of our country, such as jungles that have a low population density; therefore, low-cost solutions are required for effective telemammography. In our country, CR is only available in large cities and FFDM is only available in our hospital. Specialized equipment is available for digitizing mammogram films, and several studies have compared digital mammogram modalities to film-screen mammography [8–10], reporting no significant differences between film-screen mammography and digital mammography modalities, such as CR and FFDM [11, 12]. Nevertheless, the cost of specialized digitizers is high, which is why low-cost alternative digitization equipment, such as conventional scanners and digital cameras, is being used for teleradiology services in developing countries. While such pieces of equipment can dramatically reduce costs, their clinical performance should be determined before introducing them in telemammography.

The aim of this study was to establish and to compare the clinical performance of different alternatives to implement telemammography, such as CR, film printed from the CR, a specialized digitizer, and a digital camera. The variables used for evaluating clinical performance were the PPV, sensitivity, specificity, accuracy, the area under the receiving operating characteristic (ROC) curve (AUC), and the proportions of true negatives (TN), true positives (TP), false negatives (FN), and false positives (FP), all of which were based on the final assessment categories of the Breast Imaging Reporting and Data System (BI-RADS) [13].

No significant differences between the compared modalities have been reported in other studies designed to test the null hypothesis that the performances of different modalities are equal, but the power test was not reported, so it is not clear if these studies failed to find significant differences. In statistical hypothesis testing, failure to reject the null hypothesis does not mean the null hypothesis is true. In contrast, the present study is set to evaluate equivalence or noninferiority, in which we can conclude equivalence or noninferiority based on significant results. To establish that the performances are equal or that one modality is noninferior to the other, the null hypothesis has to be that their performances are not equal or that one is inferior to the other. Only by rejecting such a hypothesis can we conclude that the modalities under comparison are equivalent [14–17].

2. Materials and Methods

The ethics committee of our institutions approved this retrospective study, and informed consent was not required. A factorial design with repeated measures was used in this study. The design of this study applied a treatment-by-reader-by-case factorial design with 70 patients, seven radiologists, three derived images, and the reference images (i.e., CR), for a total of 1,960 observations for each variable.

2.1. The Reference Standard. The standard for positive cases was a malignant lesion confirmed by biopsy within two years of the initial mammography screening, corresponding to BI-RADS final assessment categories 4A, 4B, 4C, and 5 [9, 12, 18]. Negative cases were defined as cases without any lesions confirmed by biopsy or cases with normal follow-up mammograms within the same two-year interval, corresponding to BI-RADS final assessment categories 2 and 3. Two radiologists with more than ten years of experience in reading mammograms who had access to the clinical history of

the patients (biopsy, follow-up mammograms, etc.) established the reference standard.

2.2. Study Sample and Readers. At most rural health centers in our country, there are no mammography services [19], and where they are available, there are no mammograms repositories, so there are not available mammograms to use for a retrospective study. In addition, in these regions, there are not enough patients to develop a prospective study in a short time. For these reasons, this study was undertaken using CR screening mammograms from our hospital, which is a reference hospital for mammography screening, serving patients from remote undeserved areas of our country (approximately 8,000 mammograms interpreted per year). Mammography studies from patients who attended mammography screenings at the Fundación Santa Fe de Bogotá University Hospital (FSFBUH) were randomly selected without repetition from our screening database; the patients were all asymptomatic, and their lesions were impalpable and verified by pathology. The masses ranged in size from 6 mm to 23 mm, with a mean of 11 mm (SD = 4.2). Each case was required to include the following four standard mammographic views: mediolateral oblique, craniocaudal, left, and right, even if additional views were taken in the original screening mammograms. Cases of tomosynthesis or large masses were excluded.

To determine the sample size, we used the table proposed by Obuchowski [20] for comparisons of the AUC with the following criteria: (a) six observers, (b) small variability between radiologists, (c) moderate accuracy of the test (an AUC of approximately 0.75), (d) moderate differences suspected to be found among AUC (i.e., $\delta = 0.1$), and (e) a 1:1 ratio between malignant and benign cases. Using these criteria, minimum 60 cases were required. The final sample size was set at 70 cases, and the number of radiologists was increased to seven. Patients ranged in age from 41 to 84 years, with a mean age of 62.1 years (SD = 11.5). The cases were distributed as follows: 33 patients had cancer and 37 patients had benign lesions or normal results. The distribution of cases according to the BI-RADS final assessment categories is shown in Table 1. There were 57 cases with calcifications, 26 with masses, 35 with asymmetries, and 11 with architectural distortions and associated features. Four patients with prostheses were included in the sample. The detailed lesion classification of the cases is presented in Table 2. In terms of composition, the distribution of cases was as follows: 17 of the breasts were almost entirely fatty, 32 had scattered areas of fibroglandular density, 11 of the breasts were heterogeneously dense, which may obscure small masses, and 10 of the breasts were extremely dense, which lowers the sensitivity of mammography.

Seven radiologists from FSFBUH who were experienced in mammography, including four with high levels of experience (more than 10 years) and three with intermediate levels of experience (more than two years), served as observers.

2.3. Variables Observed by the Radiologists. Data collection was performed using a database and a digital form that was integrated into the image viewing software. At each interpretation, the radiologist selected the level of confidence in the presence of each selected condition, that is, calcifications,

TABLE 1: Distribution of cases in the sample according to the BI-RADS final assessment categories.

BI-RADS final assessment category[a]	Cases
2: benign	18
3: probably benign	19
4A: low suspicion for malignancy	6
4B: moderate suspicion for malignancy	14
4C: high suspicion for malignancy	3
5: highly suggestive of malignancy	10
Total	70

[a]Classification according to the American College of Radiology [13].

TABLE 2: Detailed classification of the cases in the sample.

Condition	Classification[a]	Cases
Masses	Well-defined mass	7
	Obscured edge mass	10
	Poorly defined mass	4
	Spiculated mass	5
Calcifications	Benign calcifications	33
	Solitary group of punctate calcifications	4
	Coarse heterogeneous calcification	8
	Amorphous calcification	7
	Fine pleomorphic calcifications	4
	Pleomorphic ductal pattern	1
Architectural distortions and associated features		11
Asymmetries	Asymmetry	23
	Focal asymmetry	12

[a]Classification according to the American College of Radiology [13].

nodules, asymmetries, and distortions, from the following scores: 0, definitely absent; 1, most likely absent; 2, cannot decide; 3, most likely present; and 4, definitely present. For conditions with scores of 3 or 4, the radiologist was required to classify the condition according to the value in Table 2. Next, the radiologist classified the breast composition and finally at the conclusion of this process, a BI-RADS final assessment category was selected.

2.4. Generation and Digitization of the Mammograms. The process of generating film and digital images is shown in Figure 1. The original mammograms consisted of screening CR images that were stored in the picture archiving and communication system (PACS) at FSFBUH. Routine screening digital mammograms were acquired using an Agfa CR 85-X (Agfa HealthCare NV, Belgium), hereafter referred to as CR, with a resolution of 20 pixels/mm (508 dpi), 50 μm per pixel, and a 14-bit grayscale from an 18 × 24 cm chassis and a 3,560 × 4,640-pixel matrix. The derived mammogram images were generated as follows: as we had no screen-film images, the CR images were printed under the supervision of a radiologist

on an 18 × 24 cm film with a digital Agfa Drystar 5503 printing system (Agfa HealthCare NV, Belgium) with a resolution of 508 dpi, 50 μm per pixel, and 14-bit contrast. Data that could be used to identify patients were not included in the printed mammograms. Next, the films were digitized using the following two capture devices: (1) an iCR 612SL specialized digitizer (iCR Company, Torrance, CA) that had a maximum spatial resolution of 875 dpi, a pixel spot of 29 μm, 16 bits per pixel, an optical density (OD) of 3.6, and a cost of $15,000 (hereafter referred to as ICR) and (2) a Lumix DMC-FZ28 digital camera (Panasonic Corporation, Secaucus, NJ, USA) with a 10-megapixel resolution, a focal length of 4.8 to 86.4 mm, a 1/2.33″ charge-coupled device (CCD), ISO 100–6,400, and a cost of $450 (plus $400 for support system and light box). The digital camera is hereafter referred to as LUMIX.

For each patient (case), the following four case studies were obtained: (1) the printed film, hereafter referred to as the FILM, and three images in digital form, including (2) images from the CR (3,560 × 4,640-pixel matrix and 14-bit grayscale), (3) images digitized with the ICR (2,436 × 3,636-pixel matrix and 8-bit grayscale), and (4) images digitized with the LUMIX (2,538 × 3,463-pixel matrix and 8-bit grayscale). This procedure was completed for each of the 70 sample mammograms, producing 280 case studies. DICOM-compliant software that was developed at our institution and previously tested in several studies [21–24] was used to scan, store, and display the cases (see Figure 2).

2.5. Display. At a cost of $8,500, a DICOM-compliant 3-MPixel MD213MG (NEC Display Solutions, Tokyo, Japan) medical-grade grayscale display, with a dot pitch of 0.21 mm, a spatial resolution of 2,048 × 1,536 pixels, maximum luminance of 1,450 cd/m^2, and 10-bit grayscale (i.e., 1,024 gray levels), was used as the display monitor.

2.6. Data Analysis. To compare the AUC for the detection of patients with cancer, analyses of variance (ANOVA) of the pseudovalues of the AUC were performed using DBM-MRMC 2.3 software [21]. Using the BI-RADS final assessment category as the endpoint variable, we classified all readings as negative (BI-RADS, 2 and 3) or positive (BI-RADS, 4A, 4B, 4C, and 5) [9, 12, 18], and we calculated contingency tables for these values, that is, the total true positives (tTP), the total true negatives (tTN), the total of false positives (tFP), and the total of false negatives (tFN). The common diagnostic metrics were calculated for these variables as follows: PPV = tTP/(tTP + tFP), sensitivity = tTP/(tTP + tFN), accuracy = (tTP + tTN)/(total sample), specificity = tTN/(tTN + tFP), and the area under the receiving operating characteristic (ROC) curve (AUC). In addition, we calculated the proportions of true positives TP = tTP/(total sample), the proportions of true negatives TN = tTN/(total sample), the proportions of false positives FP = tFP/(total sample), and the proportions of false negatives FN = tFN/(total sample).

These variables and the difference between the compared modalities were evaluated using generalized estimating equations (GEE) with the IBM SPSS Statistics 19 software (IBM Corp., Armonk, NY, USA). With the purpose of evaluating

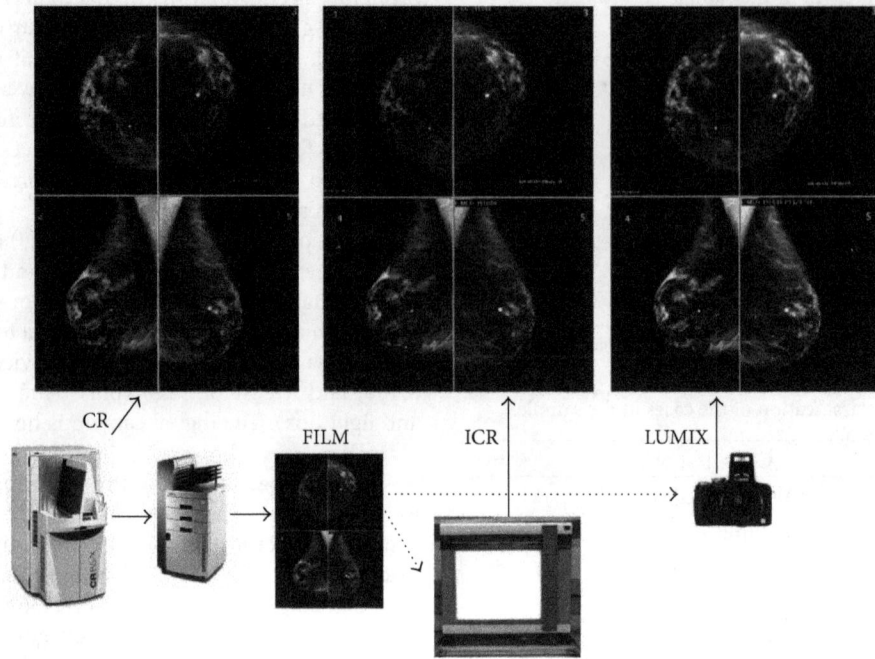

FIGURE 1: Digital image and film generation. CR: computed radiography; FILM: printed film; LUMIX: Lumix DMC-FZ28 digital camera; ICR: iCR 612SL specialized digitizer.

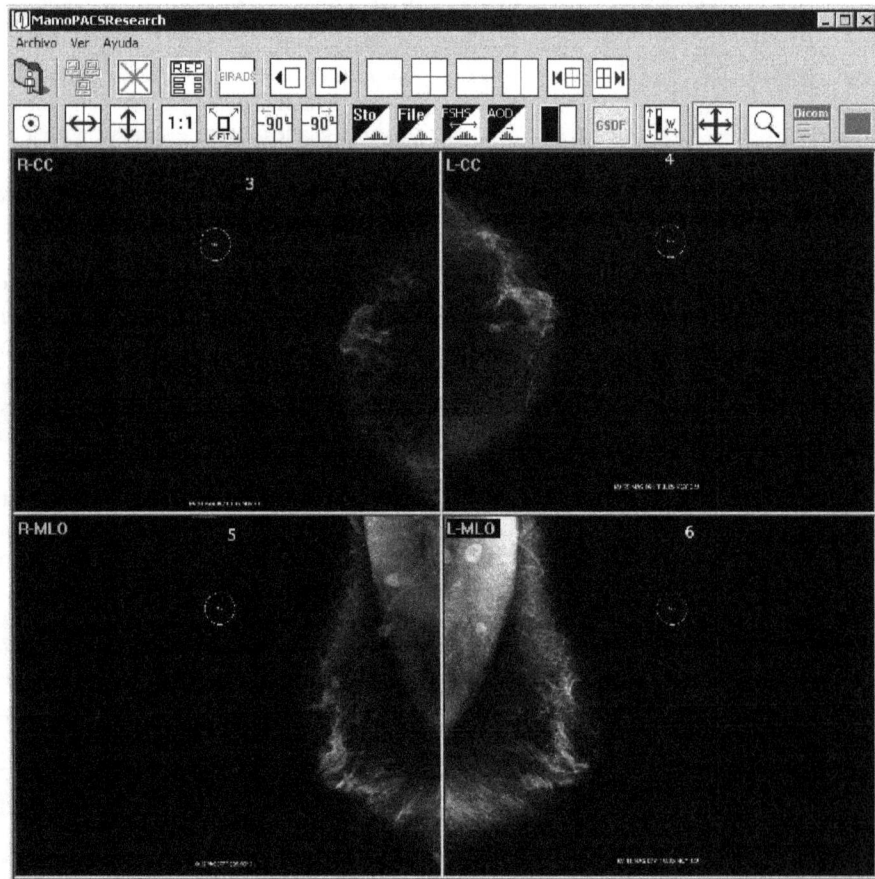

FIGURE 2: Interpretation software. This software is compliant with the Digital Imaging and Communication in Medicine (DICOM) standard.

noninferiority and equivalence, the mean differences and their standard errors were obtained from DBM-MRMC and SPSS software.

The hypothesis test for equivalence was as follows: the null hypothesis Ho was $|$Mean Difference $(I - J)| - \delta = 0$ and the alternative hypothesis Ha was $|$Mean Difference $(I - J)| - \delta < 0$, where I and J are the two modalities compared and δ (delta) is the maximum allowable difference permitted to conclude equivalence or noninferiority, as suggested by several authors in recent years [14–17]. We calculated a $(1-2\alpha)\%$ confidence interval for all comparisons, which is a method to evaluate equivalence [16, 17]. The significance level was set to 5% (i.e., $\alpha = 0.05$) and δ was set to 0.1, as this was the difference established in the sample selection to evaluate the area under the ROC curves. We were interested in evaluating equivalence using lower values for δ, in particular $\delta = 0.05$, to assess the PPV and sensitivity for screening purposes. Finally, we calculated the required value of δ to claim equivalence for each variable and the comparison.

2.7. Procedure. Each radiologist read each case using the following viewing methods: the film in a light box and three viewings on the medical display for digital cases of CR, ICR, and LUMIX. Pairs of patients and devices were presented at random by the software; hence, there were at least 30 different patients before a patient was repeated for any radiologist. At each reading, the radiologist determined the variables mentioned in the section entitled "Observed Variables." Each radiologist received training in the use of the viewer software before the readings were initiated. A pilot study was conducted to determine the usefulness of the viewer software and the interpretation form. The software provides case blinding and several image manipulation tools to adjust the window/level, brightness, and contrasts and histogram tools (e.g., the average optical density, histogram equalization, and full-scale histogram stretching). These tools may be combined with the overall zoom and the magnifying glass. These tools were available for all images and could be used at the observer's discretion to improve image quality, especially for patients with dense breasts and amorphous calcifications. The readings were performed over the course of ten months in two- or four-hour sessions by each radiologist, with no time limitations for each reading.

3. Results

3.1. Mean Values by Device. The mean values, standard error of the mean, and the 95% confidence interval for each device and each calculated variable presented in the data analysis section are shown in Table 3. Each of these means was calculated from 490 observations (70 cases and seven radiologists). The TN ranged from 0.46 to 0.48, the TP ranged from 0.30 to 0.35, the FN ranged from 0.12 to 0.17, and the FP ranged from 0.05 to 0.07. The mean values for the derived variables were as follows: accuracy ranged from 0.77 to 0.82, the PPV ranged from 0.67 to 0.68, sensitivity ranged from 0.64 to 0.74, specificity ranged from 0.87 to 0.90, and the AUC ranged from 0.87 to 0.90.

TABLE 3: Mean values for the calculated variables by device.

Variable[a]	Device	Mean	SE	95% confidence interval Lower	Upper
TN	CR	0.47	0.05	0.36	0.57
	ICR	0.47	0.05	0.36	0.57
	LUMIX	0.46	0.05	0.36	0.57
	FILM	0.48	0.06	0.37	0.59
TP	CR	0.32	0.05	0.23	0.42
	ICR	0.30	0.05	0.21	0.39
	LUMIX	0.32	0.05	0.22	0.41
	FILM	0.35	0.05	0.25	0.45
FN	CR	0.15	0.03	0.08	0.21
	ICR	0.17	0.04	0.10	0.24
	LUMIX	0.16	0.03	0.09	0.22
	FILM	0.12	0.03	0.06	0.18
FP	CR	0.06	0.02	0.03	0.09
	ICR	0.06	0.02	0.03	0.09
	LUMIX	0.07	0.02	0.03	0.10
	FILM	0.05	0.02	0.02	0.08
Accuracy	CR	0.79	0.03	0.73	0.86
	ICR	0.77	0.04	0.70	0.84
	LUMIX	0.78	0.03	0.72	0.84
	FILM	0.82	0.03	0.76	0.89
PPV	CR	0.68	0.06	0.57	0.79
	ICR	0.68	0.06	0.56	0.79
	LUMIX	0.67	0.06	0.56	0.79
	FILM	0.68	0.06	0.57	0.79
Sensitivity	CR	0.69	0.06	0.58	0.80
	ICR	0.64	0.06	0.52	0.76
	LUMIX	0.67	0.05	0.57	0.77
	FILM	0.74	0.06	0.63	0.84
Specificity	CR	0.88	0.03	0.83	0.94
	ICR	0.88	0.03	0.83	0.94
	LUMIX	0.87	0.03	0.82	0.93
	FILM	0.90	0.03	0.85	0.96
AUC	CR	0.89	0.04	0.81	0.97
	ICR	0.87	0.05	0.77	0.96
	LUMIX	0.88	0.04	0.80	0.96
	FILM	0.90	0.02	0.87	0.94

[a]Each mean was calculated from 490 observations (70 cases and seven radiologists). TN: true negative proportion, TP: true positive proportion, FN: false negative proportion, FP: false positive proportion, PPV: positive predictive value, ROC: receiver operating characteristic, AUC: area under ROC curve, SE: standard error of the mean.

3.2. Mean Difference Values and the Equivalence Test by Paired Devices in Proportion Variables. The mean values of the differences and equivalence tests for the TN, TP, FN, and FP by paired devices are shown in Table 4 (for $\delta = 0.1$) and Table 5 (for $\delta = 0.05$). The mean values of the differences

TABLE 4: Equivalence tests ($\delta = 0.1$) for TN, TP, FN, and FP by paired devices.

Variable[a]	Compared devices		Mean difference ($I - J$)	SE	(1-2α)% confidence interval for equivalence testing		z	P	H
	(I) device	(J) device			Lower	Upper			
TN	LUMIX	ICR	−0.006	0.0102	−0.023	0.011	−9.22	<0.001	Ha
	LUMIX	CR	−0.006	0.0084	−0.020	0.008	−11.20	<0.001	Ha
	LUMIX	FILM	−0.016	0.0098	−0.032	0.000	−8.53	<0.001	Ha
	ICR	CR	0.000	0.0091	−0.015	0.015	−10.96	<0.001	Ha
	ICR	FILM	−0.010	0.0097	−0.026	0.006	−9.25	<0.001	Ha
	FILM	CR	0.010	0.0067	−0.001	0.021	−13.49	<0.001	Ha
TP	LUMIX	ICR	0.016	0.0098	0.000	0.032	−8.53	<0.001	Ha
	LUMIX	CR	−0.008	0.0104	−0.025	0.009	−8.86	<0.001	Ha
	LUMIX	FILM	−0.031	0.0122	−0.051	−0.011	−5.68	<0.001	Ha
	ICR	CR	−0.024	0.0104	−0.042	−0.007	−7.26	<0.001	Ha
	ICR	FILM	−0.047	0.0135	−0.069	−0.025	−3.94	<0.001	Ha
	FILM	CR	0.022	0.0152	−0.003	0.047	−5.11	<0.001	Ha
FN	LUMIX	ICR	−0.016	0.0098	−0.032	0.000	−8.53	<0.001	Ha
	LUMIX	CR	0.008	0.0104	−0.009	0.025	−8.86	<0.001	Ha
	LUMIX	FILM	0.031	0.0122	0.011	0.051	−5.68	<0.001	Ha
	ICR	CR	0.024	0.0104	0.007	0.042	−7.26	<0.001	Ha
	ICR	FILM	0.047	0.0135	0.025	0.069	−3.94	<0.001	Ha
	FILM	CR	−0.022	0.0152	−0.047	0.003	−5.11	<0.001	Ha
FP	LUMIX	ICR	0.006	0.0102	−0.011	0.023	−9.22	<0.001	Ha
	LUMIX	CR	0.006	0.0084	−0.008	0.020	−11.20	<0.001	Ha
	LUMIX	FILM	0.016	0.0098	0.000	0.032	−8.53	<0.001	Ha
	ICR	CR	0.000	0.0091	−0.015	0.015	−10.96	<0.001	Ha
	ICR	FILM	0.010	0.0097	−0.006	0.026	−9.25	<0.001	Ha
	FILM	CR	−0.010	0.0067	−0.021	0.001	−13.49	<0.001	Ha

[a]Each comparison was calculated from 980 observations (70 cases, seven radiologists, and two devices). TN: true negative proportion, TP: true positive proportion, FN: false negative proportion, FP: false positive proportion, SE: standard error of the mean, Ho: null hypothesis, Ha: alternative hypothesis for testing equivalence, α: significance of the test (0.05), δ: difference of the means allowed to achieve equivalence, z: test for difference of compared devices, that is, $z = (|\text{Difference } (I - J)| - \delta)/\text{SE}$, H: retained hypothesis equivalence at δ level ("Ha" indicates equivalence achieved and "Ho" indicates failing to reject the null hypothes).
Ho: $|\text{difference } (I - J)| - \delta = 0$.
Ha: $|\text{difference } (I - J)| - \delta < 0$.

and the equivalence tests for accuracy, the PPV, sensitivity, specificity, and the AUC by paired devices are shown in Table 6 (for $\delta = 0.1$) and Table 7 (for $\delta = 0.05$). For both Tables 4 and 6, the equivalence test was preformed using $\delta = 0.1$ as the original setting of this study in terms of the AUC, and in addition, a value of $\delta = 0.05$ was included as explained previously. In the last column of both Tables 5 and 7, the calculated value of δ required in each variable and comparison to conclude equivalence between the compared devices is presented.

The absolute differences for the calculated variables were as follows: the TN differences ranged from 0.000 to 0.016, the TP differences ranged from 0.008 to 0.047, the FN differences ranged from 0.008 to 0.047, and the FP differences ranged from 0.000 to 0.016. For $\delta = 0.1$, all the comparisons in Table 4 showed equivalence ($P < 0.001$); for $\delta = 0.05$, most comparisons (20) showed equivalence (P values ranged from 0.0001 to 0.0347), while no significant differences were found

for the TP and the FN in LUMIX versus FILM and ICR versus FILM; nevertheless, the required δ to achieve equivalence was near 0.05 (0.051 and 0.069).

3.3. Mean Difference Values and the Equivalence Test by Paired Devices for the Derived Variables. The absolute differences for the derived variables were as follows: the accuracy differences ranged from 0.010 to 0.057, the PPV differences ranged from 0.002 to 0.009, the sensitivity differences ranged from 0.017 to 0.100, the specificity differences ranged from 0.000 to 0.031, and the AUC differences ranged from 0.009 to 0.034. For $\delta = 0.1$, all the comparisons for accuracy, the PPV, and specificity showed equivalence (P values ranged from 0.0001 to 0.004), while for sensitivity, again, the LUMIX-FILM and ICR-FILM comparisons showed no significant differences.

For $\delta = 0.1$ in the AUC tests, the comparisons showed statistical equivalence for the following pairs: LUMIX versus CR ($P = 0.008$), LUMIX versus FILM ($P = 0.04$), and FILM

TABLE 5: Equivalence tests ($\delta = 0.05$) for TN, TP, FN, and FP by paired devices.

Variable[a]	Compared devices		$(1-2\alpha)$% confidence interval for equivalence testing		z	P	H	δ_e
	(I) device	(J) device	Lower	Upper				
TN	LUMIX	ICR	−0.023	0.011	−4.31	<0.001	Ha	0.023
	LUMIX	CR	−0.020	0.008	−5.23	<0.001	Ha	0.020
	LUMIX	FILM	−0.032	0.000	−3.43	<0.001	Ha	0.032
	ICR	CR	−0.015	0.015	−5.48	<0.001	Ha	0.015
	ICR	FILM	−0.026	0.006	−4.10	<0.001	Ha	0.026
	FILM	CR	−0.001	0.021	−5.98	<0.001	Ha	0.021
TP	LUMIX	ICR	0.000	0.032	−3.43	<0.001	Ha	0.032
	LUMIX	CR	−0.025	0.009	−4.04	<0.001	Ha	0.025
	LUMIX	FILM	−0.051	−0.011	−1.59	0.06	Ho	0.051
	ICR	CR	−0.042	−0.007	−2.45	0.007	Ha	0.042
	ICR	FILM	−0.069	−0.025	−0.23	0.41	Ho	0.069
	FILM	CR	−0.003	0.047	−1.82	0.03	Ha	0.047
FN	LUMIX	ICR	−0.032	0.000	−3.43	<0.001	Ha	0.032
	LUMIX	CR	−0.009	0.025	−4.04	<0.001	Ha	0.025
	LUMIX	FILM	0.011	0.051	−1.59	0.06	Ho	0.051
	ICR	CR	0.007	0.042	−2.45	<0.001	Ha	0.042
	ICR	FILM	0.025	0.069	−0.23	0.41	Ho	0.069
	FILM	CR	−0.047	0.003	−1.82	0.03	Ha	0.047
FP	LUMIX	ICR	−0.011	0.023	−4.31	<0.001	Ha	0.023
	LUMIX	CR	−0.008	0.020	−5.23	<0.001	Ha	0.020
	LUMIX	FILM	0.000	0.032	−3.43	<0.001	Ha	0.032
	ICR	CR	−0.015	0.015	−5.48	<0.001	Ha	0.015
	ICR	FILM	−0.006	0.026	−4.10	<0.001	Ha	0.026
	FILM	CR	−0.021	0.001	−5.98	<0.001	Ha	0.021

[a]Each comparison was calculated from 980 observations (70 cases, seven radiologists, and two devices). TN: true negative proportion, TP: true positive proportion, FN: false negative proportion, FP: false positive proportion, SE: standard error of the mean, Ho: null hypothesis, Ha: alternative hypothesis for testing equivalence, α: significance of the test (0.05), δ: difference of the means allowed to achieve equivalence, z: test for difference of compared devices, that is, $z = (|\text{Difference } (I - J)| - \delta)/\text{SE}$, H: retained hypothesis equivalence at δ level ("Ha" indicates equivalence achieved and "Ho" indicates failing to reject the null hypothes).
Ho: $|\text{difference } (I - J)| - \delta = 0$.
Ha: $|\text{difference } (I - J)| - \delta < 0$.

versus CR ($P = 0.03$); in the LUMIX versus ICR comparison, equivalence was not found, but the noninferiority of LUMIX was observed ($P = 0.046$); for ICR versus CR and ICR versus FILM, neither equivalence nor noninferiority was noted, and the required values of δ to achieve equivalence were 0.133 and 0.118, respectively. However, for $\delta = 0.05$, less consistency was observed. Only paired comparisons for the PPV were all equivalent ($P < 0.001$); for specificity, the LUMIX versus FILM comparison failed to show equivalence ($P = 0.15$). For $\delta = 0.05$, in paired comparisons for the other derived variables, few tests confirmed equivalence: three showed equivalent accuracy, three showed equivalent sensitivity, and only one showed an equivalent AUC.

In general, the required values for δ to confirm equivalence ranged from 3.4% to 8.4% for accuracy, 0.7% to 1.5% for the PPV, 6.8% to 14.2% for sensitivity, 3.8% to 6.1% for specificity, and 7.3% to 13.3% for the AUC.

3.4. Evaluations of Dense Breasts. We ran the GEE analysis using only the readings of cases with heterogeneously dense and extremely dense (21 patients by 7 radiologists: 147 interpretations) breasts for the TP, TN, FP, FN, VPP, sensitivity, specificity, and accuracy evaluations (see Table 8). The best values of these variables were observed for FILM; nevertheless, the values for the digital images were very similar regardless of whether the device is of highest or lowest resolution, that is, CR or LUMIX, respectively. In pairwise comparisons between the high-resolution device (CR) and the low-resolution devices (ICR and LUMIX), the results were as follows: between CR and ICR, no significant differences were observed for the TP, TN, FP, FN, VPP, VPN, sensitivity, specificity, and accuracy; between CR and LUMIX, no significant differences were observed for the TP, TN, FP, FN, sensitivity, specificity, and accuracy. In pairwise comparisons between printed film (FILM) and the three digital devices (CR, ICR,

TABLE 6: Equivalence tests for accuracy, PPV, sensitivity, specificity, and AUC by paired devices ($\delta = 0.1$).

Variable[a]	Compared devices		Mean difference $(I - J)$	SE	$(1\text{-}2\alpha)\%$ confidence interval for equivalence testing		z	P	H
	(I) device	(J) device			Lower	Upper			
Accuracy	LUMIX	ICR	0.010	0.0142	−0.013	0.034	−6.31	<0.001	Ha
	LUMIX	CR	−0.014	0.0133	−0.036	0.008	−6.46	<0.001	Ha
	LUMIX	FILM	−0.047	0.0152	−0.072	−0.022	−3.49	<0.001	Ha
	ICR	CR	−0.024	0.0138	−0.047	−0.002	−5.46	<0.001	Ha
	ICR	FILM	−0.057	0.0162	−0.084	−0.031	−2.65	0.004	Ha
	FILM	CR	0.033	0.0164	0.006	0.060	−4.11	<0.001	Ha
PPV	LUMIX	ICR	−0.003	0.0052	−0.011	0.006	−18.69	<0.001	Ha
	LUMIX	CR	−0.007	0.0049	−0.015	0.001	−18.79	<0.001	Ha
	LUMIX	FILM	−0.009	0.0050	−0.017	−0.001	−18.28	<0.001	Ha
	ICR	CR	−0.005	0.0047	−0.012	0.003	−20.32	<0.001	Ha
	ICR	FILM	−0.007	0.0040	−0.013	0.000	−23.08	<0.001	Ha
	FILM	CR	0.002	0.0027	−0.002	0.007	−35.76	<0.001	Ha
Sensitivity	LUMIX	ICR	0.035	0.0203	0.001	0.068	−3.21	<0.001	Ha
	LUMIX	CR	−0.017	0.0219	−0.053	0.019	−3.78	<0.001	Ha
	LUMIX	FILM	−0.065	0.0246	−0.105	−0.025	−1.43	0.08	Ho
	ICR	CR	−0.052	0.0210	−0.087	−0.017	−2.28	0.01	Ha
	ICR	FILM	−0.100	0.0256	−0.142	−0.057	−0.02	0.49	Ho
	FILM	CR	0.048	0.0316	−0.004	0.100	−1.66	0.05	Ha
Specificity	LUMIX	ICR	−0.012	0.0192	−0.043	0.020	−4.60	<0.001	Ha
	LUMIX	CR	−0.012	0.0158	−0.038	0.014	−5.59	<0.001	Ha
	LUMIX	FILM	−0.031	0.0182	−0.061	−0.001	−3.79	<0.001	Ha
	ICR	CR	0.000	0.0173	−0.028	0.028	−5.79	<0.001	Ha
	ICR	FILM	−0.019	0.0182	−0.049	0.011	−4.42	<0.001	Ha
	FILM	CR	0.019	0.0124	−0.001	0.040	−6.50	<0.001	Ha
AUC	LUMIX	ICR	0.009	0.0646	−0.098	0.115	−1.412	0.08	Ho
	LUMIX	CR	−0.016	0.0350	−0.073	0.042	−2.408	0.008	Ha
	LUMIX	FILM	−0.026	0.0412	−0.093	0.042	−1.807	0.04	Ha
	ICR	CR	−0.024	0.0660	−0.133	0.084	−1.145	0.13	Ho
	ICR	FILM	−0.034	0.0508	−0.118	0.049	−1.292	0.10	Ho
	FILM	CR	0.010	0.0463	−0.066	0.086	−1.945	0.03	Ha

[a]Each comparison was calculated from 980 observations (70 cases, seven radiologists, and two devices). PPV: positive predictive value, ROC: receiver operating characteristic, AUC: area under ROC curve, SE: standard error of the mean, Ho: null hypothesis, Ha: alternative hypothesis for testing equivalence, α: significance of the test (0.05), δ: difference of the means allowed to achieve equivalence, z: test for difference of compared devices, that is, $z = (|\text{Difference} (I - J)| - \delta)/\text{SE}$, H: retained hypothesis equivalence at δ level ("Ha" indicates equivalence achieved and "Ho" indicates failing to reject the null hypotheses).
Ho: $|\text{difference } (I - J)| - \delta = 0$.
Ha: $|\text{difference } (I - J)| - \delta < 0$.

and LUMIX), the results were as follows: no significant differences were found for the TP and TN, nor for the FP, FN, VPN, specificity, and accuracy, while differences were noted for the sensitivity and VPP between FILM and CR. In comparisons between FILM and ICR and LUMIX, which are digital images with lower resolutions, differences were noted in the TP, FN, VPP, VPN, sensitivity, accuracy, and VPP, and for the specificity between FILM and LUMIX; while no differences were observed for the TP, FP, and VPN. High values for the AUC (ranging from 0.86 to 0.90), with no significant differences, were found among the four devices ($P = 0.186$).

As we found many nonsignificant differences ($P > 0.05$), we performed equivalence analyses, finding δ (delta) values for which equivalence may be claimed with significant values. In this analysis, LUMIX and CR achieved TP equivalent at 4%, while ICR and CR achieved TP equivalent at 2.2%. The TN were equivalent at 7.3% for CR-LUMIX and 6.1% for CR-ICR. Sensitivities were equivalent at 6.5% for CR-LUMIX and 3.6% for CR-ICR. The VPP values were equivalent at 7.5% for CR-LUMIX and 1.8% for CR-ICR. Only for specificity comparisons were the equivalence values larger than 10%. In this analysis, LUMIX and CR achieved AUC values equivalent at 4.9%, while ICR and CR achieved AUC values equivalent at

TABLE 7: Equivalence tests for accuracy, PPV, sensitivity, specificity, and AUC by paired devices ($\delta = 0.05$).

Variable[a]	Compared devices		$(1-2\alpha)\%$ confidence interval for equivalence testing		z	P	H	δ_e
	(I) device	(J) device	Lower	Upper				
Accuracy	LUMIX	ICR	−0.013	0.034	−2.80	0.003	Ha	0.034
	LUMIX	CR	−0.036	0.008	−2.69	0.004	Ha	0.036
	LUMIX	FILM	−0.072	−0.022	−0.20	0.42	Ho	0.072
	ICR	CR	−0.047	−0.002	−1.84	0.03	Ha	0.047
	ICR	FILM	−0.084	−0.031	0.44	0.67	Ho	0.084
	FILM	CR	0.006	0.060	−1.06	0.14	Ho	0.060
PPV	LUMIX	ICR	−0.011	0.006	−9.10	<0.001	Ha	0.011
	LUMIX	CR	−0.015	0.001	−8.68	<0.001	Ha	0.015
	LUMIX	FILM	−0.017	−0.001	−8.20	<0.001	Ha	0.017
	ICR	CR	−0.012	0.003	−9.68	<0.001	Ha	0.012
	ICR	FILM	−0.013	0.000	−1.71	<0.001	Ha	0.013
	FILM	CR	−0.002	0.007	−17.47	<0.001	Ha	0.007
Sensitivity	LUMIX	ICR	0.001	0.068	−0.76	0.22	Ho	0.068
	LUMIX	CR	−0.053	0.019	−1.49	0.07	Ho	0.053
	LUMIX	FILM	−0.105	−0.025	0.61	0.73	Ho	0.105
	ICR	CR	−0.087	−0.017	0.09	0.54	Ho	0.087
	ICR	FILM	−0.142	−0.057	1.94	0.97	Ho	0.142
	FILM	CR	−0.004	0.100	−0.08	0.47	Ho	0.100
Specificity	LUMIX	ICR	−0.043	0.020	−2.00	0.023	Ha	0.043
	LUMIX	CR	−0.038	0.014	−2.43	0.008	Ha	0.038
	LUMIX	FILM	−0.061	−0.001	−1.05	0.15	Ho	0.061
	ICR	CR	−0.028	0.028	−2.90	0.002	Ha	0.028
	ICR	FILM	−0.049	0.011	−1.68	0.05	Ha	0.049
	FILM	CR	−0.001	0.040	−2.47	0.007	Ha	0.040
AUC	LUMIX	ICR	−0.098	0.115	−0.638	0.26	Ho	0.115
	LUMIX	CR	−0.073	0.042	−0.980	0.16	Ho	0.073
	LUMIX	FILM	−0.093	0.042	−0.592	0.28	Ho	0.093
	ICR	CR	−0.133	0.084	−0.387	0.35	Ho	0.133
	ICR	FILM	−0.118	0.049	−0.308	0.38	Ho	0.118
	FILM	CR	−0.066	0.086	−0.865	0.19	Ho	0.086

[a]Each comparison was calculated from 980 observations (70 cases, seven radiologists, and two devices). PPV: positive predictive value, ROC: receiver operating characteristic, AUC: area under ROC curve, SE: standard error of the mean, Ho: null hypothesis, Ha: alternative hypothesis for testing equivalence, α: significance of the test (0.05), δ: difference of the means allowed to achieve equivalence, z: test for difference of compared devices, that is, $z = (|\text{Difference} (I - J)| - \delta)/\text{SE}$, H: retained hypothesis equivalence at δ level ("Ha" indicates equivalence achieved and "Ho" indicates failing to reject the null hypotheses).
Ho: $|\text{difference } (I - J)| - \delta = 0$.
Ha: $|\text{difference } (I - J)| - \delta < 0$.

7.3%. Compared to FILM, AUC values of LUMIX and ICR were equivalent at 3.8% and 5.2%, respectively, while CR was equivalent at 6.8%.

3.5. The Evaluation of Amorphous Calcifications. To evaluate this point, we ran the GEE analysis using only the readings of cases with amorphous calcifications (7 patients evaluated by 7 radiologists, with a total of 49 interpretations for each device) for the TP, TN, FP, FN, VPP, sensitivity, specificity, and accuracy. There were no true negatives nor false positives, and thus the mean value of the VPP was 1.0 and the sensitivity, TP, FN, and accuracy values were all equal to 0.63, while the VPN,

specificity, TN, and FP were 0.0. There were no significant differences in the sensitivity, TP, and FN ($P = 0.133$). The results of the comparisons of TP for LUMIX and ICR versus CR (i.e., the original reference image) were as follows: a larger TP mean for LUMIX (0.65) compared to CR (0.63), but with no significant difference ($P = 0.053$). The CR was greater than the ICR, but again with no significant difference ($P = 1.0$). The results of comparisons of the TP for LUMIX and ICR versus FILM (which is a derived image printed from the original CR) were as follows: larger TP were observed for FILM (0.71) but with no significant differences among CR, ICR, or LUMIX (this is an expected result, as the overall analysis was

TABLE 8: Evaluation of dense breasts. Mean values, pairwise comparisons, and observed delta for equivalence for TP, TN, FP, sensitivity, specificity, accuracy, VPP, VPN, and AUC.[a]

	TP	TN	FP	FN	SEN	SPE	ACC	VPP	VPN	AUC
Device (resolution)										
CR ($3,560 \times 4,640$)	0.46	0.33	0.05	0.16	0.74	0.86	0.78	0.77	0.53	0.86
ICR ($2,436 \times 3,636$)	0.46	0.30	0.08	0.16	0.74	0.79	0.76	0.76	0.53	0.90
LUMIX ($2,538 \times 3,463$)	0.45	0.29	0.10	0.17	0.73	0.75	0.73	0.73	0.53	0.88
FILM	0.51	0.33	0.05	0.11	0.82	0.88	0.84	0.86	0.53	0.90
Tests of model effects										
Chi-square	26.01	7.25	7.25	9.26	12.70	16.52	24.84	10.23	10.02	4.82
Degree of freedom	3	3	3	3	3	3	3	3	3	3
P value	0.026	0.064	0.064	0.026	0.005	0.001	0.000	0.017	0.018	0.186
Pairwise comparisons										
CR versus ICR										
Bonferroni's significance	1.000	1.000	1.000	1.000	1.000	0.944	1.000	0.568	1.000	0.304
Delta for equivalence	0.022	0.061	0.061	0.022	0.036	0.0155	0.068	0.018	0.0	0.073
CR versus LUMIX										
Bonferroni's significance	1.000	0.223	0.223	1.000	1.000	0.063	0.518	0.011	0.424	1.000
Delta for equivalence	0.040	0.073	0.073	0.040	0.065	0.0176	0.093	0.075	0.001	0.049
FILM-CR										
Bonferroni's significance	0.094	1.000	1.000	0.094	0.048	1.000	0.078	0.009	0.380	0.532
Delta for equivalence	0.091	0.026	0.026	0.091	0.0144	0.068	0.0102	0.0134	0.0	0.068
FILM-ICR										
Bonferroni's significance	0.045	0.662	0.662	0.045	0.016	0.449	0.005	0.009	1.000	1.000
Delta for equivalence	0.083	0.069	0.069	0.083	0.0138	0.0172	0.0133	0.0139	0.0	0.038
FILM-LUMIX										
Bonferroni's significance	0.042	0.193	0.193	0.042	0.014	0.046	0.000	0.010	0.147	1.000
Delta for equivalence	0.097	0.084	0.084	0.097	0.0154	0.0197	0.0154	0.0199	0.001	0.052

[a]Each mean was calculated from 147 observations (21 cases and seven radiologists). TP: true positive proportion, TN: true negative proportion, FN: false negative proportion, FP: false positive proportion, PPV: positive predictive value, SEN: sensibility; SPE: specificity; ACC: accuracy, ROC: receiver operating characteristic, AUC: area under ROC curve, δ: difference of the means allowed to achieve equivalence (i.e., to claim equivalence with a significant value).

not significant). As we found no significant differences ($P > 0.05$), we performed equivalence analyses, finding δ values for which equivalence may be claimed with significant values. In this analysis, the LUMIX was equivalent to CR at 10.8% and ICR was equivalent to CR at 14.1%. With respect to the printed FILM, δ (delta) value was lower for LUMIX (14%) while the CR (the original and the larger digital image) delta value was 19.7%.

4. Discussion

The values observed for the AUC for each device ranged from 0.87 to 0.90. These accuracies were higher than the assumed value accuracy used in the sample size calculation for this study (i.e., 0.75). In the paired comparisons, low differences were observed for most derived variables; for PPV, which is one of the most important variables in mammography [4–6], all values were inferior to 0.9% (0.009). In contrast, the largest differences identified among the paired comparisons were 10.0% (0.1) for sensitivity in a comparison of ICR and FILM. Readings from the LUMIX, which was the lowest-cost device in this study, were equivalent to CR in terms of accuracy, the PPV, sensitivity, specificity, and the AUC for $\delta = 0.1$. This is

important because the LUMIX images were obtained after printing CR images on film and digitizing them with the camera, which may deteriorate the quality of these images. Comparing LUMIX with ICR (which is approximately 30 times more expensive than LUMIX), equivalence was observed in terms of the accuracy, the PPV, sensitivity, specificity, and noninferiority in the AUC for $\delta = 0.1$.

In this study, we used a value of $\delta = 0.1$ (10%) to evaluate equivalence, which was the value used in this study and in our previous studies to calculate sample size [22, 25, 26]. With this value, global equivalence was observed. As a post hoc evaluation, $\delta = 0.05$ was used to be more conservative with respect to sensitivity. With this value, fewer comparisons showed equivalence or noninferiority at a cutoff significance level of 0.05. The value of the required δ to achieve equivalence may be useful in further calculations of the required sample size for similar studies.

Our results regarding dense breasts suggest that the lower digital images of the digital camera LUMIX and especially ICR are still good quality low-cost alternatives, even for heterogeneously dense and extremely dense breasts, with better performance observed for ICR than LUMIX. The results provide support for the hypothesis that there are no significant differences between the interpretations of CR mammography examinations and soft copy examinations produced by a specialized film digitizer or a digital camera. In the same sense, our results suggest that the lower quality digital images of the digital camera LUMIX are still of adequate quality even for amorphous calcifications.

A limitation of our study, as explained before, is that all of the mammography images in this study were obtained from a referral hospital with high standards and quality equipment. Therefore, the results of this study should be revisited using film-screen mammography images obtained at rural hospitals with equipment and technical standards of varying quality. Another limitation of this study is the variability between radiologists. Consequently, it was more difficult to obtain significant results when less-than-10% non-inferiority or equivalence margins were selected. A third limitation was the selection procedure to establish this margin, which must be a predetermined clinically meaningful limit. The researchers of this study did not agree when to set the value at 5% or 10%, or another more appropriate value, for the inferiority or equivalence margin, and of course, this value may be different for each calculated variable (e.g., sensitivity, specificity, the PPV, and the AUC). This disagreement is due to ignorance regarding the actual values that these variables take on when our radiologists interpret routine mammograms. In this sense, this study is a first estimation of these values and can be used to improve sample size calculations in further studies at our hospital.

In our analysis, the specificity and AUC values were high, whereas the accuracy and PPV were moderate, and the sensitivity values were relatively low. Other studies have compared film-screen mammography with digitized film [8–10, 12] and reported no significant differences in their diagnostic accuracy, but these studies were not equivalence or noninferiority evaluations, and no report about the power test was presented. In our study, we measured mean AUC values that were similar to or higher than those reported by Powell et al. [8], Gitlin et al. [9], and Pisano et al. [10] and by Lewin et al. using FFDM [18]. To our knowledge, no previous study has evaluated the equivalence or noninferiority performance of observers reading mammograms that were captured with a digital camera.

Screening may have side effects associated with false positives. Previous studies have shown that one in three test results leads to biopsy, which often turns out to be negative for cancer. Even when cancer is ruled out by the pathology results, high rates of testing generate a 33% cost overrun for screening [27] and cause permanent anxiety in patients [1]. Moreover, 50% of cancer patients survive regardless of whether they were enrolled in a screening program [2]. The risk of false positives should be maintained below 10% by comparing successive screening mammograms at intervals of 12 to 18 months until the patient's life expectancy is less than 10 years [22]. In our study, low FP were noted (<6.7%) for all devices, which is important for reducing stress in patients and the health system costs.

The principal difference of our study with respect to previous studies is that in this evaluation an equivalence or

noninferiority study was performed, instead of a conventional two-sided hypothesis test setting for the nonequivalence testing as was the case in many previously published articles, in which no statistical differences were reported without reporting the power test.

5. Conclusion

In conclusion, our findings suggest that telemammography screening programs may be provided to underserved populations at a low cost, using a film digitizer or a digital camera, with differences of 10% in terms of the sensitivity, specificity, positive predictive value, accuracy, and the area under the receiver operating characteristic curve. To increase the power in equivalence or noninferiority tests for margin differences of 5%, more images or more observers must be included in the study.

Competing Interests

The authors declare that there is no conflict of interests regarding the publication of this paper.

Acknowledgments

The authors thank the radiologists who carried out the readings, their institutions, and the National Department of Science, Technology and Innovation for funding this study (Grant 1204-545-31353).

References

[1] L. L. Humphrey, M. Helfand, B. K. S. Chan, and S. H. Woolf, "Breast cancer screening: a summary of the evidence for the U.S. Preventive Services Task Force," *Annals of Internal Medicine*, vol. 137, no. 5, part 1, pp. 347–360, 2002.

[2] S. W. Fletcher and J. G. Elmore, "Mammographic screening for breast cancer," *The New England Journal of Medicine*, vol. 348, no. 17, pp. 1672–1680, 2003.

[3] R. Shyyan, S. Masood, R. A. Badwe et al., "Breast cancer in limited-resource countries: diagnosis and pathology," *Breast Journal*, vol. 12, no. 1, pp. S27–S37, 2006.

[4] D. B. Kopans, "The positive predictive value of mammography," *American Journal of Roentgenology*, vol. 158, no. 3, pp. 521–526, 1992.

[5] K. Kerlikowske, D. Grady, J. Barclay, E. A. Sickles, A. Eaton, and V. Ernster, "Positive predictive value of screening mammography by age and family history of breast cancer," *The Journal of the American Medical Association*, vol. 270, no. 20, pp. 2444–2450, 1993.

[6] L. Liberman, A. F. Abramson, F. B. Squires, J. R. Glassman, E. A. Morris, and D. D. Dershaw, "The breast imaging reporting and data system: positive predictive value of mammographic features and final assessment categories," *American Journal of Roentgenology*, vol. 171, no. 1, pp. 35–40, 1998.

[7] A. Venkatesan, P. Chu, K. Kerlikowske, E. A. Sickles, and R. Smith-Bindman, "Positive predictive value of specific mammographic findings according to reader and patient variables," *Radiology*, vol. 250, no. 3, pp. 648–657, 2009.

[8] K. A. Powell, N. A. Obuchowski, W. A. Chilcote, M. M. Barry, S. N. Ganobcik, and G. Cardenosa, "Film-screen versus digitized

mammography: assessment of clinical equivalence," *American Journal of Roentgenology*, vol. 173, no. 4, pp. 889–894, 1999.

[9] J. N. Gitlin, A. K. Narayan, C. A. Mitchell et al., "A comparative study of conventional mammography film interpretations with soft copy readings of the same examinations," *Journal of Digital Imaging*, vol. 20, no. 1, pp. 42–52, 2007.

[10] E. D. Pisano, E. B. Cole, E. O. Kistner et al., "Interpretation of digital mammograms: comparison of speed and accuracy of soft-copy versus printed-film display," *Radiology*, vol. 223, no. 2, pp. 483–488, 2002.

[11] T. Kamitani, H. Yabuuchi, H. Soeda et al., "Detection of masses and microcalcifications of breast cancer on digital mammograms: comparison among hard-copy film, 3-megapixel liquid crystal display (LCD) monitors and 5-megapixel LCD monitors: an observer performance study," *European Radiology*, vol. 17, no. 5, pp. 1365–1371, 2007.

[12] E. D. Pisano, C. Gatsonis, E. Hendrick et al., "Diagnostic performance of digital versus film mammography for breast-cancer screening," *The New England Journal of Medicine*, vol. 353, no. 17, pp. 1773–1783, 2005.

[13] E. A. Sickles, C. J. D'Orsi, and L. W. Bassett, "ACR BI-RADS® mammography," in *ACR BI-RADS® Atlas, Breast Imaging Reporting and Data System*, A. C. O. Radiology, Ed., American College of Radiology, Reston, Va, USA, 5th edition, 2013.

[14] W. Chen, N. A. Petrick, and B. Sahiner, "Hypothesis testing in noninferiority and equivalence MRMC ROC studies," *Academic Radiology*, vol. 19, no. 9, pp. 1158–1165, 2012.

[15] H. Jin and Y. Lu, "A non-inferiority test of areas under two parametric ROC curves," *Contemporary Clinical Trials*, vol. 30, no. 4, pp. 375–379, 2009.

[16] J.-P. Liu, M.-C. Ma, C.-y. Wu, and J.-Y. Tai, "Tests of equivalence and non-inferiority for diagnostic accuracy based on the paired areas under ROC curves," *Statistics in Medicine*, vol. 25, no. 7, pp. 1219–1238, 2006.

[17] N. A. Obuchowski, "Testing for equivalence of diagnostic tests," *American Journal of Roentgenology*, vol. 168, no. 1, pp. 13–17, 1997.

[18] J. M. Lewin, C. J. D'Orsi, R. E. Hendrick et al., "Clinical comparison of full-field digital mammography and screen-film mammography for detection of breast cancer," *American Journal of Roentgenology*, vol. 179, no. 3, pp. 671–677, 2002.

[19] S. Velasco, O. Bernal, A. Salazar, J. Romero, Á. Moreno, and X. Díaz, "Availability of mammography services in Colombia," *Revista Colombiana de Cancerología*, vol. 18, no. 3, pp. 101–108, 2014.

[20] N. A. Obuchowski, "Sample size tables for receiver operating characteristic studies," *American Journal of Roentgenology*, vol. 175, no. 3, pp. 603–608, 2000.

[21] A. J. Salazar, D. A. Aguirre, J. Ocampo, X. A. Diaz, and J. C. Camacho, "Diagnostic accuracy of digitized chest X-rays using consumer-grade color displays for low-cost teleradiology services: a multireader-multicase comparison," *Telemedicine and e-Health*, vol. 20, no. 4, pp. 304–311, 2014.

[22] A. J. Salazar, D. A. Aguirre, J. Ocampo, J. C. Camacho, and X. A. Díaz, "DICOM gray-scale standard display function: clinical diagnostic accuracy of chest radiography in medical-grade gray-scale and consumer-grade color displays," *American Journal of Roentgenology*, vol. 202, no. 6, pp. 1272–1280, 2014.

[23] A. J. Salazar, J. Romero, O. Bernal, A. Moreno, S. Velasco, and X. Díaz, "Evaluation of low-cost telemammography screening configurations: a comparison with film-screen readings in vulnerable areas," *Journal of Digital Imaging*, vol. 27, no. 5, pp. 679–686, 2014.

[24] A. J. Salazar, J. Romero, O. Bernal, A. Moreno, S. Velasco, and X. Díaz, "Effects of the DICOM grayscale standard display function on the accuracy of medical-grade grayscale and consumer-grade color displays for telemammography screening," in *Proceedings of the 9th International Seminar on Medical Information Processing and Analysis*, vol. 8922 of *Proceedings of SPIE*, Mexico City, Mexico, November 2013.

[25] A. J. Salazar, J. C. Camacho, and D. A. Aguirre, "Agreement and reading time for differently-priced devices for the digital capture of X-ray films," *Journal of Telemedicine and Telecare*, vol. 18, no. 2, pp. 82–85, 2012.

[26] A. J. Salazar, J. C. Camacho, and D. A. Aguirre, "Comparison between differently priced devices for digital capture of X-ray films using computed tomography as a gold standard: a multireader-multicase receiver operating characteristic curve study," *Telemedicine and e-Health*, vol. 17, no. 4, pp. 275–282, 2011.

[27] J. G. Elmore, M. B. Barton, V. M. Moceri, S. Polk, P. J. Arena, and S. W. Fletcher, "Ten-year risk of false positive screening mammograms and clinical breast examinations," *The New England Journal of Medicine*, vol. 338, no. 16, pp. 1089–1096, 1998.

23

Characterizing the Use of Telepsychiatry for Patients with Opioid Use Disorder and Cooccurring Mental Health Disorders in Ontario, Canada

Brittanie LaBelle,[1] **Alexandra M. Franklyn,**[1] **Vicky PKH Nguyen,**[1] **Kathleen E. Anderson,**[1] **Joseph K. Eibl,**[1] **and David C. Marsh** (ID)[1,2]

[1]*Northern Ontario School of Medicine, 935 Ramsey Lake Rd., Sudbury, ON, Canada P3E 2C6*
[2]*Canadian Addiction Treatment Centers, 13291 Yonge St., Ste. 403., Richmond Hill, ON, Canada L4E 4L6*

Correspondence should be addressed to David C. Marsh; dmarsh@nosm.ca

Academic Editor: Malcolm Clarke

Rural patients with opioid use disorder (OUD) face a variety of barriers when accessing opioid agonist therapy (OAT) and psychiatric services, due to the limited supply of physicians and the vast geographic area. The telemedicine allows for contact between patients and their physician—regardless of physical distance. *Objective.* We characterize the usage of telemedicine to deliver psychiatric services to patients with OUD in Ontario, as well as traits of treatment-seeking patients with opioid dependence and concurrent psychiatric disorders. *Methodology.* A retrospective cohort study was conducted using an administrative database for patients who received psychiatric services via telemedicine between 2008 and 2014 and who also had OUD. *Results.* We identified 9,077 patients with concurrent opioid use and other mental health disorders who had received psychiatric services via telemedicine from 2008 to 2014; 7,109 (78.3%) patients lived in Southern Ontario and 1,968 (21.7%) in Northern Ontario. Telemedicine was used more frequently to provide mental health services to patients residing in Northern Ontario than Southern Ontario. *Conclusion.* Telemedicine is increasingly being utilized throughout Ontario for delivering mental health treatment. There is an opportunity to increase access to psychiatric services for patients with opioid dependence and concurrent psychiatric disorders through the use of the telemedicine.

1. Introduction

Nonmedical use of prescription opioids is a major public health crisis across North America [1]. From 2010 to 2011, 6% of the adult population reported nonmedical prescription opioid use, making opioids the second most prevalent nonprescribed drug following cannabis. This rate becomes further inflated among high-school students (15%–20%) and in marginalized populations [2, 3]. In Canada alone, opioid use disorder (OUD) and opioid-related overdoses account for 12% of deaths in patients between the ages of 25 and 34 [4]. Furthermore, in Ontario, opioid-related overdoses are responsible for higher death rates than all other nonprescribed drugs combined [1, 5].

Methadone and buprenorphine are long-acting synthetic opioid agonists prescribed to treat OUD [6]. Health Canada's Best Practice Guideline on Methadone Maintenance Treatment identifies opioid agonist therapy (OAT) with methadone or buprenorphine as key treatment and prevention strategies to manage OUD and its associated consequences [6]. OAT is associated with a reduction in the use of other substances, criminal activity, mortality, and risk behaviors for blood-borne pathogens [6]. Moreover, OAT leads to improvements in physical and mental health, social functioning, and quality of life among people with OUD [6].

In Ontario, patients who initiate OAT require supervised daily dosing of methadone or buprenorphine in a specialized addiction clinic, family physician's office, or pharmacy [7]. Patients residing in Northern Ontario face a variety of barriers when accessing these healthcare services, such as a lack of primary care physicians and the need to travel long distances to access care [7]. Considering the long-lasting nature of OAT, patients are required to stay connected with healthcare providers over an extended period of time and, consequently, patients receiving OAT are even more affected by the barriers of living in Northern Ontario.

The barriers experienced by patients seeking OAT mirror those experienced by patients seeking psychiatric services in Northern Ontario. As of 2009, the overall psychiatrist supply in Ontario was 15.7 psychiatrists per 100,000 people [8]. Delivery of health care in Ontario is provided across fourteen Local Health Integration Networks (LHINs). Southern Ontario is comprised of LHIN 1–12, and Northern Ontario is comprised of LHIN 13-14. Of the fourteen LHINs, Northern Ontario LHINs are far below average; North Western Ontario (LHIN 14) had the third lowest psychiatrist supply (approximately 7 per 100,000) and North Eastern Ontario (LHIN 13) had the sixth lowest psychiatrist supply (approximately 8.5 per 100,000) [8]. This problem is compounded by the vast geographic landscape of Northern Ontario, where many communities are isolated from larger urban centers. This—combined with the chronic shortage of physicians—leaves many Northern Ontario mental health patients without access to treatment.

To address these barriers, the provincial government invested in the Ontario Telemedicine Network (OTN), which is now one of the largest telemedicine networks in the world [9]. Telemedicine allows for the exchange of health information between providers and their patients from various locations across the province through two-way secure videoconferencing [9, 10]. The Ministry of Health and Long-Term Care reports that 49% of total telemedicine activity is used to service Northern Ontario [9]. According to the OTN, mental health and addiction medicine accounted for 72% of total patients served by telemedicine from 2012 to 2013 [11].

With a high prevalence of mental health disorders and many patients' needs being unmet, more research is required to better understand how access to mental health treatment can be improved, particularly for those patients seeking treatment in geographically isolated regions. In this study, we characterize patients with mental health disorders and concurrent OUD who receive psychiatric services via OTN. We also quantify resource usage by region, with a focus on Northern Ontario versus Southern Ontario.

2. Methods

2.1. Cohort Definition. We conducted a retrospective cohort study of all patients with OUD (as defined by having been engaged in OAT at some point during the study period) who also received psychiatric services for a mental health diagnosis other than substance use disorder via telemedicine from 2008 to 2014. Patients were at least 15 years or older and were residents of Ontario. Due to the nature of data collection (primarily derived from physician billing data), undiagnosed patients were not captured.

2.2. Data Sources. Data was accessed through the Institute for Clinical and Evaluative Sciences (ICES) through the Data Access Services division. The Ontario Drug Benefit (ODB) database was used to identify all patients engaged in OAT

and to determine their past medication use of methadone or buprenorphine. The ODB database contains detailed records of all prescriptions dispensed to Ontario residents eligible for public drug coverage. In Ontario, residents are eligible for public drug coverage if they are aged 65 or older, reside in a long-term care facility, are disabled, are receiving social benefits for income support, or have high prescription drug costs relative to their net household income. Health system utilization was identified using the Canadian Institute for Health Information (CIHI) and the National Ambulatory Care Reporting System, and hospital admissions were identified using the CIHI Discharge Abstract Database. All diagnosis information from physician visits was determined using billing data from the physician Ontario Health Insurance Plan (OHIP) database. OHIP covers physician services for all permanent residents of Ontario. We obtained patient location of residence and demographic information from the Ontario Registered Persons Database, which contains a unique entry for each resident who has ever received insured health services. Patient information was linked anonymously across databases using encrypted 10-digit health card numbers. The linking protocol has been described extensively elsewhere [12, 13] and is used routinely for health system research in Ontario [14–16].

2.3. Telemedicine Definition. Patients' data were irrevocably stripped of personal identifiers before being made available for analysis. Telemedicine care via the OTN was identified by physician OHIP billing codes, which are specific to telemedicine appointments. Patients were included in the observational cohort if they had received a psychiatric diagnosis between 2008 and 2014 (listed in Table 1) from a psychiatrist via OTN (billing codes listed in Table 1) and if they were also diagnosed with OUD, as defined by having engaged in OAT at some point during the study period. It is worth noting that the treatment of OUD may or may not have involved physician care by OTN for the purposes of this study. Only patient data files with attachment to one of the 14 LHINs in Ontario were included in the analysis to aid subcohort analysis.

2.4. Methadone/Buprenorphine Subgroups. Patients with OUD were identified as any patient with a prescription for methadone or buprenorphine for the treatment of OUD during the study window. Patients receiving methadone or buprenorphine for whom the cost of medication was covered by the patient through direct payment or through private insurance or federal government insured health benefits were not identifiable in the data set. Previous research has demonstrated that the vast majority of patients treated with OAT in Ontario utilize the Ontario Drug Benefit program and therefore would be included in this analysis [17]. All patients were at least 15 years or older (to exclude data entry errors for newborns; patients < 18 years of age accounted for <1% of cohort) and were eligible for public drug coverage through the ODB plan. In Ontario, methadone is dispensed exclusively in liquid formulation, with very few exceptions; therefore, patients prescribed methadone in a tablet formulation (with a medication possession ratio

TABLE 1: ICD-9 mental health classifications.

291: alcoholic psychosis, delirium tremens, Korsakov's psychosis

292: drug psychosis

295: schizophrenia

296: manic depressive psychosis, involutional melancholia

297: paranoid states

298: other psychoses

300: anxiety neurosis, hysteria, neurasthenia, obsessive compulsive neurosis, reactive depression

301: personality disorders (e.g., paranoid personality, schizoid personality, obsessive compulsive personality)

302: sexual deviations

303: alcoholism

304: drug dependence, drug addiction

305: tobacco abuse

307: habit spasms, tics, stuttering, tension headaches, anorexia nervosa, sleep disorders, enuresis

309: adjustment reaction

311: depressive or other nonpsychotic disorders, not elsewhere classified

313: behaviour disorders of childhood and adolescence

314: hyperkinetic syndrome of childhood

greater than 20% over a one-year period) were excluded due to the likelihood that methadone was being administered for chronic pain management, despite being coded for addiction therapy in the billing records. We also excluded patients with missing information regarding place of residence, age, or gender. For evaluation of response to OAT, all patients were followed from their date of OAT initiation to the date of treatment discontinuation (patient did not receive a prescription for methadone or buprenorphine within 30 days of their last prescription), death, one-year follow-up, or end of the study period (December 31st, 2014).

2.5. Geographical Definition. Patient's postal codes were used to determine location of residence. Ontario is divided into 14 health care planning areas called Local Health Integration Networks (LHINs) for administrative, funding, and planning purposes. For geographic comparisons, patient data files with attachment to the North East (LHIN 13) or North West LHINs (14) were included in the Northern Ontario group for analysis compared to the remaining LHINs for Southern Ontario.

2.6. Costing. In order to calculate costs of OTN, the following variables were considered: inpatient hospitalization, same day surgery, National Ambulatory Care Reporting System (visits to ED, dialysis clinics, and cancer clinics), ODB, rehabilitation, complex and continuing care cost, home care services, OHIP physician billing, OHIP lab billings, OHIP nonphysician billings, OHIP shadowing billings, Family Health Organization/Family Health Network physician capitation cost, long-term care cost, Ontario Mental Health Reporting System Metadata admissions to designated mental health beds, and assisted device costs.

2.7. Analysis. Descriptive statistics were summarized for baseline characteristics of patients, and standardized differences were used to compare characteristics between Northern

Ontario and Southern Ontario patients. Standardized differences < 0.1 are generally not considered to be meaningful [18]. All statistical analyses were carried out using SPSS (V.22). We used ArcGIS to produce maps illustrating the distribution of telemedicine delivery and distance between patients and their provider for each LHIN. Geographic boundaries by LHIN were retrieved from Statistics Canada [19].

2.8. Ethics Review. This study was approved by the Research Ethics Board of Laurentian University, Sudbury, Ontario, and by Sunnybrook Hospital, Toronto, Ontario.

3. Results

From 2008 to 2014, we identified 9,077 publicly insured patients who had received OAT and who received a mental health diagnosis from a psychiatrist through telemedicine. Of these, 7,109 (78.3%) lived in Southern Ontario and 1,968 (21.7%) lived in Northern Ontario. Patient characteristics by geographic location are summarized in Table 3. When comparing patients residing in Northern Ontario to those in Southern Ontario, it was found that Northern Ontario contains a concurrent disorder patient cohort with higher percentage of females (52.74% versus 45.17%), less education (23% high school completion rate versus 27%), greater impoverishment (47.46% in lowest income quintile versus 42.90%), and less enrolment in primary care (46.70% versus 51.68%).

Telemedicine is used more frequently to deliver psychiatric services in Northern Ontario than Southern Ontario for patients with concurrent OUD (Figure 1). In fact, telemedicine accounts for 26% to 40% of all psychiatry delivery to patients with concurrent disorders living in Northern Ontario LHINs; this number ranges from 1% to 30% in Southern Ontario LHINs (Figure 1). Overall, when moving from Southeastern Ontario towards Northwestern Ontario, there

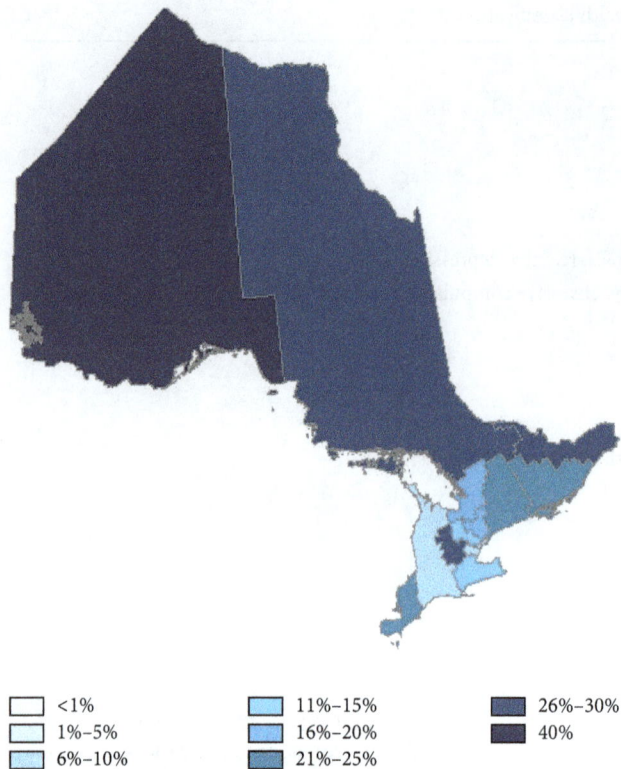

☐ <1%		☐ 11%–15%		■ 26%–30%	
☐ 1%–5%		■ 16%–20%		■ 40%	
☐ 6%–10%		■ 21%–25%			

FIGURE 1: Percent of patients with concurrent disorders receiving psychiatric services via telemedicine.

is increased telemedicine usage for delivering psychiatry to patients with concurrent disorders.

Concurrent disorder patients residing in Northern Ontario live farther away from their physicians (Figure 2) (median distance 341 km; interquartile range 73 km–901 km) compared with patients residing in Southern Ontario (median distance 75 km; interquartile range 33 km–142 km) (Table 1). Moreover, patients live a greater distance from their psychiatrist when they are receiving their services through telemedicine. In fact, LHIN 14 has the largest median distance between patients receiving mental health services and their provider (median distance 900 km), followed by LHIN 11 (median distance 322 km), LHIN 2 (median distance 136 km), and LHIN 13 (median distance 122 km) (Figure 2). LHIN 7, Toronto Central, has a median distance of only 4 km between patients and psychiatrists when receiving psychiatric services via telemedicine and it also has less than 1% of its patients serviced by telemedicine.

The number of concurrent disorder patients receiving psychiatry via telemedicine has increased from 347 to 5,879 over a period of six years (Table 2). The mean cost per patient of delivering psychiatric services to patients via telemedicine has also increased during this period; therefore, the total cost to the health care system of using telemedicine for mental health services has increased as well. However, we are not able to describe the costs avoided through the provision of care by telemedicine compared to transportation of patients to see the psychiatrist in person within the data utilized for this analysis.

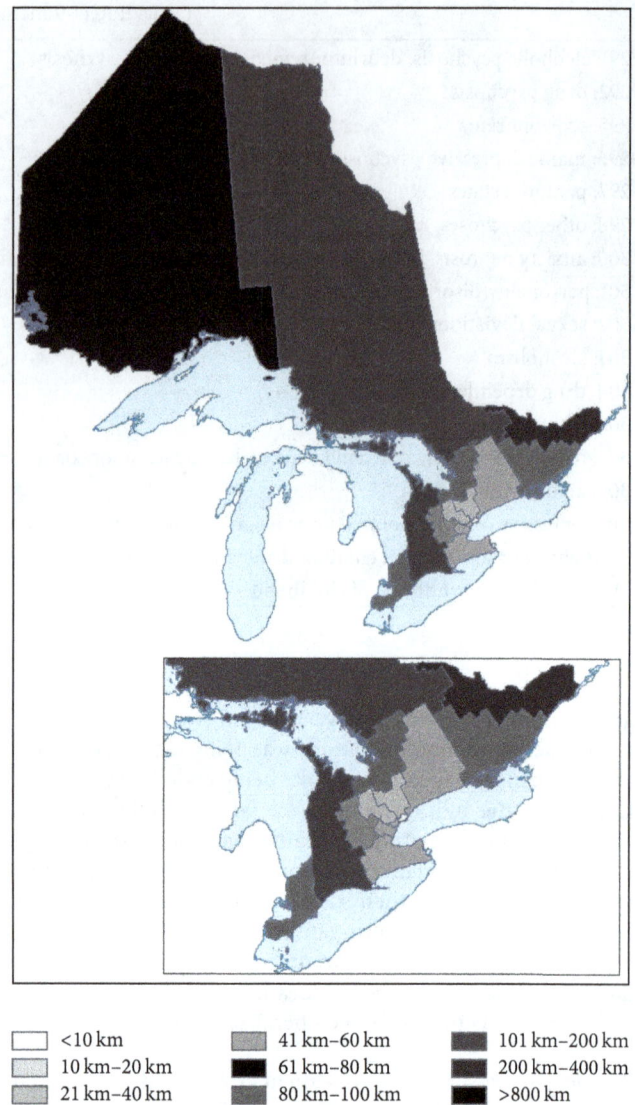

☐ <10 km		■ 41 km–60 km		■ 101 km–200 km	
☐ 10 km–20 km		■ 61 km–80 km		■ 200 km–400 km	
■ 21 km–40 km		■ 80 km–100 km		■ >800 km	

FIGURE 2: Median distances (km) between the residence of patients receiving psychiatry via telemedicine and their provider.

4. Discussion

In the present study, we found that patients with concurrent disorders receive psychiatric services via OTN more often than patients who do not have OUD. Overall, telemedicine is currently heavily utilized for psychiatric service delivery, particularly in Northern and rural regions of Ontario. Notably, OTN is utilized more frequently in the geographically dispersed regions of Northern Ontario.

In Ontario, opioid agonist therapy can be delivered remotely via telemedicine where the physician is remote and a nurse, pharmacist, or clinic staff interact with the patient and dispense observed or carried methadone or buprenorphine doses. While there are no set determinants where virtual addiction medicine clinics can be established, historically, Northern, rural, and remote regions were almost exclusively serviced by telemedicine [7]. More recently, virtual clinics are also being established in urban centers due to the enhanced

TABLE 2: Utilization of telemedicine for psychiatry and mean cost to the health care system.

Year	Total number of patient visits	Number of unique patients	Mean (± SD) cost to the system per patient
2008	1,588	347	6,455.64 ± 11,268.20
2009	4,768	943	7,255.15 ± 12,189.21
2010	11,507	1,748	7,852.72 ± 12,868.25
2011	22,998	3,175	8,417.49 ± 13,189.38
2012	46,150	4,300	9,003.45 ± 15,719.65
2013	56,261	5,254	9,605.53 ± 17,107.52
2014	58,863	5,879	-

TABLE 3: Characteristics of patients receiving psychiatry via telemedicine by geographic location.

Variable	Overall N = 9,077	Southern Ontario N = 7,109	Northern Ontario N = 1,968
Age, yr			
Median (IQR)	36 (29–45)	36 (29–45)	35 (28–44)
Gender, N (%)			
Female	4,249 (46.81%)	3,211 (45.17%)	1,038 (52.74%)
Male	4,828 (53.19%)	3,898 (54.83%)	930 (47.26%)
Median (IQR) distance between patient residence and physician address (km)	86 (36–262)	75 (33–142)	341 (73–901)
Median percentage of high school completion, % (IQR)	26 (21–31)	27 (22–32)	23 (19–27)
Number enrolled in primary care, N (%)	4,593 (50.60%)	3,674 (51.68%)	919 (46.70%)
Income quintile, N (%)			
Missing	23 (0.25%)	15 (0.21%)	8 (0.41%)
1	3,984 (43.89%)	3,050 (42.90%)	934 (47.46%)
2	2,058 (22.67%)	1,664 (23.41%)	394 (20.02%)
3	1,385 (15.26%)	1,089 (15.32%)	296 (15.04%)
4	981 (10.81%)	789 (11.10%)	192 (9.76%)
5	646 (7.12%)	502 (7.06%)	144 (7.32%)

efficiency of allowing a single physician to service multiple clinic locations regardless of the clinic location or setting.

The heightened demand for telemedicine in isolated regions indicates a need to provide a model of care that overcomes geographical isolation. For this reason, telemedicine is particularly important in Northern Ontario, where there are geographic barriers to accessing services due to the uneven distribution of limited physician supply in a vast geographic area. Similar to patients enrolled in OAT [7], the concurrent disorder cohort residing in Northern Ontario live a greater median distance from their physicians than patients in Southern Ontario. To address this issue, telemedicine can provide a platform for physicians to provide psychiatric care to patients living further away with little to no travel for both the physician and patients.

We also found that the number of patients receiving psychiatry via telemedicine increased from 2008 to 2014. This can be explained by a number of factors, including the increased demand for psychiatry and the billing incentive [20] that is associated with providing treatment via telemedicine. The increase in OTN has resulted in better access to mental health services—including OAT—throughout Northern and Southern Ontario and a decrease in travel time for patients [10, 21]. In addition, the Ontario Ministry of Health and Long-Term Care have reported that Northern travel costs have been reduced by an estimated $25,000,000 annually [9].

Telemedicine is a key solution for increasing access to mental health services for patients with concurrent disorders, particularly for those patients living in isolated regions. A recent review found not only that telemedicine increases access to psychiatric services, but that it is effective from the perspective of the patient, provider, program, and society as a whole [22]. Patients across diverse clinical populations and receiving a wide-range of services have reported high levels of satisfaction with telemedicine [23]. For example, Lindsay et al. (2015) reported that psychotherapy delivered via telemedicine has similar results as traditional in-person treatment with regard to treatment outcomes, therapeutic relationship, and retention [24]. Moreover, mental health services provided via telemedicine are clinically superior to reduced or no mental health services [23]. A recent study on treatment outcomes in OAT found that patients receiving services via telemedicine had levels of substance use, time to abstinence, and treatment retention rates that were equal to patients receiving OAT face-to-face [25].

Altogether, as many as 55% of patients receiving OAT have a concurrent mental health disorder [26]. Importantly, without treatment that targets both OUD and other psychiatric symptoms, patients have higher rates of continued substance use and overdose, as well as decreased occupational functioning and quality of life [27–29]. Studies have demonstrated that telemedicine-delivered OAT for OUD is an effective treatment modality [20]; therefore, it is reasonable to conclude that telemedicine may also be an effective platform to coordinate mental health care and OAT for patients with concurrent mental health and OUD.

Our study has some limitations that should be noted. Using the data from ICES, we were able to obtain an accurate and complete picture of telemedicine usage for psychiatry delivery; however, because Ontario's publically funded drug benefit plan only covers patients aged 18–65 who are on social assistance, we did not capture patients whose methadone or buprenorphine medication cost was covered by the patient directly or through private insurance or federal government funded insured health benefits. Considering that this study only includes patients who are provincially insured, the lowest income quintiles may be inflated and, consequently, may not entirely represent the clinical population of patients with OUD and concurrent mental health diagnoses. We were also limited in capturing the true opioid dependent population, as only treatment-seeking patients would be captured in our definition. Patients were only included if they had received a prescription for methadone or buprenorphine within the timeframe; however, a patient with OUD who was not seeking treatment would not have met these criteria. Additionally, given the nature of secondary data, we were unable to evaluate the patient experience, including whether the patient was satisfied with OTN care that they received.

This study also has many strengths, one of which being its large sample size. With over 9,000 patients in our study, we were able to characterize the use of telemedicine to care for patients with OUD and concurrent mental health disorders, further contributing to the existing literature on telemedicine in Ontario. More specifically, we have focused our study on patients who are accessing psychiatry in Northern Ontario, an area that is not well studied. Given the psychiatrist shortage in this region of the province—and the common cooccurrence of OUD in this population—it is important to better understand how telemedicine is being utilized to provide psychiatric care to patients with concurrent disorders throughout the province. Patients in Northern Ontario are often faced with a variety of barriers when accessing treatment; understanding the utilization of telemedicine in this geographic area may enhance care for this patient population.

Telemedicine is increasingly being applied throughout Ontario for delivering mental health treatment to patients with concurrent disorders. Increasing the access to psychiatric care delivered via telemedicine may improve clinical outcomes for patients with OUD and concurrent psychiatric disorders. This is especially true of Northern and rural areas, where physician supply is limited. Future qualitative studies

may aid in measuring telemedicine care outcomes, including patient's perspective of whether OTN achieves the same results as face-to-face care.

The application of telemedicine-delivered mental health and addiction services are very well suited in rural and remote settings. In Ontario, virtual clinics are often employed to service remote communities and include some clinics operating on First Nation reserves in collaboration with the First Nation leadership. While the present study is based on the Ontario context, we believe the findings are generalizable due to high quality video conferencing options being widely available with broadband Internet. It is important to note that not all remote communities will have access to broadband service, and in those instances alternative models may be more appropriate.

Acknowledgments

This study was funded by a Northern Ontario Academic Medicine Association grant and by the Canadian Observational Cohort Collaboration.

References

[1] P. Madadi, D. Hildebrandt, A. E. Lauwers, and G. Koren, "Characteristics of Opioid-Users Whose Death Was Related to Opioid-Toxicity: A Population-Based Study in Ontario, Canada," *PLoS ONE*, vol. 8, no. 4, Article ID e60600, 2013.

[2] B. Fischer, A. Ialomiteanu, A. Boak, E. Adlaf, J. Rehm, and R. E. Mann, "Prevalence and key covariates of non-medical prescription opioid use among the general secondary student and adult populations in Ontario, Canada," *Drug and Alcohol Review*, vol. 32, no. 3, pp. 276–287, 2013.

[3] B. Brands, "Nonmedical use of opioid analgesics among Ontario students," *Can Fam Physician*, vol. 56, no. 3, pp. 256–262, 2010.

[4] T. Gomes, M. M. Mamdani, I. A. Dhalla, S. Cornish, J. M. Paterson, and D. N. Juurlink, "The burden of premature opioid-related mortality," *Addiction*, vol. 109, no. 9, pp. 1482–1488, 2014.

[5] O. o. t. C. C. o. Ontario, *Office of the Chief Coroner Report for 2009-2011*, Ministry of Community Safety and Correctional Services Toronto, 2012.

[6] B. Brands et al., *Best practicesmethadone maintenance treatment*, Health Canada, Ottawa, Canada, 2002.

[7] J. K. Eibl, T. Gomes, D. Martins et al., "Evaluating the Effectiveness of First-Time Methadone Maintenance Therapy Across Northern, Rural, and Urban Regions of Ontario, Canada," *Journal of Addiction Medicine*, vol. 9, no. 6, pp. 440–446, 2015.

[8] P. Kurdyak, *Universal coverage without universal access: a study of psychiatrist supply and practice patterns in Ontario. Open Med*, vol. 8, p. e87-99, 8(3, 2014.

[9] O. M. o. H. a. L.-T. Care, "Telemedicine - Improving access to care through technology," 2008, http://www.health.gov.on.ca/en/pro/programs/ecfa/action/primary/pri_telemedecine.aspx.

[10] T. Molfenter, M. Boyle, D. Holloway, and J. Zwick, "Trends in telemedicine use in addiction treatment," *Addiction science & clinical practice*, vol. 10, p. 14, 2015.

[11] S. Stein, *Mental Health Addictions... an OTN Overview*, Centre for Addiction and Mental Health, 2012.

[12] S. Hall, K. Schulze, P. Groome, W. Mackillop, and E. Holowaty, "Using cancer registry data for survival studies: The example of the Ontario Cancer Registry," *Journal of Clinical Epidemiology*, vol. 59, no. 1, pp. 67–76, 2006.

[13] A. R. Levy, "Coding accuracy of administrative drug claims in the Ontario Drug Benefit database," *Can J Clin Pharmacol*, vol. 10, no. 2, pp. 67–71, 2003.

[14] D. N. Juurlink, "Editorial: Proton pump inhibitors and clopidogrel: Putting the interaction in perspective," *Circulation*, vol. 120, no. 23, pp. 2310–2312, 2009.

[15] D. N. Juurlink, T. Gomes, L. L. Lipscombe, P. C. Austin, J. E. Hux, and M. M. Mamdani, "Adverse cardiovascular events during treatment with pioglitazone and rosiglitazone: population based cohort study," *British Medical Journal*, vol. 339, Article ID b2942, 2009.

[16] M. Mamdani, P. Rochon, D. N. Juurlink et al., "Effect of selective cyclooxygenase 2 inhibitors and naproxen on short-term risk of acute myocardial infarction in the elderly," *JAMA Internal Medicine*, vol. 163, no. 4, pp. 481–486, 2003.

[17] J. K. Eibl, K. Morin, E. Leinonen, and D. C. Marsh, "The state of opioid agonist therapy in canada 20 years after federal oversight," *The Canadian Journal of Psychiatry*, vol. 62, no. 7, pp. 444–450, 2017.

[18] M. Mamdani, K. Sykora, P. Li et al., "Reader's guide to critical appraisal of cohort studies: 2. assessing potential for confounding," *British Medical Journal*, vol. 330, no. 7497, pp. 960–962, 2005.

[19] LHIN, "Ontario's LHINs," http://www.lhins.on.ca.

[20] J. K. Eibl, J. Daiter, M. Varenbut, D. Pellegrini, and D. C. Marsh, "Evaluating the effectiveness of telehealth-delivered opioid agonist therapy across Ontario, Canada," *Drug and Alcohol Dependence*, vol. 156, p. e63, 2015.

[21] W. A. Hart, Report of the Methadone Maintenance Treatment Practices Task Force.

[22] D. M. Hilty, D. C. Ferrer, M. B. Parish, B. Johnston, E. J. Callahan, and P. M. Yellowlees, "The effectiveness of telemental health: A 2013 review," *Telemedicine and e-Health*, vol. 19, no. 6, pp. 444–454, 2013.

[23] L. K. Richardson, B. C. Frueh, A. L. Grubaugh, L. Egede, and J. D. Elhai, "Current directions in videoconferencing tele-mental health research," *Clinical Psychology: Science and Practice*, vol. 16, no. 3, pp. 323–338, 2009.

[24] J. A. Lindsay, M. R. Kauth, S. Hudson et al., "Implementation of Video Telehealth to Improve Access to Evidence-Based Psychotherapy for Posttraumatic Stress Disorder," *Telemedicine and e-Health*, vol. 21, no. 6, pp. 467–472, 2015.

[25] W. Zheng, M. Nickasch, L. Lander et al., "Treatment outcome comparison between telepsychiatry and face-to-face buprenorphine medication-assisted treatment for opioid use disorder: A 2-year retrospective data analysis," *Journal of Addiction Medicine*, vol. 11, no. 2, pp. 138–144, 2017.

[26] M. Krausz, P. Degkwitz, A. Kühne, and U. Verthein, "Comorbidity of opiate dependence and mental disorders," *Addictive Behaviors*, vol. 23, no. 6, pp. 767–783, 1998.

[27] J. S. Cacciola, A. I. Alterman, M. J. Rutherford, J. R. McKay, and F. D. Mulvaney, "The relationship of psychiatric comorbidity to treatment outcomes in methadone maintained patients," *Drug and Alcohol Dependence*, vol. 61, no. 3, pp. 271–280, 2001.

[28] K. L. Mills, M. Teesson, J. Ross, S. Darke, and M. Shanahan, "The costs and outcomes of treatment for opioid dependence associated with posttraumatic stress disorder," *Psychiatric Services*, vol. 56, no. 8, pp. 940–945, 2005.

[29] P. J. Carpentier, P. F. M. Krabbe, M. T. van Gogh, L. J. M. Knapen, J. K. Buitelaar, and C. A. J. de Jong, "Psychiatric comorbidity reduces quality of life in chronic methadone maintained patients," *American Journal on Addictions*, vol. 18, no. 6, pp. 470–480, 2009.

24

Use of Expectation Disconfirmation Theory to Test Patient Satisfaction with Asynchronous Telemedicine for Diabetic Retinopathy Detection

Christina I. Serrano,[1] **Vishal Shah** (iD),[2] **and Michael D. Abràmoff** (iD)[3]

[1]*Department of Computer Information Systems, Colorado State University, Fort Collins, CO, USA*
[2]*Department of Business Information Systems, Central Michigan University, Mt. Pleasant, MI, USA*
[3]*Department of Ophthalmology and Visual Sciences, University of Iowa, Iowa City, IA, USA*

Correspondence should be addressed to Vishal Shah; vishal.shah2784@gmail.com

Academic Editor: Max E. Stachura

Objective. The purpose of the study is to extend research on patient satisfaction with telemedicine services by employing the theoretical framework of Expectation Disconfirmation Theory (EDT) for diabetic retinopathy screenings focusing on rural patients. *Method.* Adult subjects (n=220) with diabetes were recruited from a single family practice office in rural Iowa. Subjects completed a "pre" survey concerning their forward-looking perceptions of telemedicine prior to using telemedicine for detection of diabetic retinopathy and a "post" survey after they received recommendations from the distant ophthalmologists. *Results.* All hypotheses of the EDT model were supported. Patient satisfaction is influenced by both patients' expectations ($P<.001$) and disconfirmation of expectations ($P<.001$), and patient satisfaction has a positive impact on patient preference for telemedicine services ($P<.001$). Overall, patients who received telemedicine services were highly satisfied with telemedicine and developed a favorable disposition towards telemedicine services. *Conclusions.* The EDT model is a viable framework to study patient satisfaction of telemedicine services. While previous feasibility studies have shown that telemedicine for diabetic retinopathy screenings yields diagnostic efficacy, this study applies a theoretical framework to demonstrate the viability of telemedicine for diabetic retinopathy screenings in rural areas.

1. Introduction

In the United States (US), diabetic retinopathy is the main cause of blindness among individuals who are 20 to 74 years old [1, 2], and its estimated prevalence is approximately 29 percent among adults with diabetes [3]. Early detection and effective treatment of diabetic retinopathy can prevent blindness and visual loss in almost all cases, but most patients are symptomless until the retinopathy has reached advanced stages [4, 5]. Therefore, the American Diabetes Association, the American Academy of Ophthalmology, and other scientific organizations recommend regular or annual screenings for diabetic retinopathy; however, a significant proportion of people with diabetes do not undergo such examinations [4, 5]. Prior studies show that patient satisfaction is critical in improving patients' decisions to seek appropriate healthcare [6, 7] and this extends to diabetic retinopathy exams [8]. In fact, recent work suggests that telemedicine shows promise for diabetic retinopathy screening, with the potential to increase patient adherence with prescribed disease management practices (e.g., blood sugar control, office visits, and medication compliance), all of which can help prevent end-organ damage [7]. Thus, it becomes important to investigate factors driving patients' satisfaction and preferences, as they are important consumers of healthcare services. To this end, we develop a research model of patients' preference for diabetic retinopathy exams using an asynchronous telemedicine service.

Telemedicine involves the use of telecommunication networks to enable information exchange between healthcare providers and patients who are geographically separated. The two primary modes of telemedicine delivery are store-and-forward, which is asynchronous, and real-time, which is synchronous. With increasing advances in telecommunications networks and technology, telemedicine has shown promise in providing healthcare services to patients remotely [9, 10], particularly to patients in rural areas, who have limited access to many healthcare services locally [11]. In rural areas, access to eye care specialists is limited; thus, applications of telemedicine that enable rural patients to access diabetic retinopathy screenings in their local primary care setting may facilitate their compliance with annual eye exams [12, 13]. Telemedicine has been successfully used to detect asymptomatic retinal abnormalities in Spain [14]. A recent meta-analysis showed that the use of telemedicine for type 2 diabetes mellitus (DM) patients showed promising results for self-management of the disease [15]. Thus, it becomes important to understand the disposition of diabetic patients towards telemedicine. Recent research [7] suggests designing telemedicine systems for diabetic retinopathy screening as well advocates studying patients' perceptions.

For this application of telemedicine to be successful, patients with diabetes will need to have positive perceptions concerning the actual experience of using telemedicine services for these screenings. Research has shown that the application of telemedicine for diabetic retinopathy screenings is both feasible and efficacious [12, 13, 16–20], not only in the US, but also in other countries, such as India [21], South Africa [22], and China [23]. Although some studies have shown that patients reported high levels of satisfaction with using telemedicine for diabetic retinopathy screenings [20, 21, 24–27], none of these studies investigate changes in patient perceptions over time, before and after usage of telemedicine. Furthermore, no studies to date concerning telemedicine patient satisfaction have employed a theoretical framework to investigate patient satisfaction for diabetic retinopathy screenings. Thus, the purpose of this study is to examine the antecedents and consequences of patient satisfaction with telemedicine for diabetic retinopathy screenings by employing the theoretical framework of Expectation Disconfirmation Theory (EDT) with a longitudinal field study design (assessing "pre" and "post" service encounter beliefs) to gain a deeper understanding of this phenomenon.

We concentrate on patient satisfaction for two primary reasons. First, patient satisfaction is considered an important component of the quality of care a patient receives [28, 29] and is linked to improved treatment adherence and clinical outcomes [26, 30]. Second, existing studies of patient satisfaction have been criticized for their lack of conceptual unity and theoretical development [6], particularly within the context of telemedicine [31, 32]. In fact, many telemedicine patient satisfaction studies conflate the concept of satisfaction with related but conceptually distinct factors, such as telemedicine acceptance and perceived quality of care [31, 32]. A recent systematic review of the impact of medical informatics (including telemedicine) on patient satisfaction found that, though most studies report improvements in patient satisfaction, results are largely inconsistent across studies, and few studies focused on patient satisfaction

[33]. Another recent systematic review focused on patient satisfaction with telemedicine for cardiology and found that none of the existing studies provided a clear definition or used the same measures for patient satisfaction [34]. There is a need to conduct scholarly research that grounds the empirical assessment of patient satisfaction within valid theoretical frameworks as scholars and practitioners alike generally agree that patient satisfaction is an important component of healthcare quality [35]. Otherwise, it becomes difficult to synthesize findings across patient satisfaction studies and to build on existing research in this domain.

Some healthcare studies have leveraged the well-established consumer satisfaction literature in the marketing discipline to conceptualize patient satisfaction [36], one of the most prominent theories being EDT [37, 38]. Studies in marketing have applied EDT to predict consumer preferences [39], repurchase intentions [40, 41], and customer loyalty [40, 42]. Furthermore, EDT has been used in the information systems literature to predict technology users' intentions to continue using information technologies [43, 44]. In healthcare, the EDT model also has been adapted in patient satisfaction studies across a variety of contexts, such as medication-related services [45], surgical treatment outcomes [46], waiting times for surgery [47], emergency department services [48], and eHealth Website users [49]. Although several telemedicine studies concerning patient satisfaction exist [50, 51], they are largely atheoretical in nature [31, 32, 35].

We address this gap by building on existing research related to patient satisfaction with telemedicine [50, 51], specifically employing the theoretical framework of EDT to conceptualize and empirically investigate patient satisfaction with telemedicine for diabetic retinopathy screenings. Our goal is to develop a nomological model for patients' preference behavior. Because our research stems from the behavioral psychology paradigm, our focus is on perceptions; i.e., various constructs/variables in the model represent patients' perceptions of reality. It has been well established that perceptions offer valuable insights in studying human behavior, as is the case for this study [52, 53].

Although EDT has been leveraged in patient satisfaction studies, it is important to note that some scholars criticize research that employs theories of consumer behavior in the healthcare context. The criticism stems from the notion that market conditions in the US healthcare industry differ from markets that are traditionally studied in economically driven models [54]. At the same time, some scholars note that healthcare in various countries is increasingly becoming commoditized [55, 56] and patients can be regarded as consumers who make choices about their healthcare [57]. Given these rising shifts in healthcare, it becomes even more important to study patient perceptions and experiences, particularly because patient experiences and satisfaction are core components of the Triple Aim framework aimed at guiding healthcare improvements [58]. Furthermore, from a service point of view, it is important to understand what makes patients satisfied with a specific service. This need is more pronounced when trying to understand the feasibility of implementing telemedicine in rural areas. If potential patients do not "buy in" to the proposed method of medical

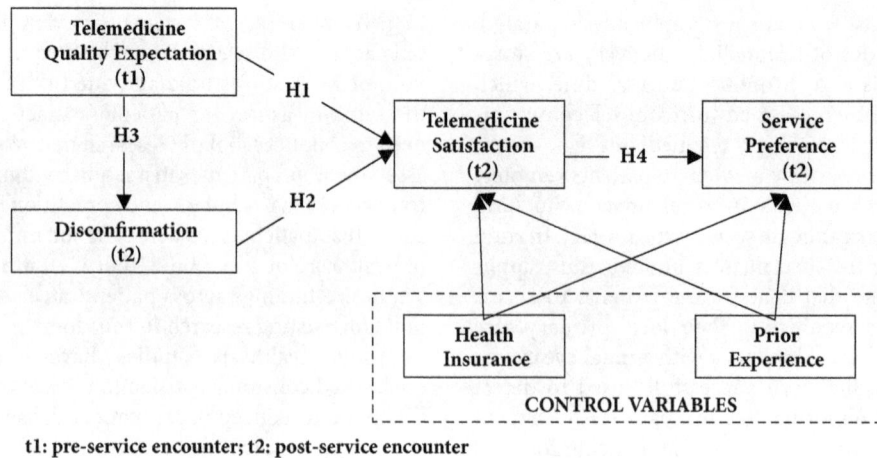

t1: pre-service encounter; t2: post-service encounter

FIGURE 1: Research model.

delivery (in this case, telemedicine), then the exercise of rolling out such a service may be futile. Thus, there is merit to examining patient perceptions. Theories such as EDT provide an overarching framework to examine patient satisfaction and preferences systematically. This pilot study is a step in the same direction.

2. Theoretical Framework and Research Hypotheses

According to EDT, satisfaction is defined as a consumer's judgment that a product or service provided a pleasurable level of consumption-related fulfillment [38]. Satisfaction is determined by consumers' preconsumption expectations about a product or service and expectation disconfirmation; each explained next. Figure 1 shows the research model (because the focus of the study is on telemedicine services, at times, we refer to telemedicine services as services).

Expectations are forward-looking beliefs concerning the service encounter and reflect patient perceptions of the telemedicine encounter prior to receiving this service. A priori expectations represent a baseline standard of comparison or comparative referent, to form postconsumption judgments. In other words, the observed performance of a service postconsumption only has meaning if it is compared to some baseline standard, the a priori expectations [38]. Expectations can be influenced by prior perceived experience and communication messages from salespeople, physicians, nurses, other personnel, and social referents [37].

Expectation disconfirmation is defined as the difference between the preconsumption expectations and postconsumption observed performance [37]. Positive disconfirmation results when the observed performance of the service exceeds preconsumption expectations (i.e., "better than expected"); negative disconfirmation results when the observed performance of the service falls below preconsumption expectations (i.e., "worse than expected"). Both expectations and disconfirmation jointly positively predict consumer satisfaction, and these relationships are explained

through two primary mechanisms: the assimilation effect and the contrast effect.

The positive relationship between expectations and satisfaction is explained through an assimilation effect. When patients observe that their postconsumption service experience performs closely to their preconsumption expectations, they tend to "assimilate" their postconsumption perceptions towards their baseline expectations (i.e., the service "meets expectations") and rely heavily on these initial expectations to form satisfaction judgments [38]. Therefore, we hypothesize the following.

H1: Patient's Preconsumption Expectations Will Positively Influence Satisfaction with Telemedicine Services. The positive relationship between disconfirmation and satisfaction is explained through a contrast effect. When individuals observe postconsumption experiences that deviate notably from their preconsumption expectations, they tend to exaggerate these differences such that service performance observed to be better than expected is considered exceptionally good, whereas service performance that is worse than anticipated is regarded as exceptionally bad [38]. When service performance is perceived as exceptionally good (i.e., positively disconfirmed), individuals are more satisfied as compared to when service performance is perceived as exceptionally bad (i.e., negatively disconfirmed), the latter leading to dissatisfaction.

H2: Patient's Expectation Disconfirmation Will Positively Influence Satisfaction with Telemedicine Services. The relationship between expectations and disconfirmation has yielded mixed findings in empirical studies that have tested EDT [38, 43]. Typically, this relationship has been modeled as negative [42, 59]. Most commonly, the negative relationship between expectations and disconfirmation is explained through a ceiling/floor effect [38]. The "ceiling effect" refers to situations in which the actual performance of the service will be incapable of reaching extremely high (i.e., ceiling) expectation levels, leading to negative disconfirmation. The same applies to low levels of expectations, the lowest level possible representing "the floor." There is a lower likelihood that the actual performance will reach these extreme low (i.e., floor) expectation levels, resulting in positive disconfirmation. In our telemedicine context, this means that the higher the patients' expectations of the telemedicine service, the greater the likelihood of negative disconfirmation (i.e., perceptions of the telemedicine service being "worse than expected"), due to the ceiling effect. Alternatively, the lower the patients' expectations of the telemedicine service, the greater the likelihood of positive disconfirmation (i.e., perceptions of the telemedicine service being "better than expected"), due to the floor effect.

H3: Patient's Preconsumption Expectations Will Negatively Influence Expectation Disconfirmation. The EDT framework has been extended to include cognitive outcomes of satisfaction, including consumer preference, which is positively influenced by satisfaction [60]. In our study, this means that the more satisfied patients are with the telemedicine service, the higher their preference for consuming telemedicine.

H4: Patient Satisfaction Will Positively Influence Preference for Receiving Telemedicine Services. Two control variables, health insurance and prior perceived experience with ophthalmologist exams, which may influence patient satisfaction and patient preference, are included in the research model to control for rival explanations. Though these control variables are outside the scope of the EDT framework, they have been proposed as predisposing and enabling factors that influence patients' utilization of health services and ultimately patient satisfaction [61].

3. Method

3.1. Sample and Procedure. Subjects were recruited from a single family practice office in rural Iowa. In this rural location, patients did not have an alternative to telemedicine, other than refusal of the service, because there were no available ophthalmologists within a reasonable driving distance of the rural community. The study protocol and consent procedures were approved by the Institutional Review Board of the University of Iowa and the family practice office. Written informed consent was obtained from all participants, and the study was performed according to the tenets of the Declaration of Helsinki. One week prior to the start of the study, the family practice office was equipped with a digital camera and other types of equipment required for Internet-based remote diabetic retinopathy screening using telemedicine. This equipment and the system, operational in the Netherlands as well as in the Midwest US, have been described previously [17].

To participate in the study, the patients had to be at least 18 years of age and must have had a diagnosis of diabetes 1 or 2 by the American Diabetes Association criteria. Patients were excluded if they had a documented dilated retinal exam within the last 12 months or had ever utilized telemedicine. By precluding patients with any previous experience with

telemedicine, we attempted to ensure that we indeed measured expectations of first-time users.

Consecutive patients with diabetes that visited the primary care clinic for diabetes follow-up were identified and consented by one of the practice nurses. After explaining the nature of the study and the process of digital photography and remote detection, the "pre" survey was administered. Participants were then photographed by the same nurse with the Topcon NW-200 "nonmydriatic" digital fundus camera (Topcon, Paramus, NJ), with pharmacological dilation if deemed necessary by the nurse. Pharmacological dilation was done for certain patients to ensure sufficient image quality. The nurse entered the digital retinal images and clinical data including Haemoglobin A1c, (HbA1C), duration of diabetes, and any risk factors on a secure Internet website. Within two working days, the images were reviewed electronically by retina fellowship-trained ophthalmologists at the University of Iowa. The International Clinical Diabetic Retinopathy Disease Severity Scale was used to document the severity of diabetic retinopathy and the recommended course of action: annual follow-up with telemedicine or referral to an ophthalmologist for follow-up or treatment [62]. The subject then returned for a follow-up appointment, during which the nurse accessed the subject-specific report via the Internet website and explained the report to the subject. After this interaction, the subject completed the "post" survey. Both "pre" and "post" surveys were paper-based.

3.2. Measures and Descriptive Statistics. Variables used for the analysis were captured before consumption via the presurvey and after consumption via the post survey. Table 1 describes the variables measured in the study and specifies which are included in the research model and post hoc analysis. Given the behavioral perspective of this study, all constructs in this study are perceptual measures. Patients' expectations (preusage) and their preference for telemedicine service prior to (preusage) and after its use (postusage) were measured. The difference between patients' expectations of the quality of the retinal exam (preusage) and their postusage perceptions of the actual quality of the exam is referred to as "disconfirmation." Expectations, disconfirmation, and satisfaction constitute the core ideas of EDT. Because the study is anchored in behavioral psychology, we used Likert scales to measure the various constructs in the study. Expectations about service are a construct that is relevant prior to using the service and hence only measured before use (i.e., pre). Patients' preference for a particular service can change based on their actual experiences with the service; thus, patient preference is measured before and after use of a telemedicine retinal exam (i.e., pre and post). Satisfaction with the service is measured after use (i.e., post). Because we precluded participants with telemedicine experience from participating in the study, we did not measure satisfaction with telemedicine prior to its consumption. According to EDT, expectations and disconfirmation are the primary drivers of satisfaction.

Most scales were measured using a 5-point Likert scale. The two control variables were measured using a binary scale (yes/no), and the disconfirmation variable was computed using a difference score, which is one of two main approaches

TABLE 1: Summary of variables included in the study.

Time	Variable	Description and role in the research model	Scale	Included in Research Model	Included in Post Hoc Analysis
Pre (t1)	Service Quality Expectation	Forward-looking belief concerning the quality of the health service that provides a baseline value of expectations.	Likert scale of 1-5, ophthalmologist's office to telemedicine	Yes	Yes
Pre (t1)	Service Preference	Pre-consumption inclination for face-to-face or telemedicine service that provides a baseline value of service preference. This variable is used in the post-hoc analysis.	Likert scale of 1-5, ophthalmologist's office to telemedicine	No	Yes
Control (t1)	Health Insurance	Possession of health insurance, used as a control variable in the research model.	Binary scale, Yes/No (0=no, 1=yes)	Yes	No
Control (t1)	Prior Service Experience	Prior experience (in the last five years) with ophthalmologist exams, used as a control variable in the research model	Binary scale, Yes/No (0=no, 1=yes)	Yes	No
Post (t2)	Service Quality Performance	Post-consumption judgment that the actual service delivered quality outcomes. This variable is used in the post-hoc analysis.	Likert scale of 1-5, ophthalmologist's office to telemedicine	No	Yes
Post (t2)	Service Preference	Post-consumption preference for face-to-face or telemedicine service.	Likert scale of 1-5, ophthalmologist's office to telemedicine	Yes	Yes
Post (t2)	Disconfirmation	The difference between pre-consumption expectation and post-consumption performance. It may be positive or negative.	Calculated difference score between Service Quality Expectation (t1) and Service Quality Performance (t2)	Yes	No
Post (t2)	Satisfaction	A patient's overall satisfaction with the telemedicine service.	Likert scale of 1-5, Terrible to Very good	Yes	No

a. Four of the variables were measured using a Likert scale of 1-5, ophthalmologist's office to telemedicine, which represents a continuous scale according to the richness of medium (ophthalmologist's office=richer medium; telemedicine=leaner medium).

TABLE 2: Descriptive statistics of variables (n=220).

Time	Variable	Mean	Std. Dev.	Min	Max
Pre (t1)	Service Quality Expectation	3.02	1.19	1	5
Pre (t1)	Service Preference	3.43	1.26	1	5
Control (t1)	Health Insurance	0.95	0.22	0	1
Control (t1)	Prior Service Experience	0.60	0.49	0	1
Post (t2)	Service Quality Performance	4.01	1.16	1	5
Post (t2)	Service Preference	4.22	1.09	1	5
Post (t2)	Disconfirmation	0.99	1.43	-3	4
Post (t2)	Satisfaction	4.50	0.77	2	5

TABLE 3: Post hoc assessment of self-selection bias.

Variable	Study sample		Dropped cases		T-Test	
	Mean	Std. Dev.	Mean	Std. Dev.	t-Stat.	Sig.
Service Quality Expectation (pre)	3.02	1.19	3.4	1.30	1.29	$P=0.23$
Service Preference (pre)	3.43	1.26	3.16	1.28	0.77	$P=0.44$

to measuring disconfirmation [63]. The measure of satisfaction was an overall (global) measure that captured patients' level of satisfaction with the telemedicine service. Satisfaction can be measured at the overall service encounter level or at specific attribute levels to capture multidimensional aspects of satisfaction (e.g., wait time and staff friendliness) [27, 29, 30]. As EDT has not been employed in a telemedicine context, we opted to use an omnibus, unidimensional measure of satisfaction to improve parsimony and generalizability. Furthermore, a unidimensional measure of satisfaction is the most common approach in the consumer satisfaction literature, in which EDT is rooted [38].

A total of 247 respondents submitted both "pre" and "post" surveys. Of the 247 respondents, 101 (40.9%) were male, and 146 (59.1%) were female. Their ages ranged from 24 to 94. The vast majority of patients, 220 of the 247 patients (89.1%), were over 50 years of age, with 27 of the 247 patients (10.9%) being between 24 and 49 years of age. Because demographic data were collected separately and unpaired from the surveys, we were not able to use these variables as covariates in the data analysis. Descriptive statistics reported for age and sex reflect the total pool of respondents (n=247). Due to incomplete responses, 27 observations were dropped, yielding a final sample size of 220 patient surveys reflecting both "pre" and "post" perceptions. Descriptive statistics of the study variables are shown in Table 2. Because patients did not have an alternative to telemedicine, it precluded us from comparing results with a group that may have never wanted to use telemedicine, but our goal was not to compare two groups. Given our goal to develop a model to understand how patients' perceptions about telemedicine changed once

they consumed it firsthand, the current convenience sample served our purpose and can be considered a pilot study. Future studies can extend this work to include a group that receives the same retinopathy screening and diagnosis without the use of telemedicine (i.e., a face-to-face exam).

Because our sample included only those subjects who utilized telemedicine for remote diagnosis (as face-to-face services were not a feasible option), we investigated the extent to which our sample may be positively biased by self-selection. Using unpaired t-tests, we compared (1) answers on patient perceptions reported by subjects who participated in the first part of the telemedicine service only ("pre" survey) and never returned for the telemedicine diagnosis to (2) answers on expectations reported by subjects who experienced the full telemedicine service. This type of extrapolation method is commonly used in survey research to designate subjects who participate "less readily" (e.g., those who partially participate or require prodding to participate) as proxies for those who would choose not to participate at all [64]. Unpaired t-test results shown in Table 3 reveal that there were no significant differences between survey responses provided by subjects who received the telemedicine diagnosis and those who did not complete the study, providing some assurance that self-selection bias was not a major concern with our sample.

4. Results

To test our hypotheses, we used structural equation modeling (SEM) utilizing the partial least squares (PLS) method with SmartPLS version 2.0.M3 [65]. We used SEM because we

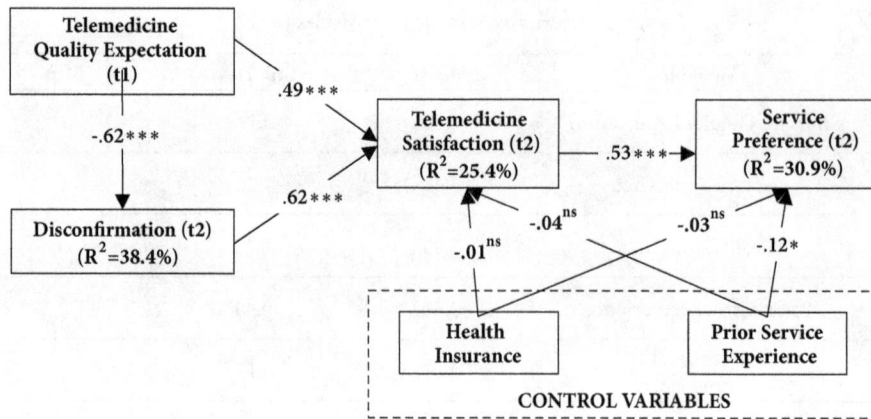

FIGURE 2: PLS analysis results.

TABLE 4: Post hoc comparison of pre- and postbeliefs (n=220).

Variable	Pre-Encounter		Post-Encounter		Paired T-Test	
	Mean	Std. Dev.	Mean	Std. Dev.	t-Stat.	Sig.
Service Quality Expectation (pre)/Actual Service Quality Performance (post)	3.02	1.19	4.01	1.16	-10.28	$P<.001$
Service Preference	3.43	1.26	4.22	1.09	-8.80	$P<.001$

want to explain the interaction of various latent variables (captured by constructs using Likert scales and difference scores) in the nomological model. Since we are proposing a model of patient satisfaction based on EDT, PLS is ideal for our theory building purposes [66–68]. PLS also has been employed in previous telemedicine research that proposes nomological models of psychological constructs [69]. Results of the PLS analysis are shown in Figure 2.

All hypotheses from our research model were supported, as illustrated in Figure 2. Both preusage expectation and disconfirmation positively predicted patient satisfaction with telemedicine (both at $P <.001$), and preusage expectation negatively influenced positive disconfirmation ($P<.001$). These factors explained 25.4% of the variance in patient satisfaction. Furthermore, patient satisfaction significantly and positively impacted patient preference for telemedicine ($P<.001$), explaining 30.9% of the variance in patient preference. The control variable of patients' possession of health insurance was a nonsignificant predictor of patient satisfaction ($P=.87$) and patients' preference for telemedicine services ($P=.62$). We surmise that since all patients had insurance, there was little variability in the data and, hence, its relationship with patient satisfaction and preference was not statistically significant. However, there was a significant negative relationship between the patients' prior experience (within the past five years) with ophthalmologist exams and patients' preference for telemedicine services ($P=.04$). In our case, the results suggest that if patients had prior experience with face-to-face ophthalmologist exams, they were less likely to prefer telemedicine services to screen for diabetic retinopathy. However, prior experience with face-to-face ophthalmologist exams had no significant

effect on patient satisfaction with telemedicine services ($P=.55$).

As a post hoc analysis, we compared "pre" and "post" telemedicine usage beliefs using paired t-tests using SPSS 20.0 [70]. The results (shown in Table 4) reveal significant increases both in patients' perceptions of the quality of telemedicine services and in patients' preferences for telemedicine services (versus face-to-face services) after the patients gained firsthand experience with telemedicine. In other words, patients' perceptions of using telemedicine for diabetic retinopathy screenings significantly improved between the "pre" and "post" periods.

Therefore, the results show that introduction of diabetic retinopathy screening using telemedicine was preferred by patients attending the rural family practice office. The post hoc analysis reveals that telemedicine also improved the perceived quality of the dilated eye exam for these patients. Both perceptions of satisfaction with and preference for telemedicine were stronger after the patients had gained firsthand experience using the service.

5. Discussion

The purpose of this study is to examine patient satisfaction with using telemedicine for diabetic retinopathy screenings leveraging reputed theories of consumer satisfaction from the marketing discipline. Reviews of the telemedicine literature have cited many challenges with patient satisfaction studies, highlighting the limited application of cohesive theories underlying satisfaction [35, 50, 51]. To address this gap, we applied the EDT model using a longitudinal study design to assess patient satisfaction with telemedicine.

Findings from our study indicate that the EDT framework can be leveraged to evaluate patient satisfaction with telemedicine. All hypotheses from the research model were supported. Further analyses of the data also reveal that patient perceptions of telemedicine significantly improved between the preusage and postusage stages. Overall, patients were satisfied with the telemedicine screenings and preferred the telemedicine service over a face-to-face visit. However, patients with prior experience with face-to-face ophthalmology exams were less likely to prefer telemedicine services, even after using telemedicine.

5.1. Contributions to the Literature. By applying the EDT framework, we contribute to the telemedicine literature by offering a new theoretical lens to study patient satisfaction of telemedicine services used to diagnose diabetic retinopathy. Furthermore, expectations, by definition, are forward-looking beliefs concerning the service encounter. Thus, an accurate account of patient expectations requires measurement of patient expectation perceptions *prior to* the telemedicine service encounter. To assess the other constructs of EDT and test the model's relationships, patient perceptions should also be measured *after* the telemedicine service encounter. Hence, this requires a longitudinal design that incorporates a "pre" and "post" assessment of perceptions [37, 43]. A few telemedicine patient satisfaction studies have measured perceptions at two points in time [71], and this study addresses this limitation as well. Furthermore, our study addresses recent calls to study patient satisfaction as a focal outcome within the context of medical informatics and specifically within the subcategory of telemedicine [32].

5.2. Contributions to Practice. The study informs practice in many ways. First, the study focuses on both the antecedents and consequences of patient satisfaction, and these factors may influence the manner in which healthcare providers and administrators deliver healthcare services to improve patient satisfaction. The success of these efforts is important because research has shown that patients who are satisfied with their healthcare services are more likely to adhere to medication and treatment advice [26, 72, 73] and return to their source of care [74].

The findings from our study suggest that both the patients' expectations of telemedicine services and the disconfirmation of these expectations (i.e., better or worse than expected) influence their perceived satisfaction with telemedicine. Thus, while it may seem counter-intuitive, one practical recommendation is that healthcare providers and administrators who wish to implement a successful telemedicine program should take into account patient expectations prior to the patients' actual service encounter and exercise caution so as not to "overhype" the service in order to avoid extreme expectations that would be difficult to positively disconfirm. This recommendation is in line with existing research in information systems that have shown the importance of accounting for preusage expectations, suggesting that those involved in system implementations should ensure they do not deliberately or inadvertently set unrealistically high

expectations when trying to "sell" the benefits of the system to management and users [75].

Recent health informatics studies support this notion as well. A study investigating medical residents' use of iPads in hospital settings found that many residents, prior to the iPad implementation, reported extremely high expectations of the benefits they would reap from using the iPads. However, four months after the deployment, a significant number of residents reported that benefits of the iPad use fell short of their initial expectations, and more residents indicated a preference for pen and paper usage to complete tasks than they did prior to the iPad deployment [76]. Another study evaluated health professionals' expectations versus actual experiences of telemonitoring and found that, although the health professionals expressed high expectations of telemonitoring benefits, they reported actual experiences that were significantly lower than their initial expectations, possibly leading to disappointment [77]. In both of these studies, a characteristic of the respondents in the preusage stage was that they had exceptionally high expectations of the health information technology. Because these extremely high expectations were difficult to positively disconfirm, the actual experiences of the health professionals in the postusage stage substantially fell short of their initial expectations, leading to negative perceptions. Had their baseline expectations been tempered, there would have been a greater likelihood of satisfaction.

Furthermore, while telemedicine has its critics, the fact that 88 out of 220 subjects (40%) with diabetes reported not seeing any eye care provider in the previous five years underscores the need for increased accessibility of the dilated eye exam for these populations, including, but not necessarily limited to, telemedicine. This study builds on existing telemedicine studies and supports the notion that telemedicine solutions for diabetic retinopathy screenings are feasible in the primary care setting [12, 17, 18]. We extend prior telemedicine research by employing the EDT framework. This framework gives researchers a way to understand the factors that drive patient satisfaction. Patient satisfaction with telemedicine has been shown to result in improved adherence to preventive screenings [26] and better clinical outcomes [30]. Hence, positive patient perceptions may enhance compliance with dilated eye exam guidelines, which has been shown to be essential for timely intervention to prevent blindness and vision loss in diabetic patients [13].

5.3. Limitations and Future Research. As with all research, our study is not without limitations. One potential limitation is that we measured variables using single items, an approach that is sometimes criticized [78, 79]. However, recent literature has revealed that single item measures have been shown statistically to be equally as reliable and valid as multiple-item measures of the same constructs [80, 81]. In the job satisfaction literature, for example, there has been growing support for the use of single item measures of satisfaction [82–85], and single items are commonly used to measure patient satisfaction with telemedicine [86, 87]. Single item measures are primarily supported when measuring *concrete* constructs, that is, concepts that respondents would clearly understand and have a similar agreement about the meaning of the concepts [81, 88, 89]. Examples of concrete concepts that are most appropriately measured with single items are likability, quality, satisfaction, and price perception [90], whereas examples of abstract concepts (requiring multiple-item measures) include creativity, power, and culture, as these latter concepts are highly complex in meaning [89]. The concepts measured in our study are all examples of concrete concepts because they are simple, well-formed ideas that are easy for respondents to understand, making them appropriate constructs for single item measures. Furthermore, unidimensional constructs, as modeled in our study, are most suitable for single item measurement [89].

The main advantages to using single item measures are that these measures are less time-intensive and taxing on the respondents and considered more flexible than multiple-item scales [81, 82]. These factors reduce respondents' refusal to participate in studies, which is of particular concern in healthcare contexts, where patients in busy clinical practices are already pressed for time [90]. In our study, the respondents were mostly elderly, which further warranted the use of a short questionnaire to reduce the participation burden. Thus, there are many valid reasons to use short scales with single items [84]. However, that being said, future research can incorporate multiple-item measures of EDT constructs within telemedicine studies, whenever it is feasible. Use of single item measures did not allow patients to differentiate between the precise components of the telemedicine service. However, that is not the goal of the study; the study measures overall patient satisfaction as a first step and the factors that lead to it. Recent research suggests that patient satisfaction can be measured as a multidimensional construct [6]. Future research can look at patient satisfaction with respect to various dimensions of the telemedicine service.

Another possible limitation of the study is that we employ the use of a difference score for the measure of disconfirmation. Difference scores have been a topic of considerable debate in the previous literature [91, 92]. However, difference scores can, in fact, represent an individual change in an unbiased manner and are well suited to measure change [92, 93], as they reduce true score variance and increase the power of the significance tests [92]. Further, difference scores may be used validly in multiple regressions on which the PLS analysis used in this study is based, and there is no reason to avoid their use when they suit the context [94]. However, as there are alternative measures of disconfirmation, future research should also investigate other disconfirmation measures within the scope of telemedicine patient satisfaction.

Furthermore, because this study uses a single cross-section of patients attending a rural family practice office in the Midwest of the US, future studies should address larger samples of rural patients and other populations, including urban underserved patients because it is possible that perceptions may differ across these populations. Additionally, though rural or underserved populations are typically the targeted groups to receive telemedicine services, as telemedicine applications diffuse and become more widespread, it will be important to explore patient perceptions across a wider cross-section of patient populations. Nevertheless, rural populations continue to need innovative solutions to improve

their access to healthcare, so future research should explore the extent to which rural patients would take advantage of telemedicine services.

Another limitation is that the study does not use a control group of patients who underwent diagnosis and treatment in a face-to-face context. The goal of this pilot study was to develop a model to understand factors that lead to telemedicine preference in and of itself based on EDT. Future research can compare two groups of patients, one using telemedicine while the other visits the ophthalmologist in person. In this study, given the sample limitations, we focus on developing a theoretical model explaining patient satisfaction and preferences once they consume/use telemedicine.

Additionally, our sample only includes patients who utilize store-and-forward (asynchronous) telemedicine for diabetic retinopathy screenings and remote diagnosis. Thus, it is not clear whether our findings will generalize to use of telemedicine in other medical specialties or for other types of telemedicine applications (e.g., interactive video telemedicine or telemonitoring). While preliminary research suggests that patients report high levels of satisfaction using both asynchronous and synchronous telemedicine for diabetes care and that the asynchronous mode is widely used for management of chronic disease such as diabetes [27, 95], future research concerning patient satisfaction with telemedicine should test the EDT framework in these different telemedicine contexts.

It is also important to note that the questionnaire asked patients about their visit specifically to an ophthalmologist in the past five years. However, because both optometrists and ophthalmologists provide routine eye care, it may be possible that patients visited an optometrist instead of an ophthalmologist and reported their past experience based on visits to either specialist. Future studies should consider recording experience with both ophthalmologists as well as optometrists.

Further, it should be noted that our study focuses on perceptions, as it is important to understand how patients perceive a new development, such as telemedicine. However, the link between a user's perception and actual behavior and outcomes is contested and largely termed the "intention-behavior" gap in various domains, such as technology use, consumer purchasing behavior, and physical activity [96–100]. Patients may form favorable perceptions of telemedicine but may not actually interact with or use the target technology. However, this concern is mitigated to a certain extent in our study, as the patients were not actively trying to manage or use the equipment but were recipients of the diagnosis. Thus, studying perceptions would be a relevant measure of whether participants will voluntarily be recipients of such asynchronous telemedicine services in the future. Additional longitudinal studies that measure patients' actual future behavior and objective clinical outcomes, to include correlations between these outcomes and patient perceptions, are needed.

Moreover, there are several caveats that researchers should be aware of when focusing on patient-reported expectations (PREM) and/or outcomes (PROM). Although there is research suggesting that patient-reported expectations and perceived outcomes are correlated with objective clinical outcomes [28, 29], this link is still contested in the literature, and some studies have presented counter evidence [101]. It may be possible that patients' perceived satisfaction would bias them towards the service regardless of the actual clinical outcomes. Furthermore, a recent metareview of telemedicine use for chronic disease management found that the majority of studies on telemedicine interventions have reported positive effects with very few studies reporting negative effects, which suggests a publication bias [102]. Future research on telemedicine interventions should consider and account for potential negative consequences of telemedicine.

Another avenue of fruitful research would be to explore additional dimensions of patient perceptions that could influence disconfirmation and patient satisfaction. While our study assessed patients' expectations and perceived preference of the quality of care provided, other dimensions, such as patient perceptions of the teleproviders' competence or the quality of information exchange via telemedicine, may also be relevant to study. Recent work on telemedicine indicates that it can detect not only diabetic retinopathy but also other visually significant eye diseases [103]. Thus, future work can consider studying telemedicine for screening a wider group of ocular diseases. Lastly, because our study is the first to test the EDT framework in a telemedicine context, we only included the key variables relevant to EDT. Future work may build on this model by investigating additional factors (such as social influence and trust in the teleprovider) that may impact patient satisfaction and telemedicine preference.

6. Conclusion

In summary, the results show that patients were very satisfied with their use of telemedicine for diabetic retinal screenings and preferred telemedicine services. Our study found that patients' satisfaction with the telemedicine service leads to a preference to use the service. The study was not aimed at making a comparison between telemedicine and face-to-face services using a randomized controlled trial—i.e., we did not have a control group (face-to-face condition). Our goal was to develop a theoretical model of telemedicine satisfaction and preferences using EDT. Previous studies of telemedicine satisfaction and preferences have been largely descriptive and atheoretical [77, 87, 104–106]. Some studies have described telemedicine implementations in detail [107], while others report a positive preference for telemedicine [108–110]. However, the theoretical mechanism that may guide patients' perceived satisfaction and preference of telemedicine has not been widely studied. This specific pilot study fills this gap in the telemedicine literature by building on the theoretical foundations of EDT.

This pilot study focused on a preliminary examination of patient perceptions. We found that the implementation approach used in this telemedicine study was perceived favorably based on patients' satisfaction with it. The results of the study suggest that telemedicine initiatives aimed at achieving this end, according to the EDT framework, should consider implementation approaches that will provide the patient with a "better than expected" telemedicine experience, which will lead to improved patient satisfaction and greater patient preference for the use of telemedicine. Offering telemedicine services for diabetic retinal screenings in primary care settings has the potential to increase compliance with routine dilated eye exams for diabetic patients. Future research can investigate this link in greater detail.

Conflicts of Interest

None of the authors have conflicts of interest that may impact the manuscript. One of the authors has been funded by the National Institutes of Health (NIH 01 EY018853, R01 EY019112, R01 EY017451, and R01 EB004640) and the Department of Veterans Affairs (I01 CX000119); is inventor on patents assigned to the University of Iowa, not the subject of this study; and is Founder, President and Director for IDx LLC, a company that has developed an autonomous diagnostic AI for diabetic retinopathy. None of these conflicts of interest are related to the subject of this study.

Acknowledgments

This study was supported by the Wellmark Foundation; National Eye Institute R01 EY017066; Research to Prevent Blindness, NY, NY; US Department of Agriculture; University of Iowa; Veteran's Administration.

References

[1] T. N. Crawford, D. V. Alfaro III, J. B. Kerrison, and E. P. Jablon, "Diabetic retinopathy and angiogenesis," *Current Diabetes Reviews*, vol. 5, no. 1, pp. 8–13, 2009.

[2] D. S. Fong, L. Aiello, T. W. Gardner et al., "Retinopathy in diabetes," *Diabetes Care*, vol. 27, no. 1, pp. S84–S87, 2004.

[3] X. Zhang, J. B. Saaddine, C.-F. Chou et al., "Prevalence of diabetic retinopathy in the United States, 2005–2008," *Journal of the American Medical Association*, vol. 304, no. 6, pp. 649–656, 2010.

[4] R. Hazin, M. Colyer, F. Lum, and M. K. Barazi, "Revisiting diabetes 2000: challenges in establishing nationwide diabetic retinopathy prevention programs," *American Journal of Ophthalmology*, vol. 152, no. 5, pp. 723–729, 2011.

[5] E. R. Schoenfeld, J. M. Greene, S. Y. Wu, and M. C. Leske, "Patterns of adherence to diabetes vision care guidelines: baseline findings from the Diabetic Retinopathy Awareness Program," *Ophthalmology*, vol. 108, no. 3, pp. 563–571, 2001.

[6] E. Batbaatar, J. Dorjdagva, A. Luvsannyam, M. M. Savino, and P. Amenta, "Determinants of patient satisfaction: A systematic review," *Perspectives in Public Health*, vol. 137, no. 2, pp. 89–101, 2017.

[7] N. G. Valikodath, T. K. Leveque, S. Y. Wang et al., "Patient attitudes toward telemedicine for diabetic retinopathy," *Telemedicine and e-Health*, vol. 23, no. 3, pp. 205–212, 2017.

[8] D.-W. Park and S. L. Mansberger, "Eye disease in patients with diabetes screened with telemedicine," *Telemedicine and e-Health*, vol. 23, no. 2, pp. 113–118, 2017.

[9] C. Dario, R. Toffanin, F. Calcaterra et al., "Telemonitoring of type 2 diabetes mellitus in Italy," *Telemedicine and e-Health*, vol. 23, no. 2, pp. 143–152, 2017.

[10] R. L. Bashshur, G. W. Shannon, E. A. Krupinski et al., "National telemedicine initiatives: essential to healthcare reform," *Telemedicine and e-Health*, vol. 15, no. 6, pp. 600–610, 2009.

[11] N. M. Hjelm, "Benefits and drawbacks of telemedicine," *Journal of Telemedicine and Telecare*, vol. 11, no. 2, pp. 60–70, 2005.

[12] J. Cuadros and G. Bresnick, "EyePACS: an adaptable telemedicine system for diabetic retinopathy screening," *Journal of Diabetes Science and Technology*, vol. 3, no. 3, pp. 509–516, 2009.

[13] C. R. Taylor, L. M. Merin, A. M. Salunga et al., "Improving diabetic retinopathy screening ratios using telemedicine-based digital retinal imaging technology: The vine hill study," *Diabetes Care*, vol. 30, no. 3, pp. 574–578, 2007.

[14] J. K. Rao, M. Weinberger, and K. Kroenke, "Visit-specific expectations and patient-centered outcomes: A literature review," *Archives of Family Medicine*, vol. 9, no. 10, pp. 1148–1155, 2000.

[15] Y. Zhai, W. Zhu, Y. Cai, D. Sun, and J. Zhao, "Clinical- and cost-effectiveness of telemedicine in type 2 diabetes mellitus: a systematic review and meta-analysis," *Medicine*, vol. 93, no. 28, article e312, 2014.

[16] J. C. Wei, D. J. Valentino, D. S. Bell, and R. S. Baker, "A web-based telemedicine system for diabetic retinopathy screening using digital fundus photography," *Telemedicine and e-Health*, vol. 12, no. 1, pp. 50–57, 2006.

[17] M. D. Abramoff and M. S. A. Suttorp-Schulten, "Web-based screening for diabetic retinopathy in a primary care population: The EyeCheck Project," *Telemedicine and e-Health*, vol. 11, no. 6, pp. 668–674, 2005.

[18] F. Gómez-Ulla, M. I. Fernandez, F. Gonzalez et al., "Digital retinal images and teleophthalmology for detecting and grading diabetic retinopathy," *Diabetes Care*, vol. 25, no. 8, pp. 1384–1389, 2002.

[19] G. Zahlmann and G. Mann, "TME6/365: Teleconsultation and telescreening for eye diseases," *Journal of Medical Internet Research*, vol. 1, p. e113, 1999.

[20] S. Luzio, S. Hatcher, G. Zahlmann et al., "Feasibility of using the TOSCA telescreening procedures for diabetic retinopathy," *Diabetic Medicine*, vol. 21, no. 10, pp. 1121–1128, 2004.

[21] P. G. Paul, R. Raman, P. K. Rani, H. Deshmukh, and T. Sharma, "Patient satisfaction levels during teleophthalmology consultation in rural south India," *Telemedicine and e-Health*, vol. 12, no. 5, pp. 571–576, 2006.

[22] B. Mash, D. Powell, F. du Plessis, U. van Vuuren, M. Michalowska, and N. Levitt, "Screening for diabetic retinopathy in primary care with a mobile fundal camera - Evaluation of a South African pilot project," *South African Medical Journal*, vol. 97, no. 12 I, pp. 1284–1288, 2007.

[23] J. Peng, H. Zou, W. Wang et al., "Implementation and first-year screening results of an ocular telehealth system for diabetic retinopathy in China," *BMC Health Services Research*, vol. 11, no. 1, 2011.

[24] P. S. Silva, J. D. Cavallerano, L. M. Aiello, and L. P. Aiello, "Telemedicine and diabetic retinopathy moving beyond retinal screening," *JAMA Ophtalmology*, vol. 129, no. 2, pp. 236–242, 2011.

[25] K. Kurji, D. Kiage, C. J. Rudnisky, and K. F. Damji, "Improving diabetic retinopathy screening in Africa: patient satisfaction with teleophthalmology versus ophthalmologist-based screening," *Middle East African Journal of Ophthalmology*, vol. 20, no. 1, pp. 56–60, 2013.

[26] P. R. Conlin, B. M. Fisch, A. A. Cavallerano, J. D. Cavallerano, S.-E. Bursell, and L. M. Aiello, "Nonmydriatic teleretinal imaging improves adherence to annual eye examinations in patients with diabetes," *Journal of Rehabilitation Research and Development*, vol. 43, no. 6, pp. 733–739, 2006.

[27] G.-H. Rotvold, U. Knarvik, M. A. Johansen, and K. Fossen, "Telemedicine screening for diabetic retinopathy: Staff and patient satisfaction," *Journal of Telemedicine and Telecare*, vol. 9, no. 2, pp. 109–113, 2003.

[28] P. Cleary and B. McNeil, "Patient satisfaction as an indicator of quality of care," *Inquiry*, vol. 25, no. 1, pp. 25–36, 1988.

[29] C. van Campen, H. Sixma, R. D. Friele, J. J. Kerssens, and L. Peters, "Quality of care and patient satisfaction: a review of measuring instruments," *Medical Care Research and Review*, vol. 52, no. 1, pp. 109–133, 1995.

[30] M. J. U. Rho, S. R. A. Kim, H.-S. Kim et al., "Exploring the relationship among user satisfaction, compliance, and clinical outcomes of telemedicine services for glucose control," *Telemedicine journal and e-health: the official journal of the American Telemedicine Association*, vol. 20, no. 8, pp. 712–720, 2014.

[31] P. S. Whitten and J. D. Richardson, "A scientific approach to the assessment of telemedicine acceptance," *Journal of Telemedicine and Telecare*, vol. 8, no. 4, pp. 246–248, 2002.

[32] L. Gill and L. White, "A critical review of patient satisfaction," *Leadership in Health Services*, vol. 22, no. 1, pp. 8–19, 2009.

[33] R. Rozenblum, J. Donzé, P. M. Hockey et al., "The impact of medical informatics on patient satisfaction: A USA-based literature review," *International Journal of Medical Informatics*, vol. 82, no. 3, pp. 141–158, 2013.

[34] I. H. Kraai, M. L. A. Luttik, R. M. De Jong, T. Jaarsma, and H. L. Hillege, "Heart failure patients monitored with telemedicine: Patient satisfaction, a review of the literature," *Journal of Cardiac Failure*, vol. 17, no. 8, pp. 684–690, 2011.

[35] P. Whitten and B. Love, "Patient and provider satisfaction with the use of telemedicine: overview and rationale for cautious enthusiasm," *Journal of Postgraduate Medicine*, vol. 51, no. 4, Article ID 16388172, pp. 294–300, 2005.

[36] P. L. Hudak, P. McKeever, and J. G. Wright, "The metaphor of patients as customers: Implications for measuring satisfaction," *Journal of Clinical Epidemiology*, vol. 56, no. 2, pp. 103–108, 2003.

[37] R. L. Oliver, "A cognitive model of the antecedents and consequences of satisfaction decisions," *Journal of Marketing Research*, vol. 17, no. 4, p. 460, 1980.

[38] R. Oliver, *Satisfaction, A Behavioral Perspective on the Consumer*, M.E. Sharpe, Inc, Armonk, NY, USA, 2nd edition, 2010.

[39] K. Diehl and C. Poynor, "Great expectations?! Assortment size, expectations, and satisfaction," *Journal of Marketing Research*, vol. 47, no. 2, pp. 312–322, 2010.

[40] H. Ha, "An integrative model of consumer satisfaction in the context of e-services," *International Journal of Consumer Studies*, vol. 30, no. 2, pp. 137–149, 2006.

[41] V. Mittal, W. T. Ross Jr., and P. M. Baldasare, "The asymmetric impact of negative and positive attribute-level performance on overall satisfaction and repurchase intentions," *Journal of Marketing*, vol. 62, no. 1, pp. 33–47, 1998.

[42] S.-J. Yoon and J.-H. Kim, "An empirical validation of a loyalty model based on expectation disconfirmation," *Journal of Consumer Marketing*, vol. 17, no. 2, pp. 120–136, 2000.

[43] A. Bhattacherjee and G. Premkumar, "Understanding changes in belief and attitude toward information technology usage: a theoretical model and longitudinal test," *MIS Quarterly: Management Information Systems*, vol. 28, no. 2, pp. 229–254, 2004.

[44] A. Bhattacherjee, "Understanding information systems continuance: an expectation-confirmation model," *MIS Quarterly*, vol. 25, no. 3, pp. 351–370, 2001.

[45] S. N. Kucukarslan and A. Nadkarni, "Evaluating medication-related services in a hospital setting using the disconfirmation of expectations model of satisfaction," *Research in Social & Administrative Pharmacy*, vol. 4, no. 1, pp. 12–22, 2008.

[46] P. L. Hudak, S. Hogg-Johnson, C. Bombardier, P. D. McKeever, and J. G. Wright, "Testing a new theory of patient satisfaction with treatment outcome," *Medical Care*, vol. 42, no. 8, pp. 726–739, 2004.

[47] B. L. Conner-Spady, C. Sanmartin, G. H. Johnston, J. J. McGurran, M. Kehler, and T. W. Noseworthy, "The importance of patient expectations as a determinant of satisfaction with waiting times for hip and knee replacement surgery," *Health Policy*, vol. 101, no. 3, pp. 245–252, 2011.

[48] T. N. Cassidy-Smith, B. M. Baumann, and E. D. Boudreaux, "The disconfirmation paradigm: Throughput times and emergency department patient satisfaction," *The Journal of Emergency Medicine*, vol. 32, no. 1, pp. 7–13, 2007.

[49] C. Koo, Y. Wati, K. Park, and M. K. Lim, "Website quality, expectation, confirmation, and end user satisfaction: the knowledge-intensive website of the korean national cancer information center," *Journal of Medical Internet Research*, vol. 13, no. 4, p. e81, 2011.

[50] F. Mair and P. Whitten, "Systematic review of studies of patient satisfaction with telemedicine," *British Medical Journal*, vol. 320, no. 7248, pp. 1517–1520, 2000.

[51] T. L. Williams, C. R. May, and A. Esmail, "Limitations of patient satisfaction studies in telehealthcare: A systematic review of the literature," *Telemedicine and e-Health*, vol. 7, no. 4, pp. 293–316, 2001.

[52] J. J. Clarkson, E. R. Hirt, L. Jia, and M. B. Alexander, "When perception is more than reality: the effects of perceived versus actual resource depletion on self-regulatory behavior," *Journal of Personality and Social Psychology*, vol. 98, no. 1, pp. 29–46, 2010.

[53] S. Jayaratne, D. Himle, and W. A. Chess, "Dealing with work stress and strain: is the perception of support more important than its use?" *The Journal of Applied Behavioral Science*, vol. 24, no. 2, pp. 191–202, 1988.

[54] M. S. Gaynor, S. A. Kleiner, and W. B. Vogt, "A structural approach to market definition with an application to the hospital industry," *The Journal of Industrial Economics*, vol. 61, no. 2, pp. 243–289, 2013.

[55] A. Liberman and T. Rotarius, "Healthcare as a commodity – a financing mechanism to control costs and ensure access," *International Journal of Public Policy*, vol. 1, no. 4, pp. 407–420, 2006.

[56] M. Grossman, *Demand for Health: A Theoretical and Empirical Investigation*, Columbia University Press, 2017.

[57] M. Al-Amin, S. C. Makarem, and R. Pradhan, "Hospital ability to attract international patients: A conceptual framework," *International Journal of Pharmaceutical and Healthcare Marketing*, vol. 5, no. 3, pp. 205–221, 2011.

[58] G. Mery, S. Majumder, A. Brown, and M. J. Dobrow, "What do we mean when we talk about the Triple Aim? A systematic review of evolving definitions and adaptations of the framework at the health system level," *Health Policy*, vol. 121, no. 6, pp. 629–636, 2017.

[59] N. Lankton, D. H. McKnight, and J. B. Thatcher, "Incorporating trust-in-technology into Expectation Disconfirmation Theory," *The Journal of Strategic Information Systems*, vol. 23, no. 2, pp. 128–145, 2014.

[60] R. Oliver and G. Linda, "Effect of satisfaction and its antecedents on consumer preference and intention," *Advances in Consumer Research*, vol. 8, pp. 88–93, 1981.

[61] R. M. Andersen, "Revisiting the behavioral model and access to medical care: does it matter?" *Journal of Health and Social Behavior*, vol. 36, no. 1, pp. 1–10, 1995.

[62] C. P. Wilkinson, F. L. Ferris III, R. E. Klein et al., "Proposed international clinical diabetic retinopathy and diabetic macular edema disease severity scales," *Ophthalmology*, vol. 110, no. 9, pp. 1677–1682, 2003.

[63] V. Prakash and J. Lounsbury, "A reliability problem in the measurement of disconfirmation of expectations," in *Advances in Consumer Research, Association for Consumer Research*, R. P. Bagozzi and A. M. Tybout, Eds., pp. 244–249, 10th edition, 1983.

[64] J. S. Armstrong and T. S. Overton, "Estimating non-response bias in mail surveys," *Journal of Marketing Research*, vol. 14, no. 3, pp. 396–402, 1977.

[65] C. Ringle, S. Wende, and A. Will, "Germany," http://www.smartpls.de [access date October 1, 2013]. Archived by WebCite® at http://www.webcitation.org/6TZXW1Ejp, 2005.

[66] V. E. Vinzi, W. W. Chin, J. Henseler, and H. Wang, *Handbook of Partial Least Squares*, Springer Handbooks of Computational Statistics, Springer, Berlin, Germany, 2010.

[67] W. W. Chin, "The partial least squares approach to structural equation modeling," *Modern Methods for Business Research*, vol. 295, no. 2, pp. 295–336, 1998.

[68] J. Henseler and G. Fassott, "Testing moderating effects in PLS path models: An illustration of available procedures," in *Handbook of Partial Least Squares*, pp. 713–735, Springer, Berlin Heidelberg, 2010.

[69] J. Y. Hwang, K. Y. Kim, and K. H. Lee, "Factors that influence the acceptance of telemetry by emergency medical technicians in ambulances: An application of the extended technology acceptance model," *Telemedicine and e-Health*, vol. 20, no. 12, pp. 1127–1134, 2014.

[70] I. Corp, *IBM SPSS Statistics for Windows*, IBM Corp, Armonk, NY, USA, 2011.

[71] P. S. Whitten and F. Mair, "Telemedicine and patient satisfaction: current status and future directions," *Telemedicine and e-Health*, vol. 6, no. 4, pp. 417–423, 2000.

[72] T. H. Wroth and D. E. Pathman, "Primary medication adherence in a rural population: The role of the patient-physician relationship and satisfaction with care," *Journal of the American Board of Family Medicine*, vol. 19, no. 5, pp. 478–486, 2006.

[73] D. E. Morisky, A. Ang, M. Krousel-Wood, and H. J. Ward, "Predictive validity of a medication adherence measure in an outpatient setting," *The Journal of Clinical Hypertension*, vol. 10, no. 5, pp. 348–354, 2008.

[74] B. C. Sun, J. Adams, E. J. Orav, D. W. Rucker, T. A. Brennan, and H. R. Burstin, "Determinants of patient satisfaction and willingness to return with emergency care," *Annals of Emergency Medicine*, vol. 35, no. 5, pp. 426–434, 2000.

[75] D. Staples, I. Wong, and P. B. Seddon, "Having expectations of information systems benefits that match received benefits: does it really matter?" *Information & Management*, vol. 40, no. 2, pp. 115–131, 2002.

[76] N. Luo, C. G. Chapman, B. K. Patel, J. N. Woodruff, and V. M. Arora, "Expectations of ipad use in an internal medicine residency program: Is it worth the hype?" *Journal of Medical Internet Research*, vol. 15, no. 5, article no. e88, 2013.

[77] A. E. de Vries, M. H. van der Wal, M. M. Nieuwenhuis et al., "Health professionals' expectations versus experiences

230   Telemedicine and Telehealth

of internet-based telemonitoring: survey among heart failure clinics," *Journal of Medical Internet Research*, vol. 15, no. 1, p. e4, 2013.

[78] T. Oshagbemi, "Overall job satisfaction: How good are single versus multiple-item measures?" *Journal of Managerial Psychology*, vol. 14, no. 5, pp. 388–403, 1999.

[79] V. Scarpello and J. P. Campbell, "Job satisfaction: are all the parts there?" *Personnel Psychology*, vol. 36, no. 3, pp. 577–600, 1983.

[80] R. E. Lucas and M. B. Donnellan, "Estimating the reliability of single-item life satisfaction measures: results from four national panel studies," *Social Indicators Research*, vol. 105, no. 3, pp. 323–331, 2012.

[81] L. Bergkvist and J. R. Rossiter, "The predictive validity of multiple-item versus single-item measures of the same constructs," *Journal of Marketing Research*, vol. 44, no. 2, pp. 175–184, 2007.

[82] M. S. Nagy, "Using a single-item approach to measure facet job satisfaction," *Journal of Occupational and Organizational Psychology*, vol. 75, no. 1, pp. 77–86, 2002.

[83] C. L. Dolbier, J. A. Webster, K. T. McCalister, M. W. Mallon, and M. A. Steinhardt, "Reliability and validity of a single-item measure of job satisfaction," *American Journal of Health Promotion*, vol. 19, no. 3, pp. 194–198, 2005.

[84] J. P. Wanous, A. E. Reichers, and M. J. Hudy, "Overall job satisfaction: how good are single-item measures?" *Journal of Applied Psychology*, vol. 82, no. 2, pp. 247–251, 1997.

[85] S. Emani, M. Healey, D. Y. Ting et al., "Awareness and use of the after-visit summary through a patient portal: evaluation of patient characteristics and an application of the theory of planned behavior," *Journal of Medical Internet Research*, vol. 18, no. 4, p. e77, 2016.

[86] Y. M. Chae, J. H. Lee, S. H. Ho, H. J. Kim, K. H. Jun, and J. U. Won, "Patient satisfaction with telemedicine in home health services for the elderly," *International Journal of Medical Informatics*, vol. 61, no. 2-3, pp. 167–173, 2001.

[87] L. Edwards, C. Thomas, A. Gregory et al., "Are people with chronic diseases interested in using telehealth? A cross-sectional postal survey," *Journal of Medical Internet Research*, vol. 16, no. 5, p. e123, 2014.

[88] J. R. Rossiter, "The C-OAR-SE procedure for scale development in marketing," *International Journal of Research in Marketing*, vol. 19, no. 4, pp. 305–335, 2002.

[89] C. Fuchs and A. Diamantopoulos, "Using single-item measures for construct measurement in management research," *Die Betriebswirtschaft*, vol. 69, no. 2, pp. 195–210, 2009.

[90] M. Zimmerman, C. J. Ruggero, I. Chelminski et al., "Developing brief scales for use in clinical practice: the reliability and validity of single-item self-report measures of depression symptom severity, psychosocial impairment due to depression, and quality of life," *Journal of Clinical Psychiatry*, vol. 67, no. 10, pp. 1536–1541, 2006.

[91] D. Griffin, S. Murray, and R. Gonzalez, "Difference score correlations in relationship research: A conceptual primer," *Personal Relationships*, vol. 6, no. 4, pp. 505–518, 1999.

[92] D. Chan, "Data analysis and modeling longitudinal processes," *Group & Organization Management*, vol. 28, no. 3, pp. 341–365, 2016.

[93] D. Rogosa, D. Brandt, and M. Zimowski, "A growth curve approach to the measurement of change," *Psychological Bulletin*, vol. 92, no. 3, pp. 726–748, 1982.

[94] D. R. Thomas and B. D. Zumbo, "Difference scores from the point of view of reliability and repeated-measures ANOVA: In defense of difference scores for data analysis," *Educational and Psychological Measurement*, vol. 72, no. 1, pp. 37–43, 2012.

[95] F. Verhoeven, K. Tanja-Dijkstra, N. Nijland, G. Eysenbach, and L. van Gemert-Pijnen, "Asynchronous and synchronous teleconsultation for diabetes care: a systematic literature review," *Journal of Diabetes Science and Technology*, vol. 4, no. 3, pp. 666–684, 2010.

[96] A. Bhattacherjee and C. Sanford, "The intention-behaviour gap in technology usage: The moderating role of attitude strength," *Behaviour & Information Technology*, vol. 28, no. 4, pp. 389–401, 2009.

[97] M. J. Carrington, B. A. Neville, and G. J. Whitwell, "Why ethical consumers don't walk their talk: Towards a framework for understanding the gap between the ethical purchase intentions and actual buying behaviour of ethically minded consumers," *Journal of Business Ethics*, vol. 97, no. 1, pp. 139–158, 2010.

[98] E. Boulstridge and M. Carrigan, "Do consumers really care about corporate responsibility? Highlighting the attitude—behaviour gap," *Journal of Communication Management*, vol. 4, no. 4, pp. 355–368, 2000.

[99] B. Lane and S. Potter, "The adoption of cleaner vehicles in the UK: exploring the consumer attitude-action gap," *Journal of Cleaner Production*, vol. 15, no. 11-12, pp. 1085–1092, 2007.

[100] R. E. Rhodes and G.-J. De Bruijn, "How big is the physical activity intention-behaviour gap? A meta-analysis using the action control framework," *British Journal of Health Psychology*, vol. 18, no. 2, pp. 296–309, 2013.

[101] Y. J. Choi and H. J. Ra, "Patient satisfaction after total knee arthroplasty," *Surgery & Related Research*, vol. 28, no. 1, 2016.

[102] R. Wootton, "Twenty years of telemedicine in chronic disease management—an evidence synthesis," *Journal of Telemedicine and Telecare*, vol. 18, no. 4, pp. 211–220, 2012.

[103] G. T. Petito, "The evolution of telemedicine in eye care," *Advances in Ophthalmology and Optometry*, vol. 2, no. 1, pp. 1–14, 2017.

[104] J. W. Mcgillicuddy, A. K. Weiland, R. M. Frenzel et al., "Patient attitudes toward mobile phone-based health monitoring: Questionnaire study among kidney transplant recipients," *Journal of Medical Internet Research*, vol. 15, no. 1, article no. e6, 2013.

[105] M. Price, D. Williamson, R. McCandless et al., "Hispanic migrant farm workers' attitudes toward mobile phone-based telehealth for management of chronic health conditions," *Journal of Medical Internet Research*, vol. 15, no. 4, p. e76, 2013.

[106] E. Seto, K. J. Leonard, C. Masino, J. A. Cafazzo, J. Barnsley, and H. J. Ross, "Attitudes of heart failure patients and health care providers towards mobile phone-based remote monitoring," *Journal of Medical Internet Research*, vol. 12, no. 4, p. e55p.10, 2010.

[107] V. Mohan, M. Deepa, R. Pradeepa et al., "Prevention of diabetes in rural India with a telemedicine intervention," *Journal of Diabetes Science and Technology*, vol. 6, no. 6, pp. 1355–1364, 2012.

[108] C. L. Lowery, J. M. Bronstein, T. L. Benton, and D. A. Fletcher, "Distributing medical expertise: The evolution and impact of telemedicine in Arkansas," *Health Affairs*, vol. 33, no. 2, pp. 235–243, 2014.

[109] T. M. Petitte, G. L. Narsavage, Y.-J. Chen, C. Coole, T. Forth, and K. D. Frick, "Feasibility study: Home telemonitoring for patients with lung cancer in a mountainous rural area," *Oncology Nursing Forum*, vol. 41, no. 2, pp. 153–161, 2014.

25

Introducing Videoconferencing on Tablet Computers in Nurse–Patient Communication: Technical and Training Challenges

Lisbeth O. Rygg ⓘ, Hildfrid V. Brataas, and Bente Nordtug

Faculty of Nursing and Health Sciences, Nord University, Bodø, Norway

Correspondence should be addressed to Lisbeth O. Rygg; lisbeth.o.rygg@nord.no

Academic Editor: Cristiana Larizza

Background. This article examines personnel and patient experiences of videoconferencing (VC) trials on tablet computers between oncology certified nurses (OCNs) and patients with cancer who live at home. The study points to organizational pitfalls during the introduction process. In many different arenas, the use of VC has increased recently owing to improved Internet access and capacity. This creates new opportunities for contact between patients living at home and their nurses. Video conferencing presupposes knowledge about Internet access, training, and usability of technological equipment. The aim of this pilot study was to illuminate patients' and nurses' experiences of the technical functionality, usability, and training of tablet use in VC in primary cancer care. The results point to the drawbacks concerning the introduction of VC. *Method.* A pilot study with an explorative design was used to describe patients' and OCNs' experiences of technical functionality and usability of VC on tablet computers. After a three-month trial, data were gathered, focusing on both patients' and nurses' perspectives. Individual interviews with four female OCNs, aged 32–65 (mean 46), and six patients with cancer, two men and four women aged 49–78 (mean 69), were content-analyzed. *Results.* The analysis revealed two main categories: *network connectivity and tablet usability* and *training and educational pitfalls.* *Conclusion.* When planning VC implementation, the organizational leadership should consider network access and stability, as well as individualized VC training on tablets. Ensuring patient safety should also be a priority. Further research should provide knowledge of technological and educational pitfalls, and possible implications of VC on the care quality of nursing.

1. Introduction

The article examines personnel and patient experiences of videoconferencing (VC) trials on tablet computers between oncology certified nurses (OCNs) and patients with cancer who live at home, determining organizational pitfalls during the introduction process.

Cancer is a major health problem worldwide. In 2015, the prevalence and incidence rates in Norway were 262.900 and 32.800, respectively [1]. Many patients with cancer have high symptom burdens during and after therapy [2]. In addition, access to healthcare in rural environments can be challenging [3, 4]. To overcome such follow-up challenges for care, VC may be a solution.

Quality work, i.e., concerns and work on ensuring quality health services and quality improvement, is not new, but has evolved over the last 50 years [5, 6]. To ensure quality services, it is necessary to employ several quality approaches and measures at a variety of levels [5, 7]. Some examples are organizational, technical, and professional approaches, which promote a culture that focuses on patients' perspectives and the best ways to meet their nursing needs and the needs of their families [5]. Therefore, both nurses' and patients' perspectives should be considered when introducing new technology. In addition, patients' safety requirements should also be emphasized [8]. When implementing tele-oncology, the aim should be to deliver high-quality medical care to rural areas [9].

The use of information and communication technology (ICT) has a long history [10]. Although ICT like VC are more commonly used in surgical treatment, there are few studies on the use of VC as a tool in primary cancer care

[11–13]. Accessibility to healthcare can be promoted by VC [12–14]. Knowledge of benefits and pitfalls is needed when introducing VC in primary cancer care.

Implementing the use of VC in cancer care may benefit both patients and nurses; however, there may be a need for support and training in the use of the technical equipment. Introducing VC on tablets challenges the traditional nursing organization, as well as patient safety. Sheridan (2013) points to structures, processes, and people as framework factors in the work to prevent safety risks in cancer care [15].

The aim of this pilot study was to illuminate patients' and nurses' experiences of the technical functionality, usability, and training of tablet use in VC in primary cancer care in order to determine pitfalls concerning the introduction of VC.

2. Methods

A pilot study with an explorative design was used to describe patients' and OCNs' experiences of the technical functionality and usability of VC on tablet computers. The pilot study [16] is a small scale study used as part of planning a major study on the use of VC on tablets in the care for patients with cancer living at home. Individual interviews were conducted from autumn 2016 to spring 2017 and analyzed by traditional content analysis methods.

2.1. Sample and Sampling. This pilot study was performed in three rural municipalities in Norway. The three municipalities have about 7500 inhabitants and cover an area of 3842.1 km^2. The sample was informative [17]. Participants were recruited among OCNs and patients with cancer. Inclusion criteria of patients comprised being aged $\geq$ 18 years, living at home, physically and mentally able to communicate using VC on a tablet, being diagnosed with cancer, and currently receiving cancer home care. OCNs working in the three municipalities were included: the heads of the healthcare administration in each municipality selected experienced OCNs. There were four OCNs that were included, and they were asked to then select the patients. During the project period, eight patients who met the inclusion criteria were asked to voluntarily participate. Two of them did not want to participate because they felt too sick, so a total of four women and two men were included (aged 49–78 years). One was single, and five lived with their spouses. One was employed, three were retired, and two were receiving a disability pension. The mean time since diagnosis was 27 months (range = 2–87 months). The cancer diagnoses varied, and prognoses also varied from possibly being cured to a life-long or recurrent life-threatening disease.

2.2. Ethics. Throughout the research process, research ethics were considered in line with the Helsinki Declaration [18]. All included patients and nurses received oral and written information from the researchers about confidentiality and anonymity and provided written consent before the interviews took place. Results were presented anonymously. The Regional Committee for Medical and Health Research

Ethics in Southern Norway (ref. no. 2016/968) and the Data Inspectorate (ref. no. 49571) assessed and approved this study.

2.3. Intervention. A VC with sound and picture between OCNs and patients using tablets was utilized during a three-month trial period. Patients and their OCN each received a tablet that had the program "Skype" installed. As the regular Skype version was not accepted by the firewall IT-security in the municipalities' healthcare systems, the program "Skype for Business" was installed on the tablets [19]. Using this program, the patient can see on the tablet if the nurse is present [20, 21]. Skype for Business does not protect health information using firewalls [22]; patients and nurses were aware of this limitation. Both the OCNs and the patients initiated contact using VC.

An IT employee affiliated with this project provided the OCNs with oral instructions about the technical use of tablet computers and Skype. Each OCN then gave patients instructions. The IT technician also assisted to ensure the VC functioned optimally. The OCNs were free to organize their work using the VC, for example, using VC at specific times or when they felt they had the opportunity. Patients were informed that the OCNs were available during work hours from 7:00 am to 3:00 pm Monday through Friday.

2.4. Data Collection. Data were collected through in-depth individual interviews using a semistructured interview guide [17]. Participants were asked about their Internet connection, training, use of tablets, how they organized their tablet interface, experiences with the confidentiality of using tablets, and whether they had other experiences learning how to use tablets. All interviews were audio-recorded and transcribed verbatim.

2.5. Analyses. Data were analyzed using traditional content analysis [23, 24]. Analyses included repeated examinations of the text: first, the authors read the transcribed text from the interviews several times to obtain a sense of the content. Two researchers began coding the material to reach a common understanding of the meaning units, condensed meaning, and code designation. Then, the researchers analyzed coded material for relevance under each category. Next, the nursing material, followed by the patient material, was coded. Materials were compared for novel information, which led to a draft of categories. All researchers reviewed the saturation of categories and subcategories and discussed the results considering the research question, theory, and previous research.

3. Results

The analysis revealed two main categories, *network connectivity and tablet usability* and *training and educational pitfalls,* as well as four subcategories (Table 1).

3.1. Network Connectivity and Tablet Usability. This category had two subcategories.

TABLE 1: Experiences using videoconferencing during primary care.

Category	Sub-category
Network connectivity and tablet usability	Connection issues
	The usability of VC on tablet
Training and educational pitfalls	Importance of previous experience with VC on tablets
	Inadequate individualized VC training

3.1.1. Connection Issues. In all three municipalities, OCNs and patients faced some obstacles connecting the tablets to the Internet. The OCNs experienced external IT assistance to be very helpful and they connected their tablets to the Internet easily when they followed instructions provided by the project's IT technician. OCNs also highlighted some problems with online connectivity of the patients' tablets due to the use of various networks in their homes. Connection problems came from firewalls and virus problems; patients also experienced this problem. "*It was difficult because of the firewall that we could not get through*" (patient). Some patients were given online access with help from family members or the project IT employee. One patient did not have network access installed in their home. With a simcard that was installed in the patients' tablets, network connections were possible; however, such network access could be unstable over time. There was poor network coverage in some rural areas. One patient reported, "*...on the day they came with the tablet...just then there was no net...that was strange, because it worked before they came.*"

3.1.2. The Usability of VC on Tablets. When the technology worked properly, the VC on tablets positively contributed to contact between patients and nurses. Initially, the nurses were present in the patients' homes, where they handed over the tablet and provided VC training. Later, OCNs called the patients on the tablet from their office to test the web contact, voice quality, and picture quality. The usability of VC was then tested with varying amounts of conversations.

For one patient, only two VC sessions were completed because the patient avoided using the tablet. Other patients found the tablets to be easy and usable. The most frequent testing of usability occurred with several conversations weekly between the patient and the OCN during the project period.

Some patients felt that having the OCNs available was a beneficial feature: "*Just a quick conversation... I noticed when I got access to VC on a tablet that (availability) was so great.*" The technology made it possible for patients to see whether the nurses were available for a call. One patient checked on the nurses' availability every morning.

One OCN stated, "*We have somehow tried to have a systematic online sign when we are available. It lights up green.*"

For patients who preferred VC on tablets to the telephone, communication that included sound and picture was experienced as if one were talking with the OCN face-to-face. VC also helped a patient with hearing loss understand what the nurse was saying by reading nonverbal clues: "*I hear a bit poorly; it's good to be able to see the person also.*" Using

VC, OCNs also received the benefit of patients' nonverbal expressions, and they could, for instance, see the patients' skin. The latter was helpful, since one patient had wounds: "*Sometimes, I had some rashes and the OCN immediately saw what my condition was.*"

One of the OCNs experienced VC with a patient who was on vacation. VC was helpful in her contact with her patient.

> "*Then I was on Skype with one of them when he was on vacation...he had gotten a bad message while he was on that trip. He had been on a medical checkup. The VC was nice to use then...My experience with VC was better than using a phone. The best would have been a meeting at his home, but when this was not possible, VC was a better option than just talking on the phone.*"

This situation explores the usability of VC on tablet.

3.2. Training and Educational Pitfalls. This category comprised two subcategories.

3.2.1. Importance of Previous Experiences with VC on Tablets. The amount of previous experiences with VC on tablets varied among both nurses and patients. They had varied experiences of Internet use and VC on tablets, as well as varying views on VC as a natural communication tool. Two of the four nurses were unfamiliar with use of VC on tablet computers while one had used VC to some extent, and one was familiar with VC on tablets.

Of the patients, two out of the six had used VC on tablets and one of those was familiar with the use. Three were familiar to some extent with the use of Internet and one had used a tablet computer before. The OCNs worked with older patients over 70 years of age who were less experienced with the use of the Internet than the younger ones. Several of the patients had family members who gave them support for connection and use of the Internet. One patient who only had experience with paying bills over the Internet recalled support from a grandchild: "*... just calling one of the grandchildren....*"

3.2.2. Inadequate Individualized VC Training. There was no individual mapping of the need for training among either nurses or patients. The IT technician for the project who met the nurse participants at their office gave the OCNs one to two hours of individual training. He was also available for questions by both phone and network. Two nurses trained on the use of VC on tablets by communicating with each other:

"We had a quick tryout here—me and another OCN—because the other one had used VC before, and I had not used it that much. But it was easy to learn, and I quickly got into it when I began to try it out."

The other two nurses did not have any VC training before starting VC on tablets with patients.

"...it is a little unusual; so I think it's much easier for me to take the phone and call—because I'm used to that ... and it certainly has something to do with age in a way, because I think that young people are much more accustomed to communicating online."

Regarding patient education, two nurses started the training with the patients soon after Internet access was in place, while one of the nurses took a long time before starting training. She reported that she spent a considerable amount of time teaching one patient how to use VC. Another patient with no Internet experience avoided use of the tablet computer even though she had received training. Patients who had used a tablet or computer to pay their bills found it easy to learn how to use Skype on the tablet. One of the oldest patients, who had little experience using electronic devices, stated: *"It is very easy to use such a tablet computer; it is just pressing the buttons."* She grew very fond of the tablet.

4. Discussion

Regarding the technical nature of the VC, while there were some occurrences of unstable network access, it generally functioned well. VC on tablets contributed positively to the contact between patients and nurses. Nurses and patients had very varying previous experience of Internet use and VC on tablets, but there was no mapping of individual training needs. When considering introducing VC on tablets, the research findings point to technical and human needs for quality work. Quality work should focus on measures at both technical and professional levels, as well as on patients and their needs [5, 6].

4.1. Network Connectivity and Usability of VC on Tablet. Technological challenges must be solved at an organizational level [5], because they can affect the communication between patient and health personnel [25]. Health personnel have emphasized the importance of well-functioning technology, which is required in order to have a usable VC encounter [26]. Even in 2018, in Norway, we found that broadband Internet, which is necessary for the use of high-quality VC, might be less available in some rural areas, similar to rural areas of Australia and the US [27, 28]. Patient safety as a structural factor in ensuring quality of health services requires secure networking [15].

After the training, VC on tablet was considered easy to use and participants were satisfied with it, which was consistent with a prior study [21]. Seen from the participants' perspective, VC was experienced satisfactorily by both patients and nurses. This was despite some problems with Internet connections. The existence of sound and picture together makes communication more comprehensive compared to just sound.

4.2. Training and Educational Pitfalls. The study demonstrated that there were varying types of experiences with VC on tablets among both nurses and patients. The results revealed that training and educational pitfalls revolved around participants' previous experiences with VC, as well as with the individualization of VC training. New skills that will be required are the use of tablets.

Securing user competence is a key organizational factor [5]. The study showed that it can be a challenge for some nurses and their patients to use tablets because of their lack of experience with electronic communication tools. Using computers may require mass training; therefore, nurses should participate in organized training before using VC. They should also receive guidance on how to effectively implement VC with their patients.

Some OCNs felt that they had insufficient experience in using telehealth. They needed more training than other OCNs who had such experience. Nevertheless, all OCNs saw telehealth as a facilitator, rather than a barrier, for communication [29].

Our results revealed that patients enjoyed knowing nurses' availability. Easy accessibility to healthcare personnel is of critical importance to patients living with cancer in rural areas [27, 30]. Further, the quality of the picture and sound is vital for efficient communication [31, 32]. When introducing VC as an aid in nursing, nurses should be aware of quality assurance.

4.3. Work Changes and Organizational Quality Assurance Work. Implementing VC on tablet as a new tool implies work changes, and accordingly new qualitative indicators that can be measured and evaluated should be developed [7].

Patient safety must always be safeguarded. The fact that patients cannot always connect to VC can be a threat to care quality. Problematically, nurses might assume that a patient is doing well simply because he/she is not reaching out to the nurse through VC; however, the silence may be caused by a poor network connection, not a lack of need. These drawbacks regarding the quality of care require further consideration.

Adopting VC on tablets for communication between patients with cancer living at home and their nurses can improve primary health service in rural municipalities. However, the implementation of quality safeguards is required before introducing VC.

4.4. Study Limitations. In sum, gathering data from both patients and nurses provided rich information. However, this study had a small sample size of ten participants including only two men. The study was conducted in three rural Norwegian municipalities. The results are not generalizable, and further studies should include more participants from more widely varied areas. Reliability and validity are endeavored through accurate work and collaboration between three researchers throughout the entire research process.

Risk assessments regarding the use of such a communication system were not conducted. A counterweight to this was nurses' awareness of privacy matters: they did not use the tablets in rooms where other people were present or could be listening.

5. Conclusion

When planning VC implementation, organizational leadership should consider network access and stability, as well as individualized training for VC on tablets. Ensuring patient safety should also be a priority. Further research should provide knowledge of technological and educational drawbacks, as well as possible implications of VC on the quality of care in nursing.

Acknowledgments

We express our sincere thanks to the 10 participants, the heads of the healthcare administrations in the three municipalities, and Nord University's ICT technician, who helped facilitate the use of VC on tablets. We would like to thank Editage (https://www.editage.com/) for English language editing. This work was supported by the Regionale Forskningsfond Midt-Norge https://www.forskningsradet.no/servlet/web/prognett-midtnorge/Forside/1253953730477 [grant numbers 269236, 2016]; Fylkesmannen i Nord-Trøndelag (County Governor of North Trondelag) [2016/2324]; and the Nord University.

References

[1] Cancer Registry of Norway, *Cancer in Norway 2016 - Cancer Incidence, Mortality, Survival And Prevalence in Norway*, Cancer Registry of Norway, Oslo, Norway, 2016.

[2] H.-S. Wu and J. K. Harden, "Symptom burden and quality of life in survivorship: a review of the literature," *Cancer Nursing*, vol. 38, no. 1, pp. E29–E54, 2015.

[3] P. N. Butow, F. Phillips, J. Schweder, K. White, C. Underhill, and D. Goldstein, "Psychosocial well-being and supportive care needs of cancer patients living in urban and rural/regional areas: A systematic review," *Supportive Care in Cancer*, vol. 20, no. 1, pp. 1–22, 2012.

[4] F. Brundisini, M. Giacomini, D. DeJean, M. Vanstone, S. Winsor, and A. Smith, "Chronic disease patients' experiences with accessing health care in rural and remote areas: A systematic review and qualitative meta-synthesis," *Ontario Health Technology Assessment Series* , vol. 13, no. 15, pp. 1–33, 2013.

[5] Helsedirektorat [Directorate of Health], *Og bedre skal det bli! Nasjonal strategi for kvalitetsforbedring i sosial- og helsetjenesten [And better it will be! National Strategy for Quality Improvement in Health and Social Services 2005-2015]*, vol. IS1162, Helsedirektorat, Oslo, Norway, 2005.

[6] L. M. Connelly, "overview of Quality Improvement," *Medical-Surgical Nursing*, vol. 27, no. 2, pp. 125-126, 2018.

[7] W. Deming, *Out of the Crisis*, Massachusetts Institute of Technology, Center for Advanced Engineering Study, Cambridge, UK, 1986.

[8] K. Walshe and N. Offen, "A very public failure: Lessons for quality improvement in healthcare organisations from the Bristol Royal Infirmary," *Journal for Healthcare Quality*, vol. 10, no. 4, pp. 250–256, 2001.

[9] E. Maserat, "Information communication technology: New approach for rural cancer care improvement," *Asian Pacific Journal of Cancer Prevention*, vol. 9, no. 4, pp. 811–814, 2008.

[10] H. Alami, M. P. Gagnon, R. Wootton, J. P. Fortin, and P. Zanaboni, "Exploring factors associated with the uneven utilization of telemedicine in Norway: A mixed methods study," *BMC Medical Informatics and Decision Making*, vol. 17, no. 1, 2017.

[11] B. Lindberg, C. Nilsson, D. Zotterman, S. Söderberg, and L. Skär, "Using Information and Communication Technology in Home Care for Communication between Patients, Family Members, and Healthcare Professionals: A Systematic Review," *International Journal of Telemedicine and Applications*, vol. 2013, Article ID 461829, 31 pages, 2013.

[12] K. M. Augestad and R. O. Lindsetmo, "Overcoming distance: Video-conferencing as a clinical and educational tool among surgeons," *World Journal of Surgery*, vol. 33, no. 7, pp. 1356–1365, 2009.

[13] B. Nordtug, H. Brataas, and L. Rygg, "The Use of Videoconferencing in nursing for people in their homes: A Review," *Nursing Reports*, 2018.

[14] A. M. Johansson, I. Lindberg, and S. Söderberg, "The views of health-care personnel about video consultation prior to implementation in primary health care in rural areas," *Primary Health Care Research & Development*, vol. 15, no. 2, pp. 170–179, 2014.

[15] C. A. Sheridan, "The science of patient safety: Implications for oncology nursing practice," *Clinical Journal of Oncology Nursing*, vol. 17, no. 6, pp. 601–603, 2013.

[16] B. Resnick, "The definition, purpose and value of pilot research," *Geriatric Nursing*, vol. 36, no. 2, pp. S1–S2, 2015.

[17] D. Polit and C. Beck, *Nursing Research: Generating and Assessing Evidence for Nursing Practice*, Wolters Kluwer Health — Lippincott Williams & Wilkins, Philadelphia, Pennsylvania, 2012.

[18] World Medical Association, "WMA Declaration of Helsinki: ethical principles for medical research involving human subjects," *The Journal of the American College of Dentists*, vol. 81, no. 3, pp. 14–18, 2014.

[19] "Microsoft Skype for Business Basic," https://www.microsoft.com/en-us/download/details.aspx?id=49440.

[20] "How much bandwidth does Skype need?" https://support.skype.com/en/faq/FA1417/how-much-bandwidth-does-skype-need.

[21] A. Gund, B. A. Sjöqvist, H. Wigert, E. Hentz, K. Lindecrantz, and K. Bry, "A randomized controlled study about the use of eHealth in the home health care of premature infants," *BMC Medical Informatics and Decision Making*, vol. 13, no. 1, 2013.

[22] A. M. Edmundson, *Privacy Infrastructure for Content and Communications Doctors Dissertation*, Princeton University, Princeton, NJ, USA, 2018.

[23] H. F. Hsieh and S. E. Shannon, "Three approaches to qualitative content analysis," *Qualitative Health Research*, vol. 15, no. 9, pp. 1277–1288, 2005.

[24] M. Vaismoradi, H. Turunen, and T. Bondas, "Content analysis and thematic analysis: implications for conducting a qualitative

descriptive study," *Nursing & Health Sciences*, vol. 15, no. 3, pp. 398–405, 2013.

[25] L. Skär and S. Söderberg, "The Use of Information and Communication Technology to Meet Chronically Ill Patients' Needs when Living at Home," *The Open Nursing Journal*, vol. 5, pp. 74–78, 2011.

[26] A. M. Johansson, I. Lindberg, and S. Söderberg, "Healthcare personnel's experiences using video consultation in primary healthcare in rural areas," *Primary Health Care Research & Development*, vol. 18, no. 1, pp. 73–83, 2017.

[27] M. Charlton, J. Schlichting, C. Chioreso, M. Ward, and P. Vikas, "Challenges of rural cancer care in the United States," *Oncology (Williston Park)*, vol. 29, no. 9, pp. 633–640, 2015.

[28] L. H. Schwamm, "Telehealth: Seven strategies to successfully implement disruptive technology and transform health care," *Health Affairs*, vol. 33, no. 2, pp. 200–206, 2014.

[29] M. Koivunen and K. Saranto, "Nursing professionals' experiences of the facilitators and barriers to the use of telehealth applications: a systematic review of qualitative studies," *Scandinavian Journal of Caring Sciences*, vol. 32, no. 1, pp. 24–44, 2018.

[30] M. Jansson, K. Dixon, and D. Hatcher, "The palliative care experiences of adults living in regional and remote areas of Australia: A literature review," *Contemporary Nurse*, vol. 53, no. 1, pp. 94–104, 2017.

[31] A. M. Johansson, I. Lindberg, and S. Söderberg, "Patients' Experiences with Specialist Care via Video Consultation in Primary Healthcare in Rural Areas," *International Journal of Telemedicine and Applications*, vol. 2014, Article ID 143824, 7 pages, 2014.

[32] L. C. Gray, N. R. Armdield, and A. C. Smith, "Telemedicine for wound care: current practice and future potential," *wound Practice and Research*, vol. 18, no. 4, pp. 158–163, 2010.

Permissions

All chapters in this book were first published in IJTA, by Hindawi Publishing Corporation; hereby published with permission under the Creative Commons Attribution License or equivalent. Every chapter published in this book has been scrutinized by our experts. Their significance has been extensively debated. The topics covered herein carry significant findings which will fuel the growth of the discipline. They may even be implemented as practical applications or may be referred to as a beginning point for another development.

The contributors of this book come from diverse backgrounds, making this book a truly international effort. This book will bring forth new frontiers with its revolutionizing research information and detailed analysis of the nascent developments around the world.

We would like to thank all the contributing authors for lending their expertise to make the book truly unique. They have played a crucial role in the development of this book. Without their invaluable contributions this book wouldn't have been possible. They have made vital efforts to compile up to date information on the varied aspects of this subject to make this book a valuable addition to the collection of many professionals and students.

This book was conceptualized with the vision of imparting up-to-date information and advanced data in this field. To ensure the same, a matchless editorial board was set up. Every individual on the board went through rigorous rounds of assessment to prove their worth. After which they invested a large part of their time researching and compiling the most relevant data for our readers.

The editorial board has been involved in producing this book since its inception. They have spent rigorous hours researching and exploring the diverse topics which have resulted in the successful publishing of this book. They have passed on their knowledge of decades through this book. To expedite this challenging task, the publisher supported the team at every step. A small team of assistant editors was also appointed to further simplify the editing procedure and attain best results for the readers.

Apart from the editorial board, the designing team has also invested a significant amount of their time in understanding the subject and creating the most relevant covers. They scrutinized every image to scout for the most suitable representation of the subject and create an appropriate cover for the book.

The publishing team has been an ardent support to the editorial, designing and production team. Their endless efforts to recruit the best for this project, has resulted in the accomplishment of this book. They are a veteran in the field of academics and their pool of knowledge is as vast as their experience in printing. Their expertise and guidance has proved useful at every step. Their uncompromising quality standards have made this book an exceptional effort. Their encouragement from time to time has been an inspiration for everyone.

The publisher and the editorial board hope that this book will prove to be a valuable piece of knowledge for researchers, students, practitioners and scholars across the globe.

List of Contributors

Pushpa Mala Siddaraju and Kaliyamoorthy Ezhilarasan
Research Scholar, JainUniversity andDepartment of Electronics and Communication Engineering, Sambhram Institute of Technology, Bangalore 560097, Karnataka, India

Devappa Jayadevappa
Department of Electronic Instrumentation, JSS Academy of Technical Education, Bangalore 560060, Karnataka, India

Adesola C. Odole
Department of Physiotherapy, College of Medicine, University of Ibadan, Ibadan 200284, Nigeria
School of Research and Postgraduate Studies, Faculty of Agriculture, Science and Technology, NorthWest University, Mafikeng Campus, Mafikeng 2735, South Africa

Oluwatobi D.Ojo
Department of Physiotherapy, College of Medicine, University of Ibadan, Ibadan 200284, Nigeria
Department of Physiotherapy, Neuropsychiatric Hospital, Aro, Abeokuta 110251, Nigeria

Sara Movahedazarhouligh
Department of Rehabilitation Management, University of SocialWelfare and Rehabilitation Sciences, Tehran, Iran

Roshanak Vameghi
Pediatric Neurorehabilitation Research Center, University of Social Welfare and Rehabilitation Sciences, Tehran, Iran

Nikta Hatamizadeh
Department of Rehabilitation Management, Pediatric Neurorehabilitation Research Center, University of SocialWelfare and Rehabilitation Sciences, Tehran, Iran

Enayatollah Bakhshi
Department of Biostatistics, University of SocialWelfare and Rehabilitation Sciences, Tehran, Iran

Seyed Muhammad Moosavy Khatat
Department of Social Welfare, University of Social Welfare and Rehabilitation Sciences, Tehran, Iran

Stephen Robert Isabalija
Department of Business Administration, Makerere University Business School, 1337 Kampala, Uganda

Victor Mbarika
International Center for Information Technology and Development, Southern University and A and M College, Baton Rouge, LA 70813-9723, USA

Geoffrey Mayoka Kituyi
Department of Business Computing, Makerere University Business School, 1337 Kampala, Uganda

Orobah Al-Momani and Khaled M. Gharaibeh
Yarmouk University, Irbid 21163, Jordan

Sharon Davidesko
Ben-Gurion University of the Negev, 84105 Beer-Sheva, Israel

Roni Peleg
Ben-Gurion University of the Negev, 84105 Beer-Sheva, Israel
The Department of Family Medicine and Siaal Research Center for Family Practice and Primary Care, Division of Community Health, Faculty of Health Sciences, Ben-Gurion University of the Negev, P.O. Box 653, 84105 Beer-Sheva, Israel

David Segal
Division of Obstetrics and Gynecology, Soroka Medical Center, P.O. Box 151, 84101 Beer-Sheva, Israel
Women Health Center, Clalit Health Services, Southern District, Henrietta Szold 1, 89428 Beer-Sheva, Israel

Deborah G. Theodoros and Trevor G. Russell
The University of Queensland, School of Health and Rehabilitation Sciences, St. Lucia, Brisbane, QLD 4072, Australia

Elizabeth C.Ward
The University of Queensland, School of Health and Rehabilitation Sciences, St. Lucia, Brisbane, QLD 4072, Australia
Centre for Functioning and Health Research, Queensland Health, Buranda, Brisbane, QLD 4102, Australia

Clare L. Burns
Speech Pathology Department, Royal Brisbane andWomen's Hospital, Herston, Brisbane, QLD 4006, Australia

Stefano Abbate
Institute of Informatics and Telematics, National Research Council, Via G. Moruzzi 1, 56124 Pisa, Italy

Marco Avvenuti
Department of Information Engineering, University of Pisa, L. Lazzarino 1, 56122 Pisa, Italy

Janet Light
Department of Computer Science and Applied Statistics, University of New Brunswick, Saint John, NB, Canada E2L 4L5

R. Eswaraiah and E. Sreenivasa Reddy
Department of Computer Science and Engineering, Acharya Nagarjuna University, Guntur 522510, Andhra Pradesh, India

Thomas J. Betjeman
Ben Gurion University of theNegev, Medical School for International Health, New York, NY 10032, USA

Samara E. Soghoian and Mark P. Foran
NYU School of Medicine, Bellevue Hospital Center, New York, NY 10016, USA

Edward O'Mahony
Department of Obstetrics and Gynaecology and Department of Perinatal Medicine, Pregnancy Research Centre, RoyalWomen's Hospital, University of Melbourne, Melbourne, VIC 3207, Australia

Adilson Cunha Ferreira
Department of Obstetrics and Gynaecology and Department of Perinatal Medicine, Pregnancy Research Centre, RoyalWomen's Hospital, University of Melbourne, Melbourne, VIC 3207, Australia
School of Medicine, University of Sᾶao Jos´e do Rio Preto, São Jos é do Rio Preto, SP, Brazil
Monash Ultrasound forWomen, Melbourne, VIC, Australia

Fabricio da Silva Costa
Department of Obstetrics and Gynaecology and Department of Perinatal Medicine, Pregnancy Research Centre, RoyalWomen's Hospital, University of Melbourne, Melbourne, VIC 3207, Australia
Monash Ultrasound forWomen, Melbourne, VIC, Australia

Antonio Hélio Oliani
School of Medicine, University of São Jos´e do Rio Preto, São Jos é do Rio Preto, SP, Brazil

Edward Araujo Júnior
Department of Obstetrics, Paulista School of Medicine-Federal University of São Paulo (EPM-UNIFESP), 05303-000 São Paulo, SP, Brazil

C. B. Barcaui
Adjunct Professor of Dermatology, Faculty of Medical Sciences, State University of Rio de Janeiro, PhD in Medicine (Dermatology), by University of São Paulo, Dermatology Department, Pedro Ernesto University Hospital, Rio de Janeiro State University, Rio de janeiro, Brazil

P.M.O. Lima
Physician Residing in Dermatology, Department of Dermatology, Pedro Ernesto University Hospital, State University of Rio de Janeiro, Rio de Janeiro, Brazil

S. Wiklund Axelsson, L. Nyberg, A. Näslund and A. Melander Wikman
Department of Health Sciences, Luleå University of Technology, 971 87 Luleå, Sweden

M. Abo-Zahhad, SabahM. Ahmed and O. Elnahas
Electrical and Electronic Engineering Department, Faculty of Engineering, Assiut University, Egypt

Lis Wagner
Research Unit of Nursing, Institute of Clinical Research, University of Southern Denmark, Campusvej 55, 5230 Odense M, Denmark

Dorthe Boe Danbjørg
Research Unit of Nursing, Institute of Clinical Research, University of Southern Denmark, Campusvej 55, 5230 Odense M, Denmark
Odense University Hospital, Department of Gynaecology and Obstetrics, Søndre Boulevard 29, 5000 Odense C, Denmark

Bjarne Rønde Kristensen
Odense University Hospital, Department of Gynaecology and Obstetrics, Søndre Boulevard 29, 5000 Odense C, Denmark

Jane Clemensen
Odense University Hospital, CIMT, University of Southern Denmark, Søndre Boulevard 29, 5000 Odense C, Denmark

AimeeM. Layton and Byron M.Thomashow
Division of Pulmonary, Allergy and Critical Care Medicine, Department of Medicine, Columbia University Medical Center, VC3-365 Center for Chest Disease NYPH-CUMC, 622W. 168th Street, New York, NY 10032, USA

James Whitworth
Department of Biobehavioral Sciences, Teachers College, Columbia University, 522W. 120th Street, New York, NY 10027, USA

James Peacock
Division of Cardiology, Department of Medicine, Columbia University Medical Center, 622W. 168th Street, New York, NY 10032, USA

Matthew N. Bartels
Department of Physical Medicine and Rehabilitation, Montefiore Medical Center, 111 E. 210th Street, Bronx, NY 10467, USA

Patricia A. Jellen
Center for Chest Disease, New York Presbyterian Hospital, 622W. 168th Street, New York, NY 10032, USA

Benedict Osei Asibey and Seth Agyemang
Department of Geography and Rural Development, Faculty of Humanities and Social Sciences, Kwame Nkrumah University of Science and Technology, Kumasi, Ghana

Augustina Boakye Dankwah
Department of Geography and Resource Development, Faculty of Social Sciences, University of Ghana, Legon, Accra, Ghana

Kerstin Kempf, Martin Röhling and StephanMartin
West-German Centre of Diabetes and Health, Düsseldorf Catholic Hospital Group, D¨usseldorf, Germany

Jürgen Könner
Occupational Health Services, Kassenärztliche Vereinigung Nordrhein, Düsseldorf, Germany

Monika Stichert
Occupational Health Services, Kassenärztliche Vereinigung Nordrhein, Düsseldorf, Germany Occupational Health Services Ärztekammer Nordrhein, Düsseldorf, Germany

Gabriele Fischer
Occupational Health Services Ärztekammer Nordrhein, Düsseldorf, Germany

Elke Boschem
Occupational Health Services Eickhoff GmbH, Bochum, Germany

Ye Zhang, Jingna Zhang and Mingguo Qiu
Department of Medical Image, College of Biomedical Engineering, Third Military Medical University, Chongqing, China

Liang Qiao
Department of Medical Image, College of Biomedical Engineering, Third Military Medical University, Chongqing, China

Department of Computer Science, College of Biomedical Engineering, Third Military Medical University, Chongqing, China

Xin Chen
College of Software and Computer, Chongqing Institute of Engineering, Chongqing, China

Yi Wu, Ying Li and Xuemei Mo
Department of Digital Medicine, College of Biomedical Engineering, Third Military Medical University, Chongqing, China

Wei Chen and Bing Xie
Department of Radiology, Southwest Hospital, Third Military Medical University, Chongqing, China

Pernille Heyckendorff Lilholt, Clara Schaarup and Ole Kristian Hejlesen
Department of Health Science and Technology, Aalborg University, Aalborg, Denmark

Harish C. Jadhav, Arun S. Dodamani, G. N. Karibasappa and Prashanth Vishwakarma
Department of Public Health Dentistry, JMF's ACPM Dental College, Dhule, Maharashtra 424001, India

Rahul G. Naik
Department of Public Health Dentistry, Dr. Hedgewar Smruti Rugna Seva Mandal's Dental College, Hingoli Maharashtra 431513, India

Mahesh R. Khairnar
Department of Public Health Dentistry, Bharati Vidyapeeth Dental College and Hospital, Sangli, Maharashtra 416416, India

Manjiri A. Deshmukh
Department of Public Health Dentistry, Swargiya Dadasaheb Kalmegh Smruti Dental College, Nagpur, Maharashtra 441110, India

Antonio J. Salazar and Xavier A. Díaz
Electrophysiology and Telemedicine Laboratory, University of Los Andes, Carrera 1 Este No. 19A-40, Bogotá 11001, Colombia

Angela P. Moreno
Department of Diagnostic Imaging, Fundación Santa Fe de Bogotá University Hospital, Calle 119No. 7-75, Bogotá 11001, Colombia

Javier A. Romero
Department of Diagnostic Imaging, Fundación Santa Fe de Bogotá University Hospital, Calle 119No. 7-75, Bogotá 11001, Colombia School ofMedicine, University of Los Andes, Carrera 1 EsteNo. 19A-40, Bogotá 11001, Colombia

Sofía C. Velasco
Department of Diagnostic Imaging, Fundaci´on Santa Fe de Bogot´a University Hospital, Calle 119No. 7-75, Bogot´a 11001, Colombia
School of Government, University of Los Andes, Carrera 1 Este No. 19A-40, Bogot´a 11001, Colombia

Oscar A. Bernal
School ofMedicine, University of Los Andes, Carrera 1 EsteNo. 19A-40, Bogot´a 11001, Colombia
School of Government, University of Los Andes, Carrera 1 Este No. 19A-40, Bogot´a 11001, Colombia

Brittanie LaBelle, Alexandra M. Franklyn, Vicky PKH Nguyen, Kathleen E. Anderson and Joseph K. Eibl
Northern Ontario School of Medicine, 935 Ramsey Lake Rd., Sudbury, ON, Canada P3E 2C6

David C. Marsh
Northern Ontario School of Medicine, 935 Ramsey Lake Rd., Sudbury, ON, Canada P3E 2C6
Canadian Addiction Treatment Centers, 13291 Yonge St., Ste. 403., Richmond Hill, ON, Canada L4E 4L6

Christina I. Serrano
Department of Computer Information Systems, Colorado State University, Fort Collins, CO, USA

Vishal Shah
Department of Business Information Systems, Central Michigan University, Mt. Pleasant, MI, USA

Michael D. Abràmoff
Department of Ophthalmology and Visual Sciences, University of Iowa, Iowa City, IA, USA

Lisbeth O. Rygg, Hildfrid V. Brataas and Bente Nordtug
Faculty of Nursing and Health Sciences, Nord University, Bodø, Norway

Index